Death or Disability?

In ancient Rome parents would consult the priestess Carmentis shortly after birth to obtain prophecies of the future of their newborn infant. Today, parents and doctors of critically ill children consult a different oracle. Neuroimaging provides a vision of the child's future, particularly of the nature and severity of any disability. The results of brain scans and other tests leave doctors and parents facing heart-breaking decisions about whether to continue intensive treatment or to allow the child to die.

Paediatrician and ethicist Dominic Wilkinson looks at the profound and contentious ethical issues facing those who care for critically ill children and infants. When should infants or children be allowed to die? How accurate are predictions of future quality of life? How much say should parents have in these decisions? How should they deal with uncertainty about the future? He combines philosophy, medicine, and science to shed light on current and future dilemmas.

Dominic Wilkinson is Professor of Medical Ethics at the Oxford Uehiro Centre for Practical Ethics, University of Oxford, research fellow at Jesus College, and a consultant neonatologist at the John Radcliffe Hospital, Oxford.

Endorsements and Praise

'His style, clear and simple for a work on a subject of considerable complexity, and yet profound in its way of dealing with issues more related to philosophy and ethics, make this book a read of great interest not only for professionals in pediatric medicine, but also for affected families and for anyone who wants to know the problems of bioethics from a multi-disciplinary perspective.'

Revista Española de Discapacidad

'this was an interesting read, comprehensive, analytical, and thought-provoking . . . Wilkinson does a good job of articulating and providing evidence to support his point of view. He successfully accomplishes what he sets out to do, while keeping the reader entertained with historical points, clinical examples, and philosophical theories and vignettes.'

Marlyse F. Haward, *The American Journal of Bioethics*

'this is an impressively serious, wise, and humane book . . . it is reflected in a deep, informed concern for all of the interests implicated in decisions about severely impaired neonates. Wilkinson's perspective is encompassing, not impersonal; he comes close to the ideal of an empathic but unsentimental Impartial Observer, displaying a rare capacity to appreciate the multiplicity of interests and values that must be taken into account in making life-and-death decisions about severely impaired neonates.'

David Wasserman, *Kennedy Institute of Ethics Journal*

Death or Disability?

The 'Carmentis Machine' and decision-making for critically ill children

Dominic Wilkinson

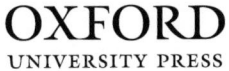

OXFORD
UNIVERSITY PRESS

Great Clarendon Street, Oxford, OX2 6DP,
United Kingdom

Oxford University Press is a department of the University of Oxford.
It furthers the University's objective of excellence in research, scholarship,
and education by publishing worldwide. Oxford is a registered trade mark of
Oxford University Press in the UK and in certain other countries

© Dominic Wilkinson 2013

The moral rights of the author have been asserted

First published 2013
First published in paperback 2017

All rights reserved. No part of this publication may be reproduced, stored in
a retrieval system, or transmitted, in any form or by any means, without the
prior permission in writing of Oxford University Press, or as expressly permitted
by law, by licence or under terms agreed with the appropriate reprographics
rights organization. Enquiries concerning reproduction outside the scope of the
above should be sent to the Rights Department, Oxford University Press, at the
address above

You must not circulate this work in any other form
and you must impose this same condition on any acquirer

Published in the United States of America by Oxford University Press
198 Madison Avenue, New York, NY 10016, United States of America

British Library Cataloguing in Publication Data
Data available

Library of Congress Cataloging in Publication Data
Data available

ISBN 978-0-19-966943-1 (Hbk.)
ISBN 978-0-19-879905-4 (Pbk.)

Links to third party websites are provided by Oxford in good faith and
for information only. Oxford disclaims any responsibility for the materials
contained in any third party website referenced in this work.

Acknowledgements

This work would not have been possible without the support of a large number of people. In particular Julian Savulescu and Tony Hope were extremely generous with their time, encouragement, and critical and constructive feedback over the course of three and a half years in Oxford. An Oxford Nuffield Medical Fellowship, Eric Burnard Fellowship, Royal Australasian College of Physicians Astra-Zeneca Medical Fellowship and Royal Children's Hospital Travelling scholarship made my stay in Oxford possible. I am very grateful to the Nuffield Dominions Trust, the Royal Australasian College of Physicians, and the Uncle Bob's Club in Melbourne.

I am indebted to those who provided invaluable feedback on related papers and projects and on versions of this manuscript including Bevan Headley, Nikki Robertson, Sudhin Thayyil, John Wyatt, Rod Hunt, Andrew Watkins, Charles Foster, Janet Radcliffe-Richards, Paul Glasziou, Angela McLean, Ray Fitzpatrick, David Archard, Mark Sheehan, Loane Skene, Neil Levy, Mike Parker, and Jeff McMahan. Rod Hunt also very kindly helped with MRI images for Figure 8.4. Special thanks are due to my former office-mates Toby Ord and Tom Douglas for their friendship, conversation, thoughtful and constructive criticisms, and inspiration.

I need to thank two people without whose support I would never have studied medicine, gone to Oxford, done a PhD. My mother and father are two of the most generous, selfless, and inspiring people I know. They taught me to love reading and thinking, debating, science and the art of caring. Finally, and most importantly, I am enormously grateful to my wife Rocci for careful proofreading and for putting up with my frequent absences and general distractedness, and to my children Sebastian, Gabriel, Penelope, and Jemima for their love and patience.

Some of the research that has gone into this manuscript has previously been published in the following papers:

Wilkinson, D. (2009). 'The window of opportunity: decision theory and the timing of prognostic tests for newborn infants', *Bioethics* 23(9): 503–14.

Wilkinson, D. (2009). 'The self-fulfilling prophecy in intensive care', *Theoretical medicine and bioethics* 30(6): 401–10.

Wilkinson, D. (2010). 'Magnetic resonance imaging and withdrawal of life support from newborn infants with hypoxic-ischemic encephalopathy', *Pediatrics* 126(2): 451–8.

Wilkinson, D. (2010). 'A life worth giving: the threshold for permissible withdrawal of treatment from disabled newborn infants', *American Journal of Bioethics* 11(2): 20–32.

Wilkinson, D. (2010). "We don't have a crystal ball': neonatologists views on prognosis and decision-making in newborn infants with birth asphyxia', *Monash Bioethics Review* 29(1): 5.1–5.19.

Wilkinson, D. (2010). 'How much weight should we give to parental interests in decisions about life support for newborn infants?', *Monash Bioethics Review* 29(2): 13.11–13.25.

Wilkinson, D. (2011). 'Should we replace disabled newborn infants?', *Journal of Moral Philosophy* 8(3): 390–414.

Wilkinson, D. (2011). 'The window of opportunity for treatment withdrawal', *Archives of pediatrics & adolescent medicine* 165(3): 211–15.

Wilkinson, D. and C. Foster (2010). 'The Carmentis machine: ethical and legal issues in the use of neuroimaging to guide treatment withdrawal in newborn infants', in M. Freeman (ed.), *Current Legal Issues: Law and Neuroscience*. Oxford: Oxford University Press, 309–34.

Contents

List of Figures and Tables   viii

Prologue 1: The Temple of Carmentis 30 AD   1
Prologue 2: The Carmentis Machine 2030 AD   5
Introduction: Neuroethics and Intensive Care   11

Part I

Death and Grief in the Ancient World   21

1. Destiny, Disability, and Death   23

   Carmentis   45

2. Best Interests and the Carmentis Machine   46
3. Starting Again   82

   Exposure and Infanticide in Ancient Rome   105

4. Competing Interests   108

Part II

Predictions and Disability in Rome   159

5. Sources of Uncertainty—Prognostic Research   162
6. Managing Uncertainty   202
7. Interests and Uncertainty   236
8. The Threshold Framework   261

Index   309

List of Figures and Tables

FIGURES

2.1	Tolerability and cognitive impairment	68
3.1	Comparing a decision to replace with a decision to conceive	92
3.2	Comparing a decision to replace with a decision to conceive (all things considered)	97
4.1	Three accounts of the harm of death	135
7.1	Decisions about life-sustaining treatment and the zero-point of well-being	244
7.2	Weighing up treatment mistakes and their implications for cut-off points for withdrawing treatment in the face of uncertainty	247
8.1	Different views about parental discretion for life-sustaining treatment	268
8.2	The threshold framework	272
8.3	Agreeing to disagree	281
8.4	The threshold framework as the basis for treatment limitation guidelines in birth asphyxia	292
8.5	The threshold framework and resources	300

TABLES

1.1	Patterns observed using conventional MRI and neurodevelopmental outcome	38
5.1	Recommendations for improving prognostic research	195
6.1	Competing values in the timing of withdrawal of life-sustaining treatment	206
6.2	Three different groups of quality of life treatment decisions	209
7.1	Different types of uncertainty	253
8.1	Patterns of imaging and treatment limitation decision in birth asphyxia	292

Prologue 1: The Temple of Carmentis 30 AD

Cassia climbed the steps slowly, cradling the warm bundle close to her breast. The sun was only just above the treetops, but already she could feel its gaze pressing down upon her back and head. Instinctively, she shielded the bundle in her arms with her shoulders. At the top, Cassia nudged the leather sandals off her feet, leaving them neatly at the base of a pillar. In a few hours these stones would be too hot to step on, but for now they still held the cool memory of the night. She walked forward towards the entrance stiffly. The burning in her groin was less today, but if she moved in the wrong way or too quickly it would rise up again suddenly as if fresh.

She had not walked about at all until this morning. Cassia had slept the whole first day, drifting in and out of consciousness, her body heavy, weighted down by the echoes of her exertions, and by the heavy, sweet draughts that her attendants forced her to drink. Tiria and Naelia brought food, water, messages from her family. Tiria had watched her pale mistress from the shadows close at hand, unsure when, or if, Cassia would wake. The older woman, Naelia, had disappeared to take on the care for the child as she had for Cassia's five older children. When Cassia woke she asked after him, but Tiria had said little; the rings below her eyes, and the creases in her brow spoke enough.

From time to time as she had lain there Cassia had heard her older children playing in the courtyard beyond the wall. Their voices would rise from some game or other, then fall suddenly as they were hushed. What day is it? She had lost track. Her last child had been quick, a few hours only, but this time something had seemed awry; the pains had continued, rising and falling like waves against the shore, beyond one day into the next, until she had no longer known where one pain began and another ended. When the infant was finally born she barely had the strength to lift her head up to look at it. Before she lapsed into blackness she had had a moment to ask herself—why is it so still?

As Cassia walked through the doorway she was struck, this time, as before, by the sudden change. The sounds of the street were still there if she listened for them: the voices of the street vendors around the corner at the market, the cries of children playing on the corner, the insistent burr of cicadas in the trees. But in the moment that it took to cross the threshold those sounds retreated, as if she had taken 200 steps, instead of just two. The air, which had been thick and heavy, was suddenly sharp and cold. She could taste the dust and the sweetness of incense.

Ahead, in the gloom, a flame burned quietly. At first, that was all that she could see, but as her eyes adjusted she could make out the edges of the room, the shapes on the wall, the flickering shadows beyond the altar, the wisps of smoke rising from the fire. She could see the figure waiting for her.

'Bring the child'

Cassia moved towards the voice. As she grew closer she could make out the face of the novitiate who had spoken. She was young, perhaps twelve or thirteen years, calm eyes, dark hair lost in the shadows of her hood. Although she was tall her cheeks still had the roundness of childhood. As Cassia approached she wondered to herself what she was doing here. 'What does this girl, what do any of these girls, know about childbirth?' There was an irony it seemed, in the steady procession of mothers who sought guidance and support from those who had never known the pain of giving birth.

She followed the girl past the flame to the back of the dark room, past a curtain, and into relative brightness. Cassia blinked. Here, light fell through a hole in the roof, dust motes silently whirling in the beam, then disappearing into shadow. The light reflected off a pool of water in the centre of the chamber, dark and smooth. In front of the water another figure, the priestess, waited, legs folded beneath her. Once her eyes had adjusted Cassia recognized the same smiling face that had greeted her following each of her previous births. The woman's eyes were creased with years of meetings and greetings like this. How many newborn infants had the priestess welcomed? How many mothers had she reassured with her visions of health, prosperity, good marriages, grandchildren? She beckoned for Cassia to approach, and motioned with her hand for Cassia to unwrap the bundle.

Cassia hesitated, then slowly, carefully, lowered herself to the ground beside the priestess. She placed the bundle on the ground and folded back the linen that encased the child. The infant stirred as the air met his face and snuffled softly, but his eyes stayed shut. His smooth face rested, and his mouth drooped a fraction. The layers of cloth were peeled back around him, revealing, bit by bit, his arms, chest, stomach, legs. His limbs were thin, and the skin over his upper legs was wrinkled. He lay on his back, and his hands rested open down by his side, legs stretched out loose and limp below him, knees splayed. As he started to get cold he stirred again, this time opening his eyes with a hint of a frown. His arms slowly lifted, his wrists curling up to his face. He started to whimper softly.

As she unveiled the infant Cassia watched closely the face of the priestess. She looked for the usual signs of pleasure, for reassurance. But the smile had vanished, and the priestess' eyes were dark and thoughtful. She paused for a moment or two, then, as if remembering what she was there to do, reached down to the pool beside her, and lifted a handful of water to her lips. She drank from her cupped hand, and scattered the remaining drops of water over the rousing infant. His whimpers grew louder, and he started for the first time to protest more vigorously. But the sound of his cry was not the harsh vibrating, echoing cry that this room had heard so many times; it was squeaky, high and soft, more like the mewling of a cat than the lusty cries of a newborn human. The priestess no longer appeared to pay any attention to the child. Her eyes were closed, and she mouthed the words of ritual,

'ipsa mone, quae nomen habes a carmine ductum, propositoque fave, ne tuus erret honor'.

She took a deep breath, then bent low over the fussing child. Her words were whispered, urgent. They pressed one into another, tumbling out, like the waters of the spring below them

'slow burnished still so then this one, deep with silence, hide away and lost from all others before were different but not to be, watching all eyes all manner, but after whispering, they point and is this because? Because stories without answer crying in shadows and darkness seek underneath the voice stolen thinness broken hold one moment then lost full fall not yet blow through him flying whither no words too to say whether what is done, there is comfort in moving past, moving not in time laughter song may hold light lost again little hope that was that once won…'

The priestess' breath ended, her last words disappearing. She opened her eyes, and Cassia could see in them the sadness that had skulked in the corners of her own mind for the last five days. The sadness in Naelia's face when she had brought her the child this morning to be taken to the temple. There were no more words that needed to be said. This was not to be a benediction and celebration of new life. Cassia gently folded again the cloths around the infant, his already soft cry muted further. She picked him up and stiffly started to rise up from the floor. She grimaced as she struggled to get up and she felt a hand at her elbow. The priestess had risen already, and the older woman held out her arm to help Cassia up. Cassia felt a sudden inexplicable anger at this woman with her nonsense words, her visions. She shook free of the proffered hand. What was the point of the temple, of the priestess if…?

She made her way to her feet by herself and turned away from the pool and the other woman. She was aware of other figures in the background, but walked back through the curtain and the main temple alone. As she went through the door into the brightness of the day Cassia paused briefly to collect her thoughts and her sandals before walking on down into the town. The anger was gone as quickly as it had come. She leaned against the pillar and looked out across the rooftops to the fields and hillsides beyond. She had known before she came this morning. The emptiness inside her rose up to the surface to claim its rightful place. The bundle was light in her arms. She knew what she must do.

Prologue 2: The Carmentis Machine 2030 AD

Behind the glass Adina sipped her lukewarm coffee and watched the box being rolled across the floor and docked into its moorings in the shadow of the machine. Over the incubator's smooth convex surface bright numbers and lines danced and jostled for prominence. A large green number over the head end was steady, but changing, 1.35, 1.36, 1.40. The number meant little to Adina, but she knew that green was reassuring. Below it there was a panel of spiking, wriggling lines. From this distance they sometimes seemed like the energetic handwriting of a dozen elderly poltergeists. Over the central curve several numbers in shades of blue floated, with other, smaller numbers above and below them, purple, orange, yellow, white. A mathematician's rainbow. At the foot end of the box two bulbous half-filled grey balloons quivered as they floated and rotated slowly.

The nurse who had pushed the incubator into the room looked behind her at Adina, then moved her hand across a panel below the main casing. The surface of the box cleared instantly, then, a moment later the numbers, shapes, and lines appeared on the left side of Adina's window. Through the now-clear surface Adina could just see a small pink shape, still, amidst snaking wires and tubes. But out of the corner of her eye to her left she could also see the shape in detail. Below the pneumographs a close up image of the infant had appeared on the window.

The nurse had disappeared from the machine room, then reappeared behind Adina. Adina turned from the glass to the desk in front of her. No more time to day-dream. She put her coffee carefully down in the arm of her chair, wiped her hands on her scrub trousers, then brushed her fingers over the surface of the desk. A series of shapes appeared. Her fingers darted across the familiar patterns, and the shapes shifted, several disappearing, one moving up to the top of the surface. Numbers and words emerged, rising to the top of the desk as they were touched, or retreating back into the dark surface if they were not chosen. Adina's hands moved, one over the other, floating and jumping in quiet choreography. On the right side of the desk the scout set appeared, and Adina pressed, pushed, and twisted the shapes until she was happy with them. Then the bagatelle was over. With one final motion of her index Adina settled back, satisfied, into her chair and looked again across the glass to the dark arch of the machine. Its concavity glowed gently, and the familiar hum rose in volume. If she had thought about it Adina could have felt its low chant rising through the chair into her spine. But the deep murmuring was so familiar now that she noticed it only by its absence, on rare occasions when the machine was shut down. The silence on those occasions was disconcerting, unsettling, loud.

Now the glass to Adina's right started to fill with bright shapes, variations on a theme. Images rolled down the glass as they appeared from the machine, each a shifting, turning palette. The same shape appeared from different sides, sometimes cut one way, sometimes another, sometimes close, sometimes further away. When she had started working here Adina used to think that they looked like nothing so much as a set of lurid iridescent walnuts. As the images rolled off the bottom of the glass they slid across the surface of the desk and collected in a set of piles below Adina's hands. From time to time she would gesture at one or more of the piles and slide it across to one side.

Ilara watched the machine steward work. When the pictures started to appear she found it hard to keep her eyes off them. She was supposed to be watching the numbers and images on the left of the window, but it was mostly unnecessary. The homeostaphin would adjust the infant's support automatically if his condition changed during the scan. Changes in regional perfusion, ventilation, metabolism would be matched with subtle changes in the cocktail of neohormones, cytokines, and neuropeptides that were trickled constantly through the infant's umbilicus. On the rare occasion that external intervention was required the displays would display a warning, and the mobinas in her pocket would vibrate to draw it to her attention. Ilara could not make sense of all of the pictures and numbers spilling down the glass. But she had been in this room enough times before to know which pictures and shapes the doctors concentrated on, which colours were good, which were worrying.

PROLOGUE 2: THE CARMENTIS MACHINE 2030 AD

The doctors were worried about this one already, she could tell. He had arrived two nights earlier, transferred by ambulance from one of the medical centres in the camp on the north edge of the city. The story wasn't unusual: a refugee family without working permits, a pregnancy concealed so that the mother could continue to work in one of the component workshops, a long, (too long) labour at home with family members tending in between work shifts. They had finally taken her to one of the volunteer-run medical clinics, where a young graduate had attempted to deliver his first infant without any of the panoply of labour modulators and monitors that had been taken for granted in the obstetric centres of his training.

He had thought it was dead when he finally managed to deliver it. The pale, limp, wet doll was warm, but otherwise seemed impossibly removed from the vigorous screaming infants whose births he had witnessed previously. More out of a sense of duty (and a sense that this was what doctors did) rather than out of any hope that it would be successful, he had carried the infant to the bench where they had earlier managed to find and set up a warming light. He could hear his own heart beating loud and frantic in his ears when he tried to listen to the infant's chest, and he vainly willed it to hush so that he could hear. Out of a routine that he half-remembered from an online simulation that he had once performed somewhere, he started to press on the infant's chest rhythmically and reached for the exbrethist with his other hand. He fumbled as he tried to fit the mask to the slippery small face and motioned to the health assistant to help him fit the mask back on to the device. His knuckles turned white as his fingers pressed the mask hard down onto the infant's face. The exbrethist, detecting the pressure, started to slowly slide in and back, a tiny silent accordion. Without enough hands to do everything at once the doctor swore, stopped his compressions briefly, and adjusted the dials on the machine to the settings that he half-remembered 50–20–21. He moved his left hand back to the chest and resumed compressions.

Several hours later the infant had arrived at the Centre. The neonatologist on call had been summoned, and together with her fellow had spent an hour or more connecting the infant to monitoring and to the ventilator, inserting umbilical lines, starting neurokines, vasopressors, bringing his temperature down. When Ilara had heard them talking to their colleagues the next morning they had been tense and downbeat. Too late, too long, too warm they had muttered.

Ilara re-entered the machine room to retrieve the infant. The scan was over. She nudged the wheel releases with the tip of her foot, and pulled the box back out from under the machine. She turned when she heard a tapping on the glass behind her. The machine steward was pointing to the numbers that she could still see (back to front) on the window. Ilara smiled, embarrassed, and reactivated the display.

As she wheeled the infant back into the unit Ilara wondered about the pictures that would now be appearing on the radiologist's screen and what the verdict would be. There had been reds and oranges marching across the display in the machine room that Ilara knew shouldn't be there. She wasn't optimistic. As she opened the door to the infant's room the parents looked up at her—anxious, hoping, questioning. Ilara tried to be non-committal.

'The scan all went fine, we'll know the results soon. You will need to speak to Dr Darina.'

As they walked through the door of her office Darina swept a hand across her desk surface, and the wall in front of her, hitherto covered with dark shapes and images, became a uniform white. The lighting in the room rose, and the window opposite the door demisted to show a view of the treetops in the park beyond. Darina smiled and gestured to the pair to sit down, turning her own chair around to face them across a low glass table. This was her fourth such meeting today, part of the routine of her work with the machine. Most days she spent about half of her time in the semi-dark decoding the images and results that poured out of the machine and annotating the automated reports that it yielded. The other half she spent talking to families about the results. Every infant that came through the Centre was scanned by the machine, usually within twenty-four or forty-eight hours of arrival. Parents were anxious to know what the future held.

Most of the time Darina's task was pleasant enough. The technology available in the newborn intensive care unit, with its liquid ventilators, homeostaphins, and neuroprots meant that the news she had to convey was usually positive. There was a group of parents who were intensely disappointed to learn from the machine that their child would only have average skills in language and mathematics, or that they would lack the necessary combination of cortical and cerebellar function for high sporting achievement. But most were pleased enough. However, once or twice a week, like now, she would have a more difficult task. She coughed drily to clear her throat, tried a sympathetic smile, and embarked on a familiar spiel

'Thank you for coming. I am sure that you are keen to find out the results of your son's scan. Before I tell you the results it is important that you understand what the machine is able to do, and what it cannot. Our machine combines detailed structural morphometry with functional assay and neurogenetic profile. It is able to give us a highly accurate assessment with very narrow confidence intervals of both the current and future neurological capacity of infants. It cannot, of course, tell us exactly what the future experience of your child will be, whether they will like tomatoes more than potatoes, football more than basketball',

Darina paused to allow her audience to share the joke, but neither of them were smiling. She went hurriedly on

'nor can it, in fact predict the future—it can't tell us, for example, whether or not your child will suffer viral encephalitis, win the lottery, be in a car accident or struck by lightning. But, absent further injury, and assuming the provision of a full range of neurorehabilitation the machine can tell us exactly what things your child will, and will not be able to do in twenty years' time.'

She paused for emphasis

'I am afraid, that for your son the machine indicates far more of the latter than the former…'

The mother heard the words, but they rolled over her like water over a stone. She looked past the doctor into the park where the tree tops were swaying gently in the breeze. Occasional words broke through, but mostly the doctor appeared to be speaking an ancient language or code. 'Intellectual disability…verbal performance IQ of thirty-two to thirty-five…less deficit in global empathic index…major functional gross motor deficit…'. The doctor had summoned images up to the wall and pointed to areas with one colour or another. This area was too bright, that one too orange, this one too small. The mother looked down from the wall to the glass table, and stared at the box of tissues unsubtly placed in the centre. She wondered if she should be crying.

'Do you have any questions?'

The mother looked up and realized that she was supposed to say something. She turned to her husband, but he was fidgeting and staring at his feet. He had never been good with doctors. The volunteers in the camps were generally friendly, but they had little equipment and few drugs. They never stayed around for long. Some of her friends had managed to see doctors inside the city by using forged identity cards, but she knew a couple who had been deported after they had tried that. There were some drugs available within the camp if you knew the right people, but she had heard bad stories about them too. Few people that she knew had ever seen the Centre, let alone been allowed inside for treatment. She still didn't understand why they had accepted her son here, but to her relief they had not been asking her for money, or for identification.

'I don't know…What do you want…what do we need to do?'

Darina tried hard to speak slowly

'Your son has very serious brain damage from lack of oxygen around the time of birth. He will be seriously disabled. We need to make a decision about the life supports that are keeping him alive. We need to know whether you want us to keep going with those treatments, or…or let him go.'

The mother looked again out of the window past the trees to the buildings on the far side of the park. She tried to translate the doctor's words into a future for her son. She saw, but did not see, the miles of streets and close-packed houses, the wall, the camp, and beyond, the hills. She thought of her other children at home, being looked after by friends in the camp, and of her hopes for this child. She thought of him in his crystal chamber, alone on the other side of the wall and wished that she could hold him in her arms. Her husband sobbed quietly beside her. She did not know what to do.

Introduction: Neuroethics and Intensive Care

In the last decade an explosion in technology and science relating to the human brain has highlighted profound ethical questions. New forms of brain imaging raise the possibility of various forms of mind-reading. Lie detection using functional magnetic resonance imaging (fMRI) or electro-encephalography (EEG) has been presented as evidence in court cases. Other brain scans appear to show that some patients, previously believed to be in a vegetative state and completely unaware of their surroundings, may in fact be conscious. Developments in brain–machine interfaces raise the possibility of restoring function to injured brain, and bring to mind the cyborgs or hybrid human/machines of science fiction novels. Still other devices and drugs are likely in the near future to substantially improve a variety of cognitive functions including memory, attention, and reasoning.

The broad array of questions raised by these technological advances has given rise to the new field of *neuroethics*. The first books in this topic started rolling off the presses in the first years of the new millennium (Gazzaniga 2005; Illes 2006; Levy 2007). Those works were devoted to addressing the ethical implications of neuroscience, but they also investigated some of the implications of neuroscience for ethics itself.

There are three recurring themes in neuroethics. The first theme is a degree of scepticism about current technology and its capacity to perform the tasks that it is claimed to do. For example, there has been considerable hype and publicity about brain lie detectors. They work in a variety of different ways, but some attempt to distinguish recollection of real memories from events that were not experienced. The idea is that if a defendant who is guilty of a murder is asked to read a description of the event, areas of the brain responsible for retrieving old memories will be active. In 2008, a woman in Mumbai was convicted of murder, at least in part on the basis of this sort of evidence. However, there has been sustained criticism of the science behind these technologies (whether it actually does what it is claimed to do) and its capacity to reliably distinguish between the guilty and the innocent (Simpson 2008).

A second recurring theme in neuroethics looks beyond the current limitations to identify those practical questions that will be raised by new technology in the years and decades ahead. Even though some of the more speculative advances may not be available for a while it is potentially worth thinking carefully about the ethical issues that will be at stake once the technology is available. What would be the implications, for example, of drugs or other interventions that improved our capacity for ethical reflection and action—forms of moral enhancement? In some cases such reflection will provide us with strong reasons to pursue such advances. In other cases it may provide us with motivation to monitor and regulate the development of technologies that have the potential for both benefits and serious harms. In still other cases, careful reflection about the problems raised by certain forms of technology may lead us to decide not to develop them.

Although there are new questions raised by neuroscience, neuroethics has also often involved a certain amount of déjà vu. Its third theme sees neuroethics revisiting or reconsidering old and difficult philosophical and ethical questions. One example is the large amount of literature now relating to the neuroscience of free will and human agency. Questions about determinism, free will, and responsibility are hardly new. However, neuroethics may bring new insights through a greater understanding of the neurological basis of volition and action; it may also simply bring back to public attention and debate old questions that still need to be solved.

The vast majority of work in the field of neuroethics has focused on adults. There are several reasons for this. The first is that one of the major developments, functional neuroimaging, is technically very difficult in babies and children. fMRI and related technologies measure acute changes in brain activity. By studying individuals in a range of situations it has been possible to identify areas of the brain that light up in response to particular stimuli, or to distinguish between the patterns of activation in different groups of individuals. In one (controversial) example, in the lead up to the 2004 US presidential election, scientists examined the response of either

INTRODUCTION: NEUROETHICS AND INTENSIVE CARE 13

Democrat or Republican voters to pictures of presidential candidates, and suggested that political allegiance triggered a differential emotional response to candidates (Kaplan, Freedman, et al. 2007). These sorts of studies are far more challenging if not impossible to perform in children or newborn infants. There are practical challenges. Children, particularly very young children, may not lie still in an MRI scanner for long periods. Indeed, young children often require an anaesthetic in order to tolerate lying still for an MRI, a procedure that would render impossible or redundant most functional imaging. There are also potential ethical challenges, since obtaining consent and ethical approval for studies in children is much harder than for adults. Furthermore, many of the potential practical applications of these technologies are far more likely to be applied in adults than in children. (Although lie detection might have some appeal to the classroom teacher or parent it is far more likely to be used in the courtroom!)

However, there have been developments in neuroscience for children and newborn infants with important practical and ethical implications. There have been developments in our understanding of the capacities of children, and their relationship to adults. There have been advances in the study of normal and abnormal development and learning. But one of the developments with the most impact has been in neurological prognostication—the prediction of future neurological outcome. New forms of imaging are able, to a far greater degree than previously possible, to identify specific areas of brain damage. It is possible with such scans to identify both the degree and type of future disability for newborn infants with congenital or acquired brain abnormalities, or older children who have suffered brain injury. Whether you are a newborn who has suffered birth asphyxia, a very premature infant who has suffered an intraventicular haemorrhage, or a child who has had a near drowning event it is highly likely that you will have an MRI of your brain performed while you are in intensive care. A neuroradiologist or neurologist will translate the results of imaging into predictions about the likely outcome if you survive intensive care, including the likelihood of serious motor, learning, or sensory impairments. Such predictions are, at least in my experience, highly influential in newborn and paediatric intensive care. They play a major role in decisions by doctors and parents to continue or to stop treatment for critically ill infants and children.

My own interest in these questions arose from working in newborn intensive care and from being involved in the care of infants and children with varying degrees of brain injury. During my clinical training there was increasing use of MRI for imaging the newborn brain, and increasing emphasis on the results of such testing for decision-making. Over a period of six or seven years MRI went from a test that was performed rarely, to one performed almost routinely in seriously ill infants and children. It became apparent to me that such testing raised a number of difficult questions in practice, and that these questions had received little or no systematic attention.

How should doctors, parents, and policy-makers respond to these technological advances, now and in the future? What are the limits of current, and future predictions? Which predictions, and which disabilities are sufficiently grave that parents and doctors may legitimately decide to withdraw treatment and allow a newborn infant or child to die? These are the three central questions of the neuroethics of prognostication in critical care, and they will be the central questions of this book. In addressing them, I will draw on science, philosophy, and clinical medicine. Scientific information will help inform the nature of prognostic information, and its limits. Philosophy will be used to develop important distinctions, and to reflect on the key values at stake, and the key arguments in favour of and against different courses of action. Throughout, I will hope to relate abstract questions back to the practical issues facing those at the bedside. As we work through these questions, the book will uncover all three of the themes of neuroethics identified above.

Currently, predictions about critically ill children are significantly limited by uncertainty. This uncertainty makes decisions more complicated, and potentially muddies the waters when it comes to reflecting on the key questions at stake. To help think clearly about predictions and decision-making, in Part I of the book we will set aside this uncertainty. We will attempt to anticipate and analyse the questions that will present themselves in the not-too-distant future once prognostic technology has advanced further. This part draws on the thought experiment of a machine (the Carmentis machine of the second prologue) that is able to provide accurate, specific, and detailed predictions of future impairment for brain injured children and infants.

In Chapter 1 I provide a context for later discussion. Intensive care has created unique ethical dilemmas by making it possible to keep alive patients who would otherwise have died (and who would still die in parts of the world with more limited health care resources). There are several different settings in which life support might be withdrawn in intensive care. There are also different types of end-of-life decision including decisions not to provide potentially life-prolonging therapies, and decisions to actively end the life of the patient. This book focuses particularly on decisions about withholding or withdrawing life-sustaining treatment, and on so-called 'quality of life' justifications for limiting treatment, since it is here that neuroimaging has the most relevance. I will look briefly at the arguments against quality of life decisions in intensive care. I will also look at the example of birth asphyxia, which will provide a useful example to return to at several points in the book.

Chapter 2 looks at the most widely recommended ethical framework for decisions about treatment in children or infants and applies these to certain predictions of impairment. Existing guidelines emphasise that treatment may be withdrawn or withheld if this is consistent with the *best interests* of the child. But what does this mean? Even if we were completely certain of the future outcome for a child, there are formidable practical and philosophical problems with performing subjective or objective assessments of their best interests. Should we use a different basis for decision-making?

An alternative ethical justification for withdrawing life-sustaining treatment is outlined in Chapter 3. Disabled newborn infants or children might be allowed to die where this would allow parents to have another (unimpaired) child. Some philosophers have argued that 'replacement' should be a legitimate and important factor for decision-making, and perhaps it does sometimes creep into clinical decisions. This chapter delves into philosophical questions relating to bringing children into existence, including the non-identity problem. (It is the most philosophical section of the book, and some readers may prefer to skip over sections of this chapter.) I suggest that the only significant moral reason to take into account replacement in decisions for newborn infants is that this would sometimes be in the interests of others, particularly parents and siblings.

The final chapter in Part I, Chapter 4, weighs up the interests of the child against the interests of other members of their family. What is at stake for each of these in the setting of known certain impairment? Family members may be profoundly affected by the need to provide care for an impaired child, though this is potentially mitigated by the amount of support provided for families. I look at the strength of the interest of the child in continued life, and at the potential difference between newborn infants and older children. Infants' interests in life are potentially somewhat less than the interest of an older child or adult because of their developmental immaturity. This may mean that decision-making in newborn intensive care is made on a different basis to decision-making in older children.

Part II of the book returns to the messy real world where predictions are imperfect, and addresses some of the practical and ethical problems relating to uncertainty. Chapter 5 looks at the different factors that contribute to uncertainty in prognosis including variations in physical and psychological susceptibility to injury, neural plasticity, and the impact of the child's environment. It also looks at research into the quality of life of children with disability. Studies have mostly been undertaken in ways that make it hard to apply predictions of quality of life to particular patients. Chapter 6 assesses one way of reducing uncertainty in prognosis, i.e. to continue treatment until more information is available, and until the patient's prognosis is clearer. But the risk with this strategy is that the child is no longer dependent on intensive forms of life support, and may survive with very severe impairment. There is sometimes a limited 'window of opportunity' to withdraw life support, and this may lead to a sense of urgency about decisions. I explore the role of the so-called doctrine of double-effect in treatment decisions of this nature. I also look at whether the option of later withdrawal of artificial nutrition would avoid the window of opportunity problem. Chapter 7 looks at how uncertainty interacts with the various interests at stake in decisions about life-sustaining treatment and the ethics of withdrawing treatment. The interests of the child and the interests of parents overlap in several different ways, partly as a result of uncertainty about outcome. We will also look at the impact of uncertainty on the interests of the child.

Chapter 8 draws together the conclusions of the earlier chapters of the book to look at policy for treatment limitation decisions in paediatric and neonatal intensive care, and at whether it is possible to define clearly when such decisions are appropriate. I argue that there should not be a single threshold for treatment withdrawal. Instead there should be several different thresholds, depending on the age of the child, on the type of treatment withdrawn, and on the type of decision. These thresholds will set out the boundaries for parental discretion in treatment decisions, including a level of impairment sufficiently severe that certain types of treatment should not be provided even if parents wish it, and at the other extreme, a level of impairment sufficiently mild that life-sustaining treatment must continue even if parents do not want this to occur. I explore how practical criteria for these thresholds might be developed and provide an example of such criteria for neonatal birth asphyxia and premature infants, and a framework for the development of local treatment guidelines.

Across both halves of the book, the fundamental questions that emerge about the treatment of critically ill newborns and children will turn out not to be new at all, but old questions that have been raised time and again over the last fifty years. Indeed, some of the questions raised by this technology for newborns are more than two thousand years old . . .

References

Gazzaniga, M.S. (2005). *The Ethical Brain.* New York: Dana Press.

Illes, J. (2006). *Neuroethics: Defining the Issues in Theory, Practice, and Policy.* Oxford: Oxford University Press.

Kaplan, J.T., J. Freedman, et al. (2007). 'Us versus them: Political attitudes and party affiliation influence neural response to faces of presidential candidates', *Neuropsychologia* 45(1): 55–64.

Levy, N. (2007). *Neuroethics.* Cambridge: Cambridge University Press.

Simpson, J.R. (2008). 'Functional MRI lie detection: too good to be true?', *J. Am. Acad. Psychiatry Law* 36(4): 491–8.

PART I

Death and Grief in the Ancient World

In developed countries today it is unusual for newborn infants to die. Parents are faced with the loss of their infant in less than five out of every 1000 live births. However, in ancient Rome birth was one of the most dangerous points in life. Almost one in ten Roman children died in early infancy, and 1/3 did not make it to one year of age (Rawson 2003).

The extremely high chance of infants dying early in life may be one reason for a Roman attitude towards infants and children that can seem callous or heartless to modern eyes. Infants achieved recognition and acceptance into the community after their naming day, which took place on day eight or nine, a delay that would have allowed time for early neonatal loss, and for parents to make an active decision to rear the child (Rawson 2003).

There was no official period of mourning for children who died before the age of three years, with a full period of mourning only observed after the age of ten. The lack of official mourning may be one reason why infants were buried rather than cremated (as was the norm for older Romans) (Harris 1994).

The attitude towards the death of infants or young children is reflected in the language of epitaphs. Death was rarely if ever described as 'untimely' for children under the age of two, though this phrase was used sometimes even for the elderly. On one Greek gravestone, of a child who died at age twelve, her parents expressed regret that she had not died at a younger age (Golden 1988).

Yet even if not officially recognized, there is evidence that the Romans grieved their lost infants and children. Cicero lamented the cruelty of infant death 'Some think that if a small child dies this must be borne with equanimity; if it is still in the cradle there should not even be a lament. And yet it is from the latter than nature has more cruelly demanded back the gift she had given' (Rawson 2003).

Historian Mark Golden, has argued that there is scant evidence that the Romans and other ancient parents failed to care for their infants, or failed to mourn their loss. In other societies parents sometimes allow infants to die, for example because of the pressure of poverty, and yet care genuinely and fully for their other children (Golden 1988).

The Roman writer and rhetorician Seneca the Elder, described the father of an exposed infant 'weeping and trembling' with grief (Harris 1994).

References

Golden, M. (1988). 'Did the ancients care when their children died?', *Greece and Rome* 35(2): 152–63.

Harris, W.V. (1994). 'Child-Exposure in the Roman Empire', *Journal of Roman Studies* 84: 1–22.

Rawson, B. (2003). *Children and Childhood in Roman Italy*. Oxford, New York: Oxford University Press.

1

Destiny, Disability, and Death

Intensive Care

The global polio epidemic that followed the Second World War caused the deaths of tens of thousands of adults and children from acute respiratory failure. Patients suffocated when they were unable to persuade the muscles of their chest to work. That epidemic contributed to the development of a vaccine for polio in the early 1950s, one of the first and most dramatic successes of widespread immunization programmes, but it also spurred the development of artificial respirators, machines to manage or assist the breathing of those unable to do it by themselves. The first generation of these machines were negative pressure ventilators—giant iron lungs that encased patients' bodies. The machines sucked on the chest wall to make it expand. They saved lives, but were heavy, cumbersome, and extremely expensive. In the mid-1950s iron lungs were followed by the development of intubation and positive pressure ventilation; tubes were manually inserted into the trachea, and patients were connected to machines that blew air forcibly into the lungs like a set of bellows.

The development of artificial ventilators led in turn to the establishment of intensive care. This new technology required dedicated units since the care of patients with single and multiple organ failure required highly specialized medical and nursing support. But the same development also gave rise to the central ethical question that has vexed doctors, nurses, and ethicists caring for critically ill patients since then. When is enough, enough? When should intensive care be provided, and when should it be stopped? When are patients too sick to benefit from treatment?

This question, relating to the benefits and risks of therapy might be, and probably has been applied to almost any medical treatment. But it is particularly important and particularly prominent in intensive care for several reasons. First, because intensive care is often provided to patients who would otherwise have died. It prevents or forestalls death, and its cessation may lead to death. A significant proportion of patients admitted to intensive care die despite treatment (usually about 1/5 of adult intensive care admissions, but a smaller proportion of paediatric or neonatal intensive care admissions). Secondly, as its name implies, intensive care often involves intensive and potentially painful interventions. An adult patient admitted with acute sepsis is likely, within a fairly short period after admission, to have a tube inserted through their mouth into their airway, to have large needles inserted into their neck and wrist, a urethral catheter inserted, another tube inserted through a nostril into their stomach. In one study, patients admitted to a neonatal intensive care unit had an average of sixty invasive interventions during their stay. (One extremely premature infant had 488 invasive procedures performed) (Barker and Rutter 1995). There is far more at stake for the patient if intensive care is continued too long than for most other treatments. Thirdly, patients who survive their acute illness following intensive care admission may be left with substantial ongoing illness and/or impairment. They may worry, or their caregivers may worry, whether their stay in intensive care was worth it.

Decisions

The easy thing to do when a patient is critically ill is to provide treatment. If their oxygen levels fall they are provided with more support from the ventilator. If their blood pressure plummets they are given vasoactive medication or more fluids. Low levels of salts or sugar in the bloodstream are treated with intravenous supplements. Appropriately, the default in intensive care is to treat the patient and the problems in front of you. But the hard thing to do is to decide *not* to provide treatment, to know when *not* to support breathing, blood pressure, or metabolism. It is hard because it requires knowledge about prognosis, the predicted outcome for the patient. As medical sociologist Nicholas Christakis argues in his book *Death Foretold,* prognosis is neglected in medical teaching (Christakis 1999). Doctors are good at *diagnosis* and *treatment*. But they are less comfortable, less familiar, often less skilled at the art of prediction. In addition, decisions not to treat are hard because they require value judgements about the benefit of treatment given a particular prognosis, and ethical judgements about decisions that may lead to the death of the patient.

There are broadly four different reasons not to provide life-sustaining treatment (LST) for a patient.

Quantity of Life

The first of these is because treatment may sustain life, but not for long. The patient will die whether or not the treatment is given. Death may be imminent, for example in a patient with overwhelming sepsis and organ failure. Perhaps the patient is already receiving maximum supportive treatment in intensive care, yet they are continuing to deteriorate. In these settings treatment is often described as *futile*. (Though this term is used in a range of different ways, and is perhaps best avoided; Wilkinson and Savulescu 2011.) In its 2004 guideline on withdrawing or withholding LST, the UK Royal College of Paediatrics and Child Health described this as a 'No Chance' situation (Royal College of Paediatrics and Child Health 2004). Alternatively, death may appear inevitable within a longer period of days, weeks, or a few months. This includes, for example, some patients with disseminated or untreatable malignancy. Intensive care will merely delay death for a short period of time, and is felt not to provide a benefit to the patient.

Quantity of life seems like a straightforward and unambiguous justification for not providing treatment. However, in practice it is extremely difficult to determine how long a patient will survive with treatment. There is a problem, to which we will return in Chapter 5, that the evidence that doctors use to determine whether treatment is not going to work is often contaminated by previous treatment limitation decisions (Wilkinson and Savulescu 2011). What is more, the chance of treatment succeeding is rarely zero. Even if all previous patients that a doctor has seen with this condition have died there is always the possibility that this patient is different in some important way, that they will buck the trend, make a miraculous recovery. The question in reality is not whether there is *no* chance of recovery, rather whether it is *sufficiently low* to warrant non-treatment. We need to know both how low this patient's chances are, as well as what counts as 'sufficiently low'. Is a 5 per cent chance of survival low enough to justify not providing intensive care? What about 1 in 100, or

1 in 1,000? Different doctors, but also different patients and families are likely to have diverging views about this. If death is inevitable, but not imminent, how long a prolongation of life is enough to outweigh the negatives of treatment? We all face 'inevitable death', so when is the quantity of life offered by intensive care too little? Finally, doctors' judgements about quantity of life are often influenced by another consideration, namely by the likely state of the patient if they do happen to survive for a period of time.

Quality of Life

The second reason not to provide LST is because of concerns about survival in a severely impaired state. Some patients survive severe head injury or an out-of-hospital cardiac arrest but are left in a persistent vegetative state. Patients with extensive burns may be left with extremely severe scarring and painful contractures (permanent shortening of their joints). Children with meningococcal sepsis sometimes develop a lack of blood supply (ischaemia) to their extremities and require amputations of all of their limbs. Infants who suffer a lack of oxygen and blood supply around the time of their birth (birth asphyxia) may develop forms of cerebral palsy rendering them unable to control any of their limbs. Faced with this prospect doctors and patients' families sometimes come to a conclusion that death is preferable to survival.

Decisions not to save the life of patients because of concerns about quality of life are relatively common in paediatric and neonatal intensive care. In two recent studies in Switzerland and the Netherlands quality of life was a significant influence on end-of-life decisions in 40–50 per cent of deaths (Berger and Hofer 2009; Verhagen, Dorscheidt, et al. 2009). In earlier studies from Australia and the United States, withdrawal of mechanical ventilation was motivated by quality of life concerns in 30–40 per cent of cases (Singh, Lantos, et al. 2004; Wilkinson, Fitzsimons, et al. 2006). The majority of neonatal physicians in a large survey across ten European countries reported having limited intensive care treatment on the basis of poor neurological prognosis (Cuttini, Nadai, et al. 2000). Furthermore, influential professional guidelines support the withdrawal of life support from newborn infants and children on the basis of predicted quality of life (Royal College of Paediatrics and Child Health 2004; American Academy of Pediatrics Committee on Fetus and Newborn 2007).

However, these decisions are also highly controversial. They are controversial because they are contrary to a long held vitalist tradition (particularly associated with Christianity and Catholicism) that views death as an absolute evil, and life as an absolute good (Finnis, Boyle, et al. 1987). However, as argued in 1974 by Catholic moral theologian Richard McCormick, vitalism is a distortion of the Judeo-Christian perspective (McCormick 1974). Life is valuable, and precious, but it is 'a relative good, and the duty to preserve it a limited one' (McCormick 1974: 174). Life is valuable because of the higher goods that it allows the individual to experience.

Controversy also arises in part because there is disagreement about which conditions are bad enough to make death preferable to continued life. In surveys, most people indicate that they would not want life-saving treatment or resuscitation if they were going to be permanently unconscious, or in a vegetative state (Emanuel, Barry, et al. 1991). However, some people *do* want treatment provided even if they were going to be in such a condition. This might be because of vitalism. But it could also be because of the value that they place on the small chance of recovery or improvement to normal function. Even if the chance is tiny it may be worthwhile from their perspective to continue life-sustaining treatment (Stone 2007). We will return shortly to the significance of patients' wishes for treatment decisions in intensive care. However, the important practical question is about what we should allow patients or their surrogate to decide if they *do* reasonably judge that survival is a worse fate than dying.

Some have concerns about the metaphysics of a comparison between life and death. They argue that it makes no sense to compare a state of existence with a state of non-existence (McMahan 1988; Glover 1990: 51). How can death *be* better than life, since if you are dead there is no you, no awareness? This question has a long history in philosophy (the Greek philosopher Epicurus argued that there was no need to fear death for this reason), and it has been covered in detail elsewhere (McMahan 1988; Grey 1999). Briefly though, there are several ways of making sense of this judgement. One is that although we cannot compare death with life directly, in some circumstances continued life might constitute a net harm, because the negative experiences that the patient will experience outweigh any positives. Secondly, although *death* might not be better than life, in some circumstances *dying* might be better than living. From the point of view of the patient still alive in intensive care the prospect of oblivion may be preferable to days or weeks or months of pain and discomfort. Alternatively, we could step back and compare two different possible versions of a life, one in which the patient dies in intensive care, and a second in which they live longer, but survive in a state of impairment and suffering. If we take a 'whole life' perspective it seems that sometimes the shorter life will be a better one than the longer life. As an analogy, we could think of a book with a good beginning and middle, but then a very badly written final chapter. It makes some sense to think that a version of the book missing that final chapter may be a better book than another version with the bad chapter left in.

As an aside at this point it is worth briefly touching on some terminology. There are various phrases that might be used to describe a state that is judged by the individual to be so undesirable that they would rather die than experience it. For example, life might be judged to be a 'fate worse than death', or 'worse than nothing'. Both of these tempt criticism by comparing existence with non-existence. I will refer to a 'life not worth living' and a 'life worth living', though it is crucial to note that this is an internal assessment. These terms are based on a judgement *for the individual*. A 'life worth living/ not worth living' as used in this book does not denote or compare the worth of individuals to others (see Chapter 3 for a further definition of these terms).

A separate concern about quality of life decisions in intensive care arises from evidence about the views of patients with significant disabilities. Although some patients with significant illness or impairment find their lives so difficult that they attempt suicide or request help in ending their lives, most do not. Indeed, evidence from adult patients with severe illness or impairment (with conditions that would often be regarded by the non-disabled as extremely undesirable) suggests that many rate their experience of life just as positively or almost as positively as those without overt illness or impairment (Albrecht and Devlieger 1999). This finding is sometimes referred to as the 'disability paradox', and has led some to question the justification for limiting treatment on the basis of quality of life. This sort of evidence should certainly make us pause before we make judgements about the quality of life of others. However, it does not mean that we should never make such judgements. One problem with much of the available data on quality of life is that it specifically excludes both those patients who have died, and those who are unable to communicate, potentially the most important groups for such decisions. We will return to some of these problems in Chapter 5.

The strongest reason to support quality of life decisions in paediatric and neonatal intensive care is that there are some conditions where it appears that life is no longer a benefit. There are adult patients, for example those with painful and debilitating illness, who are not clinically depressed, who are able to tell us that they do not want to continue their life. For example, in 2008 French schoolteacher Chantal Sebire apparently ended her own life after a failed appeal for assisted suicide. She was suffering from an extremely rare and untreatable facial tumour (esthesioneuroblastoma) (Spooner 2009). The question of whether, in such a state, it is ethical for such patients to be given assistance in ending their lives is highly controversial. But there is almost uniform agreement that these patients have a right to decline treatment that would extend their lives, and that it would be wrong, indeed it would be a form of assault, to provide it against their wishes. We may not all agree about when life is not a benefit, some may feel that in the same circumstance they would make a different choice. But it would be egregious to force treatment on a patient who competently declines it, because we do not share their values.

If it is possible for adult patients to judge their own lives as not worth living, and it is reasonable for them to decline life saving treatment, the question is why this should not also apply to children. If treatment can be a harm to an adult then it can equally be a harm to a child or infant. Although a child or infant may not be able to make this decision by themselves, we have existing processes for making decisions on their behalf. If we refuse to make this decision, refuse to ever limit treatment on the grounds of quality of life, we will cause and prolong the suffering of a significant number of children. In fact, even those opposed to making quality of life decisions in intensive care appear to accept some cases where the quality of a child's survival is sufficiently poor to justify not providing treatment. For example, Dr Everard Koop was the US surgeon general responsible for the 'Baby Doe' rules that were introduced in the US in the 1980s in order to prevent treatment limitation on the basis of quality of life judgements. Dr Koop admitted at a court hearing on those rules that infants with anencephaly, or those with no functioning intestine should receive palliative care (Kuhse and Singer 1985: 25). The question is not whether it is acceptable to withdraw treatment on the basis of quality of life, but *when* it is acceptable.

Quantity and quality of life are the most important reasons for discontinuing treatment in paediatric and neonatal intensive care. The latter will be the focus for much of the rest of this book, since the relevance of brain imaging is almost exclusively in its ability to predict future impairment if the patient survives. With rare exceptions it is less useful at identifying patients who are not able to survive. There are, however, two other reasons to discontinue treatment in intensive care.

The Wishes of the Patient

For patients who are competent to make decisions for themselves their wishes about treatment are often the most important factor, reflecting the value placed on patient autonomy. This is perhaps the most common reason to limit treatment in adult intensive care—that the patient does not or would not want treatment to be provided. While most patients who are admitted to intensive care are too sick at the time of admission to express their wishes or to make decisions about treatment, the patient's wishes are often still relevant to decisions. They may have an advance directive that explicitly conveys their desires about treatment. Alternatively, if there is enough evidence about the desires or preferences of the patient, decisions may be made in accordance with those preferences—a process referred to as *substituted judgement*.

In paediatric and neonatal intensive care, the wishes of the patient are much less significant, since they are rarely able to be assessed. Forms of substituted judgement are sometimes applied to decisions about life-sustaining treatment for children and infants. As we will see in the next chapter, however, this is often conceptually and practically problematic.

The wishes of the patient are not divorced from considerations of quantity and quality of life since desires about treatment are frequently influenced by the chance and duration of survival with treatment, and the patient's predicted quality of life after treatment. Prognosis is still critically important. It is also worth noting that even for competent patients autonomy is not absolute. Although most legal systems respect the right of a competent patient to refuse treatment, there is often some restriction on patients' right to demand treatment (Paris 2010). This is at least partly because of the costs of providing treatment of little or no benefit.

Resources

The final factor that sometimes influences and sometimes determines decisions about the provision of intensive care is the availability of resources.

There are finite beds in intensive care, and finite funds available to provide medical care to critically ill patients. Most, if not all, intensive care units have periods of time when they reach their capacity and are unable to admit any further patients. When the intensive care unit is full elective or semi-elective surgery is cancelled, and emergency admissions have to be transferred to another hospital.

Where survival is likely if life-sustaining treatment is provided, where the quality of life of the patient if they survive is likely to be good, and where the patient (if they could choose) would want treatment provided, intensive care teams work hard not to let resource limitations influence their decision-making. However, resources may play a subliminal role in decisions—particularly where there is some uncertainty about any or all of the above factors. One place that the impact of resources can be seen is in the differences between countries in their criteria for providing intensive care. For example in the UK it is generally thought to be inappropriate to resuscitate infants who are more than seventeen weeks premature (below twenty-three weeks gestation), while at twenty-four weeks gestation resuscitation is usually provided unless parents and doctors agree that it is not in the infants' interests to do so. In other parts of Europe, for example the Netherlands, resuscitation is not usually provided for infants below twenty-five weeks. In contrast, in many parts of the developing world resuscitation is not provided for infants before twenty-eight weeks gestation. Some of these differences in practice relate to different value judgements about disability and decision-making for newborn infants. But they also reflect, to some degree, the influence of resources on decision-making for extremely premature infants.

Again, resource considerations are to some degree inseparable from the first two factors listed above. If resources are to have any role in decisions, the prognosis of patients is crucially important to determining whether or not treatment is provided, and who receives treatment.

Death

The vexed ethical question of *whether* or not to provide life-saving treatment leads inevitably on to another question—what may doctors *do* if treatment is not going to be provided. If a patient is dependent on a breathing machine to survive can the machine just be stopped? Is there a difference between a decision to take away breathing support (*withdrawing* treatment) and a decision not to start breathing support (*withholding* treatment)? If the quality of a patient's future life is judged to be so bad that death is preferable to continuing treatment is it permissible to take steps to hasten their death?

Doctors and nurses often find it much harder to stop treatment than to decide not to start it (Melltorp and Nilstun 1997; Dickenson 2000). It feels much more significant to extubate a patient (remove their breathing tube), or to switch off the machines that are supporting them, than to stand by and not provide resuscitation or breathing support when they stop breathing. However, both ethicists and the courts in most countries have argued that this difference is illusory, that withdrawing and withholding treatment are equivalent (Airedale NHS Trust v 1993; Gillon 1994; American Academy of Pediatrics Committee on Fetus and Newborn 1995; Royal College of Paediatrics and Child Health 2004). If the intention of the doctor is the same (for example to respect the patient's wishes or to avoid treatment of little benefit) and the consequences of the act (that the patient will likely die) are the same, what difference can there really be between stopping and not starting treatment? There is no difference in the ultimate cause of death in the patient who dies after having treatment withheld compared with an identical patient who has treatment withdrawn, nor any difference in the moral responsibility of the doctor for his or her decision. It would seem absurd if a doctor were inhibited or prevented from stopping treatment, but could stand by and allow the patient to die if their breathing support were accidentally disconnected. Critically ill patients sometimes develop blockages of their breathing tubes, or the tubes become dislodged when they are turned. But surely that shouldn't be the major determinant of whether they are allowed to die? Moreover, there are potential risks if doctors regard withdrawing treatment as more significant or more problematic than withholding treatment. Some patients (who could have benefited from life-sustaining treatment) may be denied treatment out of a fear that once started it could not be stopped.

There are different treatments that sustain life. One type of treatment is Cardio-Pulmonary Resuscitation or CPR: air or oxygen is provided from the mouth of a resuscitator or from a bag and mask device, and the chest is compressed to maintain circulation. For any of the reasons noted above a decision may be made not to provide CPR in the event of a cardio-respiratory arrest. Alternatively, decisions may be about the provision of intubation and positive pressure respiration or specialized forms of cardio-vascular support including drugs to maintain the patient's blood pressure (inotropes). Decisions to withhold or withdraw mechanical ventilation or cardiopulmonary resuscitation are common in newborn or paediatric intensive care. For example in neonatal units in the United States and the Netherlands more than 3/4 of all deaths were preceded by treatment limitation decisions (Verhagen, Janvier, et al. 2010). In paediatric intensive care units and paediatric hospitals 1/3–2/3 of deaths follow withdrawal or limitation of LST (Burns, Mitchell, et al. 2000; Lee, Tieves, et al. 2010).

The above treatments are in the domain of the intensive care team. It is reasonably uncontroversial that they may, at least in some circumstances, be withheld or withdrawn from critically ill patients. There are other simpler treatments, however, that also make the difference between life and death for some seriously ill patients. Providing oxygen by mask, intravenous fluids through a cannula in the patient's hand, or food through a tube in the patient's nose save the lives of patients whose oxygen levels are low, or who cannot drink or eat. Decisions not to provide these more basic treatments also take place from time to time in intensive care or on the wards of a hospital. These decisions are significantly more contentious. We will return in Chapter 6 to discuss the option of withdrawing artificial feeding from newborn infants or children with brain injury.

Allowing a patient to die by withholding or withdrawing treatment is sometimes referred to as 'Passive Euthanasia', and is generally regarded as ethically and legally justifiable. What about 'active euthanasia', or deliberate acts to hasten the death of patients? In most jurisdictions it is illegal for doctors to take such steps. That does not mean that it never happens. A significant proportion of doctors caring for newborn infants in France and the Netherlands have admitted in anonymous surveys that they sometimes give drugs with the aim of ending life (Cuttini, Nadai, et al. 2000). In the same survey a small proportion of doctors in other European countries including Spain, UK, Italy, Germany, and Sweden also reported having taken such steps. In the Netherlands, such actions are legally sanctioned in limited circumstances. Euthanasia is legal for patients older than twelve years who have a terminal illness and severe suffering (Verhagen and Sauer

2005a). In 2002, paediatricians from Groningen hospital worked with a local prosecutor to develop a set of guidelines for conditions in which euthanasia of newborn infants would not be prosecuted. According to the Groningen protocol (published in English in 2005) (Verhagen and Sauer 2005b) paediatricians would not be prosecuted for actively ending the life of a newborn infant as long as several necessary conditions were fulfilled including the presence of 'hopeless and unbearable suffering', certain diagnosis and prognosis, and parental consent. In a survey of end-of-life decisions in the Netherlands subsequent to the publication of the Groningen protocol, active euthanasia was reported to have taken place in a single infant over 12 months (Verhagen, Dorscheidt, et al. 2009). That infant had a severe (and usually lethal) disorder of bone development.

In this book I will focus mostly on questions relating to treatment withdrawal or limitation rather than active ending of life. This is firstly because in the majority of jurisdictions around the world paediatric and neonatal euthanasia remains illegal. Secondly, even in those countries where it is legal it is performed extremely rarely, whereas treatment limitation decisions occur on a regular basis and precede the majority of deaths in paediatric and newborn intensive care. Understanding the limits of those decisions will have far more potential impact on actual practice. But thirdly, the issues raised for euthanasia in newborns by advances in neuroscience are essentially the same as those raised for treatment limitation decisions. What sort of prognosis, and which patterns of neuroimaging would warrant such a decision? In the final chapter I will briefly explore whether, if we allow neonatal euthanasia, we should set different standards, different thresholds for such decisions from those that we apply to treatment withdrawal.

Destiny

The most important determinant of whether treatment is continued or discontinued in intensive care is the patient's prognosis, the outcome that is anticipated with or without treatment. How do doctors assess prognosis for critically ill patients? The details will obviously depend on the specific illness affecting the patient, it will differ significantly between extremely premature infants with intraventricular haemorrhage (bleeding in the central fluid spaces of the brain) and children with meningitis.

Interviews with doctors in intensive care suggest that they rely heavily on objective data from investigations in evaluating prognosis and establishing medical certainty (Anspach 1993; Orfali 2004). For example, doctors use published statistics on the likelihood of survival to inform quantity of life decisions. For quality of life judgements they may use clinical or imaging evidence of brain injury. On the other hand, there is also evidence of the potential *subjectivity* of prognosis. In a study of neonatal units in France and the United States neonatologists systematically differed in their evaluation of prognosis in identical cases (Orfali 2004). In the French units data that appear to reduce or erase uncertainty were valued and emphasised in justifying a decision to withdraw treatment. On the other hand, in the American unit clinical evidence that potentially contradicted the radiological evidence of brain injury was taken to preclude certainty and warrant continued treatment. One striking feature of that study was the way in which ethical judgements and apparent facts about prognosis were blurred, and the relationship between them potentially inverted. The doctors' beliefs about whether or not treatment should be continued (including the value of survival with disability and the impact of disability on families and on society) appeared to influence their assessment of the likelihood of adverse outcomes for the infant. Prognosis is always contextual and, in part, socially constructed.

To provide a richer background for some of the discussion in the ensuing chapters it will be helpful to draw on a specific example, and to look at how prognosis is determined and how this relates to treatment decisions in one specific illness.

Birth Asphyxia

Birth asphyxia, or hypoxic-ischaemic encephalopathy (HIE), affects somewhere between one to four infants out of every 1000 live births in developed countries. (In developing countries it is significantly more common, and globally it is responsible for some 900,000 deaths per year; Lawn, Cousens, et al. 2005.) The illness is diagnosed in infants who need resuscitation after birth, who subsequently manifest abnormal neurological behaviour (for example they are excessively irritable or drowsy, or have seizures), and who have some presumptive evidence of perinatal hypoxia (lack of oxygen) or ischemia (lack of blood supply).

Moderate or severe forms of HIE are associated with a high rate of mortality and morbidity. Approximately 15 per cent of cases die in the neonatal unit, 10–15 per cent develop cerebral palsy and up to 40 per cent have other impairments including blindness, deafness, autism, or global developmental delay (Volpe 2008: 441). Recently, doctors have started using a new treatment for infants with HIE, deliberately cooling the infant after birth to try to reduce the severity of brain damage. Although this treatment shows considerable promise, and reduces the chance of death or disability, almost half of the more severely affected infants still either die or are found to have significant impairment at follow up (Jacobs, Hunt, et al. 2007).

There are a variety of clinical, electrophysiological, and imaging tools that clinicians have used to help determine the prognosis of infants with HIE. The severity of encephalopathy (i.e. the degree of abnormal neurological behaviour) is among the most useful and well-studied prognostic factor. This is often used to divide HIE into categories of mild, moderate, and severe, with a poor outcome highly likely in the severe subgroup (Sarnat and Sarnat 1976; Ambalavanan, Carlo, et al. 2006). Abnormalities of background electrical patterns on electroencephalogram (EEG) are also associated with poor outcome. Two patterns are particularly worrying. Burst-suppression patterns (with very low electrical activity interspersed with bursts of abnormal activation) are a very poor prognostic sign, as are patterns of 'extreme discontinuity' (Biagioni, Mercuri, et al. 2001). Imaging of the brain provides further useful prognostic information. Changes on ultrasound predict later impairment (Rutherford, Pennock, et al. 1994). Patterns of increased cerebral blood flow and reduced vascular resistance using Doppler ultrasound have been found to be strongly associated with adverse outcome in a small number of studies (Archer, Levene, et al. 1986). Computed tomography (CT) has also been used to define the extent and site of brain injury. In recent years, however, it has largely been superseded by magnetic resonance imaging.

The above tools are able to predict the overall degree of impairment, but mostly they are not able to distinguish between different types of impairment. Certain findings or patterns of findings are associated with 'poor outcome' (often defined differently depending on the study), but that is usually as far as they are able to go. New forms of brain imaging, however, provide far more detailed assessments of damage to different areas of the brain, and potentially more gradated assessment of the severity of injury.

Nuclear magnetic resonance imaging (MRI) applies intense local magnetic fields to the body. These fields cause the protons in water molecules to line up with the magnetic field, and then return to their previous state once the magnetic field is switched off. As the protons return to their natural alignment they release energy, which is picked up by a radio receiver. Magnetic resonance images are able to provide far better soft tissue resolution than plain X-ray or CT images because variations in the amount and type of energy released are considerably greater than differences in tissue density (Edelman and Warach 1993).

Magnetic resonance (MR) technology has revolutionized imaging of the brain (Robertson and Wyatt 2004). It provides detailed structural images of the cerebrum, cerebellum, and brain-stem ('conventional' MRI). Related techniques include Diffusion Weighted Imaging (DWI), which measures the translational movement of water molecules, and which can indicate tissue oedema and Magnetic Resonance Spectroscopy (MRS), used to non-invasively assess the levels of different metabolites in tissue. Other techniques include diffusion tensor imaging, functional MRI, and MR angiography.

Several distinct patterns have been observed in infants with HIE with MRI. Some infants appear to have injury focused on deep central areas of the brain (basal ganglia and thalamus). These areas are responsible, among other things, for coordinating movement (Rutherford, Srinivasan, et al. 2006). A second distinct pattern of injury involves principally the white matter, with extension to cortex in severe cases (Miller, Ramaswamy, et al. 2005). (White matter refers to the part of the brain below the outer surface; it mainly contains myelinated nerve fibres travelling from the cortex to other parts of the brain or spinal cord, and appears macroscopically white.) Other infants have combinations of these patterns.

The different patterns of injury observed with MRI have different prognostic implications (Table 1.1). In particular, damage to the basal ganglia is associated with motor problems, and the development of severe forms of cerebral palsy. White matter injury is associated with less severe movement problems but variable problems with learning disability.

How do the results of MRI or other prognostic tests influence treatment decisions for infants with HIE? A guideline from the American Academy of

Table 1.1 Patterns observed using conventional MRI and neurodevelopmental outcome.

Pattern on conventional MRI	Usual Outcome
Normal scans, mild basal ganglia or mild-moderate white matter changes	Normal outcome (may include minor behavioural or learning problems)
Focal basal ganglia changes with bilateral signal abnormality in the PLIC	Moderate to severe motor problems (often dystonic/athetoid cerebral palsy), cognitive development may be normal
Severe white matter changes	Moderate to severe motor impairment, as well as moderate to severe cognitive impairment
Severe and diffuse basal ganglia changes	Severe motor impairment, severe cognitive impairment, microcephaly, often cortical blindness

(Rutherford, Pennock, et al. 1998; Biagioni, Mercuri, et al. 2001; Mercuri and Barnett 2003; Mercuri, Anker, et al. 2004; Jyoti, O'Neil, et al. 2006; El-Ayouty, Abdel-Hady, et al. 2007). This is not intended to represent an exhaustive list of all patterns on conventional MRI. Other patterns include cortical highlighting, or brain stem changes (Rutherford 2002: 101).

Pediatrics in 2002 recommended that all encephalopathic term infants have an MRI performed between days two and eight (Ment, Bada, et al. 2002). In one survey, a questionnaire was completed by ninety-five Australasian neonatologists about their use of prognostic tests in a hypothetical infant with HIE (Filan, Inder, et al. 2007). Almost 80 per cent of surveyed neonatologists indicated that they would order an MRI. If considering withdrawal of life support 2/3 reported that they would attempt to organize an MRI prior to that decision.

I spoke with a group of UK neonatologists about their use of prognostic tests in infants with HIE (Wilkinson 2010). They described the task of predicting outcome for infants as being like the assembly of a jigsaw puzzle. Different pieces of evidence were fitted together to try to achieve a clear picture of the future for an infant. All would use an MRI as part of that jigsaw, but several, particularly those from specialized centres with considerable experience with MRI, saw it as a large and important piece of the puzzle.

I do find brain MRIs very helpful... it is something that personally I would rely on quite heavily... I would be reluctant to prognosticate very strongly without imaging to be honest. (Consultant neonatologist, five years experience.)

Some of the neonatologists with specialized experience of MRI referred to particular patterns of MR imaging that would support treatment withdrawal:

our MRI definition for such an outcome might be clear severe basal ganglia abnormalities and almost always in conjunction with cortical abnormalities as well so that usually translates into major physical handicaps together with major mental, cognitive deficiency. And I think we are unanimous in our view that that prognosis is terrible. (Consultant neonatologist, twenty-five years experience.)

the imaging patterns that I would move towards suggesting withdrawal of care [include] ... very global grey and white matter infarction so very, very severe injury to all areas including the cortex, ... [or] the very severe white matter and partial basal ganglia problems ... I think those two fall into the area of something I would feel might be able to offer withdrawal of care. (Consultant neonatologist, fifteen years experience.)

Birth asphyxia provides an interesting case study for thinking about the ethical implications of advances in prognostication and neuroimaging for several reasons. It is the commonest single cause of death in term newborn infants (The consultative council on obstetric and paediatric mortality and morbidity 2008; Verhagen, Janvier, et al. 2010) and the majority of such deaths follow decisions to limit or withdraw treatment. Secondly, these decisions are often in practice particularly difficult and controversial (McHaffie and Fowlie 1996: 98). This is partly because they explicitly relate to quality of life predictions and judgements, and partly because of the inherent uncertainties that accompany prognosis. Finally, new forms of neuroimaging have probably been studied more in HIE than in any other defined condition in newborns or children.

How should we respond to neuroimaging and to evidence about future disability? Uncertainty makes an answer to this complicated, so in Part I of the book we will set that aside. What if we were certain of prognosis? What if we knew for sure exactly how impaired an infant or child were going to be?

References

Airedale NHS Trust v Bland. [1993] AC 789.
Albrecht, G.L. and P.J. Devlieger (1999). 'The disability paradox: high quality of life against all odds', *Social Science & Medicine* 48(8): 977–88.

Ambalavanan, N., W.A. Carlo, et al. (2006). 'Predicting outcomes of neonates diagnosed with hypoxemic-ischemic encephalopathy'. *Pediatrics* 118(5): 2084–93.

American Academy of Pediatrics Committee on Fetus and Newborn (1995). 'The initiation or withdrawal of treatment for high-risk newborns', *Pediatrics* 96(2 Pt 1): 362–3.

—— (2007). 'Noninitiation or withdrawal of intensive care for high-risk newborns', *Pediatrics* 119(2): 401–3.

Anspach, R.R. (1993). *Deciding Who Lives: Fateful Choices in the Intensive-Care Nursery*. Berkeley, Oxford: University of California Press.

Archer, L.N., M.I. Levene, et al. (1986). 'Cerebral artery Doppler ultrasonography for prediction of outcome after perinatal asphyxia', *Lancet* 2(8516): 1116–18.

Barker, D.P. and N. Rutter (1995). 'Exposure to invasive procedures in neonatal intensive care unit admissions,' *Arch Dis Child Fetal Neonatal Ed* 72(1): F47–8.

Berger, T. and A. Hofer (2009). 'Causes and circumstances of neonatal deaths in 108 consecutive cases over a 10-year period at the children's hospital of Lucerne, Switzerland', *Neonatology* 95(2): 157–63.

Biagioni, E., E. Mercuri, et al. (2001). 'Combined use of electroencephalogram and magnetic resonance imaging in full-term neonates with acute encephalopathy', *Pediatrics* 107(3): 461–8.

Burns, J.P., C. Mitchell, et al. (2000). 'End-of-life care in the pediatric intensive care unit after the forgoing of life-sustaining treatment', *Crit Care Med* 28(8): 3060–6.

Christakis, N.A. (1999). *Death Foretold: Prophecy and Prognosis in Medical Care*. Chicago: University of Chicago.

Cuttini, M., M. Nadai, et al. (2000). 'End-of-life decisions in neonatal intensive care: physicians' self-reported practices in seven European countries. EURONIC Study Group', *Lancet* 355(9221): 2112–18.

Dickenson, D.L. (2000). 'Are medical ethicists out of touch? Practitioner attitudes in the US and UK towards decisions at the end of life', *J Med Ethics* 26(4): 254–60.

Edelman, R.R. and S. Warach (1993). 'Magnetic resonance imaging (1)', *N Engl J Med* 328(10): 708–16.

El-Ayouty, M., H. Abdel-Hady, et al. (2007). 'Relationship between electroencephalography and magnetic resonance imaging findings after hypoxic-ischemic encephalopathy at term', *Am J Perinatol* 24(8): 467–73.

Emanuel, L.L., M.J. Barry, et al. (1991). 'Advance directives for medical care—a case for greater use', *N Engl J Med* 324(13): 889—95.

Filan, P., T. Inder, et al. (2007). 'Monitoring the neonatal brain: a survey of current practice among Australian and New Zealand neonatologists', *J Paediatr Child Health* 43(7–8): 557–9.

Finnis, J., J.M. Boyle, et al. (1987). *Nuclear Deterrence, Morality and Realism*. Oxford: Clarendon Press.
Gillon, R. (1994). 'Withholding and withdrawing life-prolonging treatment—moral implications of a thought experiment', *J Med Ethics* 20(4): 203–4, 222.
Glover, J. (1990). *Causing Death and Saving Lives*. Harmondsworth: Penguin.
Grey, W. (1999). 'Epicurus and the Harm of Death', *Australasian Journal of Philosophy* 77: 358–64.
Jacobs, S., R. Hunt, et al. (2007). 'Cooling for newborns with hypoxic ischaemic encephalopathy', *Cochrane Database of Systematic Reviews* (online)(4): CD003311.
Jyoti, R., R. O'Neil, et al. (2006). 'Predicting outcome in term neonates with hypoxic-ischaemic encephalopathy using simplified MR criteria', *Pediatric Radiology* 36(1): 38–42.
Kuhse, H. and P. Singer (1985). *Should the Baby Live? The Problem of Handicapped Infants*. Oxford: Oxford University Press.
Lawn, J.E., S. Cousens, et al. (2005). '4 million neonatal deaths: when? Where? Why?' *Lancet* 365(9462): 891–900.
Lee, K.J., K. Tieves, et al. (2010). 'Alterations in end-of-life support in the pediatric intensive care unit', *Pediatrics* 126(4): e859–64.
McCormick, R.A. (1974). 'To save or let die. The dilemma of modern medicine', *JAMA* 229(2): 172–6.
McHaffie, H.E. and P.W. Fowlie (1996). *Life, Death and Decisions: Doctors and Nurses Reflect on Neonatal Practice*. Hale: Hochland and Hochland.
McMahan, J. (1988). 'Death and the value of life', *Ethics* 99(1): 32–61.
Melltorp, G. and T. Nilstun (1997). 'The difference between withholding and withdrawing life-sustaining treatment', *Intensive Care Med* 23(12): 1264–7.
Ment, L., H. Bada, et al. (2002). 'Practice parameter: neuroimaging of the neonate: report of the quality standards subcommittee of the American Academy of Neurology and the practice committee of the Child Neurology Society', *Neurology* 58(12): 1726–38.
Mercuri, E., S. Anker, et al. (2004). 'Visual function at school age in children with neonatal encephalopathy and low Apgar scores', *Arch Dis Child Fetal Neonatal Ed* 89(3): F258–62.
—— and A. L. Barnett (2003). 'Neonatal brain MRI and motor outcome at school age in children with neonatal encephalopathy: a review of personal experience', *Neural Plast* 10(1–2): 51–7.
Miller, S.P., V. Ramaswamy, et al. (2005). 'Patterns of brain injury in term neonatal encephalopathy', *J Pediatr* 146(4): 453–60.

Orfali, K. (2004). 'Parental role in medical decision-making: fact or fiction? A comparative study of ethical dilemmas in French and American neonatal intensive care units', *Soc Sci Med* 58(10): 2009–22.

Paris, J.J. (2010). 'Autonomy does not confer sovereignty on the patient: a commentary on the Golubchuk case', *Am J Bioeth* 10(3): 54–6.

Robertson, N.J. and J.S. Wyatt (2004). 'The magnetic resonance revolution in brain imaging: impact on neonatal intensive care', *Arch Dis Child Fetal Neonatal Ed* 89(3): F193–7.

Royal College of Paediatrics and Child Health (2004). *Withholding and Withdrawing Life-Saving Treatment in Children: A Framework for Practice*. London: Royal College of Paediatrics and Child Health.

Rutherford, M., L. Srinivasan, et al. (2006). 'Magnetic resonance imaging in perinatal brain injury: clinical presentation, lesions and outcome', *Pediatr Radiol* 36(7): 582–92.

Rutherford, M.A. (2002). *MRI of the Neonatal Brain*. London: W.B. Saunders.

—— J.M. Pennock, et al. (1994). 'Cranial ultrasound and magnetic resonance imaging in hypoxic-ischaemic encephalopathy: a comparison with outcome', *Dev Med Child Neurol* 36(9): 813–25.

—— —— et al. (1998). 'Abnormal magnetic resonance signal in the internal capsule predicts poor neurodevelopmental outcome in infants with hypoxic-ischemic encephalopathy', *Pediatrics* 102(2 Pt 1): 323–8.

Sarnat, H. and M. Sarnat (1976). 'Neonatal encephalopathy following fetal distress. A clinical and electroencephalographic study', *Arch Neurol* 33(10): 696–705.

Singh, J., J. Lantos, et al. (2004). 'End-of-life after birth: death and dying in a neonatal intensive care unit', *Pediatrics* 114(6): 1620–6.

Spooner, M.H. (2009). 'Legal consensus eludes Europe', *CMAJ* 180(3): 282–3.

Stone, J. (2007). 'Pascal's Wager and the persistent vegetative state', *Bioethics* 21(2): 84–92.

The consultative council on obstetric and paediatric mortality and morbidity (2008). *Annual Report for the Year 2006*. Melbourne.

Verhagen, A., J. Dorscheidt, et al. (2009). 'End-of-life decisions in Dutch neonatal intensive care units', *Arch Pediatr Adolesc Med* 163(10): 895–901.

—— A. Janvier, et al. (2010). 'Categorizing Neonatal Deaths: A Cross-Cultural Study in the United States, Canada, and The Netherlands', *J Pediatr* 156(1): 33–7.

—— and P.J. Sauer (2005a). 'End-of-life decisions in newborns: an approach from The Netherlands', *Pediatrics* 116(3): 736–9.

Verhagen, E. and P.J. Sauer (2005b). 'The Groningen protocol—euthanasia in severely ill newborns', *N Engl J Med* 352(10): 959–62.

Volpe, J.J. (2008). *Neurology of the Newborn*. Philadelphia, London: Saunders.
Wilkinson, D. (2010). '"We don't have a crystal ball": neonatologists views on prognosis and decision-making in newborn infants with birth asphyxia', *Monash Bioethics Review* 29(1): 5.1–5.19.
Wilkinson, D.J., J.J. Fitzsimons, et al. (2006). 'Death in the neonatal intensive care unit: changing patterns of end of life care over two decades', *Archives of Disease in Childhood Fetal and Neonatal Edition* 91(4): F268–71.
Wilkinson, D.J.C. and J. Savulescu (2011). 'Knowing when to stop: futility in the ICU', *Current Opinion in Anesthesiology* 24(2): 160–5.

Carmentis

The Roman Goddess of childbirth Carmentis or Carmenta was said to sing prophecies of the future of newborn infants after drinking from a sacred spring. According to the poet Ovid the Romans celebrated a festival in her honour, the 'Carmentalia', on the 11th and 15th of January (Ovid 1931, Book 1, 461–542). There was a temple of Carmentis at the foot of the Capitoline hill in Rome (Richardson 1992).

'Carmenta some think a deity presiding over human birth; for which reason she is much honoured by mothers. Others say she was the wife of Evander, the Arcadian, being a prophetess, and wont to deliver her oracles in verse, and from carmen, a verse, was called Carmenta; her proper name being Nicostrata. Others more probably derive Carmenta from carens mente, or insane, in allusion to her prophetic frenzies.' (Plutarch 2008)

References

Ovid (1931). *Fasti*. Cambridge, MA: Harvard University Press.
Plutarch (2008). *Plutarch's Lives*. New York: Cosimo Inc.
Richardson, L. (1992). *A New Topographical Dictionary of Ancient Rome*. Baltimore: JHU Press.

2

Best Interests and the Carmentis Machine

Introduction

Imagine that we had a perfect prognostic machine, a machine that was able to tell us exactly what the outcome would be for a patient who was critically ill. It would tell us whether or not they would survive their acute illness, but also how they would survive, how long they would be in hospital for, whether they would be disabled, and in what ways. What then? Would such a machine make decisions about life-sustaining treatment easy? How should we use this information? When would it be permissible to withdraw treatment? When would we be ethically obliged to provide or to continue treatment?

In this chapter of the book, the aim will be to look beyond the current limitations of our technology, and to imagine a machine, like the Carmentis machine of Prologue 2, that is not limited by uncertainty in the way that current prognostic techniques are. This is what philosophers sometimes call a 'thought experiment'. It is the philosophical equivalent of a controlled trial, a way to subject our moral judgements to scrutiny. In thought experiments, as in controlled trials, it may be possible to set aside distracting or confounding factors, and to isolate particular elements of a problem.

There are several reasons for undertaking this particular thought experiment. One reason is that some guidelines and some clinicians suggest that it is only where prognosis is certain that treatment may be withdrawn (Royal College of Paediatrics and Child Health 2004: 11). There are reasons to doubt whether complete certainty is ever possible. There are also reasons to believe that it is sometimes appropriate to limit treatment in the face of uncertainty.

But in any case, a fairly high degree of certainty about prognosis is possible for at least some patients. Surely we should be able to answer the question of when treatment may be withdrawn for this subgroup of patients? A second reason is that it is possible that further advances in imaging technology and science may diminish the problem of uncertainty. One important task for medical ethics is to anticipate future developments in technology, the impact that they may have on medical practice, and the potential ethical issues that they may generate. So it will be useful to know what decisions may be made if and when this improved prognosis is available. But thirdly, and more importantly, it is only possible to develop an approach to decision-making in the face of uncertainty if we know how to make decisions in the face of *certain* prognosis. This does not necessarily mean that there need be a single accepted or correct response to certain prognosis. There may be, indeed there are likely to be, competing answers to this question. We then have to determine an appropriate response to moral uncertainty (i.e. uncertainty that arises not from problems predicting the outcome, but from knowing how we ought to behave, what we ought to do) (Lockhart 2000). We will discuss moral uncertainty in more detail in Chapter 7. But first we need to understand which impairments, if certain to occur, would be sufficiently severe to justify treatment withdrawal and which would not.

In this chapter I want to examine one frequently encountered answer to the problem of treatment limitation for incompetent patients—the idea that we should be guided by the *best interests of the patient*. This principle is found in guidelines in a number of different countries. We will look at a small group of example cases through the lens of current treatment guidelines and case law, and try to assess whether or not treatment withdrawal should be allowed. The aim will not be to provide a detailed analysis of current law as it relates to treatment decisions in children and infants. Rather, we will look at two different ways of interpreting best interests that emerge from these guidelines and from past legal cases. Many of these cases and guidelines come from the UK, but the basic analysis is applicable in any part of the world that uses the best interests of the child as a touchstone to determine whether or not life-sustaining treatment may be limited. I will argue that current guidelines are vague, and this is at least partly because the best interests principle is unable to provide a clear answer to this question in many cases.

Best Interests

And if we actually concluded... [that] this baby is going to be very, very severely disabled, unable to sit up, very likely to have severe learning problems,... this is the point where we think that actually it is not in the baby's best interest [to continue]. (Wilkinson 2010: 5.9)

This quote, from an interview with an experienced neonatologist illustrates the way that the concept of the best interests of the child has penetrated into clinical practice. But, while this concept has emerged as a core principle in medical ethics, what does it actually mean?

At first glance 'acting in a patient's best interests' can appear to be a tautology, since doing what is best for the patient and acting in their interests ought to be the same thing, surely? (Brody and Bartholome 1988). One way of understanding it is that perhaps there are multiple different courses of action that are in the interests of the patient (i.e. benefit them), but the best interests principle invites us to seek that course which will maximally promote their interests overall, or the one that will promote their most important interest at stake. (Here immediately we encounter one of the problems with best interests, since these two different interpretations may lead us in different directions.)

The phrase 'best interests' comes originally from custodial decision-making about children. Prior to the 1970s in the United States and in other parts of the world there was a judicial presumption that young children (under the age of 13) would remain in the custody of their mother if their parents divorced (this was the so-called 'Tender Years Doctrine'). In the 1970s it was recognized that this was not always the most appropriate course, and the Tender Years Doctrine was replaced by the 'Best Interests' standard. Decisions were now to be guided by what was felt to be best for the child; children might therefore end up in the care of either parent (Roth 1976).

In medical ethics the 'Best Interests' standard draws on the principle of beneficence. There is a medical decision-making hierarchy. At the top of the tree is Autonomy—for competent patients we should act in accordance with their wishes. Western medical ethics has raised autonomy to a position of pre-eminence. We usually think that doctors should respect a patient's wishes even if the patient is clearly mistaken about what would be best for them, unless they are mentally ill or otherwise incompetent to make a decision. Below this principle is Substituted Judgement. For patients who are not able to express their wishes, but who were previously competent we should be guided by what we believe they would have wanted. This is the basis for the use of advance directives, and is one of the reasons why families are involved in decision-making for adults—they are often a good source of information about the desires and preferences of the patient. Finally, at the lowest level of the tree lies Best Interests. For patients who are incompetent and whose wishes are either unknown or unknowable (as is the case for infants, and young children) we should be guided by what would be best for them.

Although the idea of acting in the patient's best interests seems self-evidently the right thing to do (at least when we can't ask them what they would like us to do), it has been the subject of some criticism. Some bioethicists have criticized the best interests principle as incoherent, unrealistic, unknowable, or overly individualistic (Brody and Bartholome 1988; Engelhardt 1989; Veatch 1995). It is all very well in theory to say that we should do what is best for the patient, but what if a doctor has multiple patients to care for, or what if it isn't clear what would be best for the patient? What about the interests of others, are they to be ignored? Should we really hold doctors and parents to this standard of always making the very best choice for the child? There are plenty of occasions when parents may not do what would be best for the child, but we don't usually think that the state should interfere each and every time that they do make a choice other than the best one. Think for example of parents who give their children junk food, or fail to take them to the dentist for regular check-ups. The parents are not really acting in the best interests of their child, but should we intervene? Other ethicists have distinguished between different uses of the concept. US philosopher Loreta Kopelman has argued that 'best interests' is used appropriately in different ways in different contexts. So in some circumstances it is used to express an ideal to aim for—doctors and parents should aspire to do the best for children (even if we cannot always achieve this). In other settings, 'best interests' is used as a minimum threshold. Is a parent's choice bad enough for the child that it should not be allowed? This interpretation applies when parents are seeking to decline standard medical interventions for their child, perhaps because of religious or other beliefs. In other settings again, when the court is asked to arbitrate between the views of different parties Kopelman suggests that it be used as a pragmatic 'standard of reasonableness' to determine which of available choices would be better for the child (Kopelman 1997).

Cases

It may be helpful to have some concrete hypothetical cases in mind when we are looking at guidelines and case law. For each of them, the practical question is: given the prognosis, may treatment be withdrawn if parents wish it?

Case 1: Baby Amelia was unexpectedly delivered in very poor condition following a planned home birth. She received resuscitation from ambulance officers when they arrived at fifteen minutes of age, but had early evidence of hypoxic brain damage with severe encephalopathy and seizures that were refractory to treatment. Neuroprotective interventions were commenced on arrival in intensive care, but despite this she remains ventilator-dependent and neurologically abnormal. The Carmentis machine predicts that she will have profound motor impairment with severe spastic quadriplegic cerebral palsy and mild intellectual impairment (IQ 68). She will be permanently wheelchair-bound, but able to control an electric wheelchair. Expressive language will be limited by her degree of physical impairment but communication will be possible.

Case 2: Angelos is a one-year-old child who was noted before birth to have polyhydramnios (excess amniotic fluid) and to be growth restricted (unusually small). After delivery he was noted to have abnormal facial features, contractures of his joints (inability to straighten them), and an appearance of general weakness—he moved his arms and legs very little. Angelos was subsequently diagnosed with a severe congenital myopathy (a disorder of muscles). He has been dependent on a mechanical ventilator for the whole of his first year of life, and had a surgical tracheostomy performed. The Carmentis machine predicts that Angelos will remain dependent on the mechanical ventilator throughout life. He will be moderately intellectually impaired with an IQ of 45 (he is likely to be socially interactive and to understand basic language, albeit expressive language will be limited by weakness). He will have severe muscle weakness and limited voluntary movements. He will develop progressive scoliosis (curvature of the spine) and restrictive lung disease without major surgery in mid-childhood.

Case 3: Phillip is a six-year-old child who suffered a severe head injury after running out on to a road and being hit by a car. He was brought in to hospital, resuscitated, and treated in the intensive care unit. On day three of his intensive care stay the Carmentis machine identifies widespread diffuse axonal injury. The machine predicts that Phillip will remain in an apparent vegetative state for six months. He will subsequently develop some neurological improvement, but will be severely cognitively impaired with a predicted IQ of 30. He will have moderately difficult to control epilepsy. Phillip will eventually have up to ten words of expressive language, but will be able to walk independently.

Case 4: Baby Chloe developed abnormal movements in the first days after birth. She is found to have an inherited form of bilateral fronto-parietal polymicrogyria (a congenital abnormality of brain development). The machine predicts profound intellectual impairment (IQ unmeasurable but less than 20). She will only be able to achieve even rudimentary self-care tasks with extensive training, and will require total supervision and care. She is not predicted to have major separate motor impairment, sensory impairment, or epilepsy.

These cases obviously do not encompass all possible combinations of impairments. The aim is that they represent a spectrum of realistic cases involving substantial cognitive or motor deficits. With these cases in mind we will now turn to existing guidelines to see what they indicate that we should do with the predictions of the Carmentis machine.

Guidelines

UK: Royal College of Paediatrics

One of the most influential and detailed guidelines for treatment decisions comes from the UK Royal College of Paediatrics and Child Health (RCPCH) (2004). In 2004 the College's 'Ethics Advisory Committee' published a revised framework for decisions about withdrawal of life-sustaining treatment. This framework has been cited by the UK courts (e.g. An NHS Trust v D 2000, para 77; K (A minor) 2006, para 37–39; Re OT 2009: 29–30) and is used by clinicians (Street, Ashcroft, et al. 2000), at least in the UK.

The cornerstone of the approach advocated by the RCPCH is a determination of the best interests of the child. However, the guidelines go further and delineate five settings where treatment limitation decisions could be appropriate: The 'Brain Dead Child', The 'Permanent Vegetative State', The 'No Chance' situation, The 'No Purpose' situation, and The 'Unbearable' situation. Of these, the fourth, the so-called 'No-Purpose' situation, is most relevant to treatment withdrawal decisions on the basis of quality of life. The guidelines apply this label to situations where survival is possible but the degree of physical or mental impairment will be so great that it is 'intolerable'.

In the RCPCH guideline this justification for withdrawing or withholding treatment is linked to an English High Court judgement, the case of Re J (1991) (see below). The guideline suggests two possible interpretations of intolerable: 'that which cannot be borne' or 'that which an individual should not be asked to bear', though it seems to favour the latter (RCPCH 2004: 11). Usefully, the RCPCH guideline also provides some examples of what the committee believes this to refer to in practice, e.g. 'when there is little or no prospect of meaningful interaction with others or the environment' (RCPCH 2004: 24), and suggests that spastic quadriplegia (a severe form of cerebral palsy affecting all four limbs) combined with severe associated cognitive and sensory deficits may be one such condition. Does this exclude withdrawal of treatment from Amelia (Case 1) who is predicted to have severe physical, but only mild cognitive impairment? What about Chloe (Case 4), with severe cognitive impairment, but mild or no physical impairment? The guidelines are unclear.

Although the RCPCH guidelines are reasonably specific, some difficulty in interpretation remains. For example, we might ask when interaction with the environment becomes 'meaningful'. Is it the capacity to communicate that confers meaning, or would the recognition of faces or voices be sufficient? Consider Phillip (Case 3) for example, who is predicted to develop rudimentary communication skills. Does his life have meaning? (We may also wonder who it is that we are judging to be obtaining meaning from the interaction—is it Phillip, or his caregivers, or someone else?)

Disability, Impairment, and Handicap: Language, Causation, and Discrimination

There are various words used to describe disabling conditions or illnesses. These words have come in and out of fashion, and have a variety of potential connotations. The language used may imply the cause or the consequences of a child's condition. Some words have been used in a pejorative way, and are now seen as offensive, though were once used as forms of neutral description. For example, the word 'cretin' used to be used to describe growth restriction and cognitive impairment due to congenital hypothyroidism. Similarly, the term 'handicap' is nowadays usually avoided because of potential offence.

In the 1980s and 1990s researchers drew attention to two different models, or ways of thinking about disability. The so-called 'medical model' of disability emphasises the physical or structural abnormalities that leads individuals to experience difficulties in everyday life. This is the way that doctors have traditionally thought about disability and often still do. There is a defined problem or abnormality in a body system, which leads to a particular loss of normal function. Interventions to fix or ameliorate the underlying problem are sought in order to improve function as far as possible. In contrast, the 'social model' of disability, which has emerged from the work of sociologists and disability activists, points to the major contribution of the social environment to the disadvantages experienced by those with illness or impairment. One reason why people who live in London and who are wheelchair-bound might find it difficult to obtain employment is because the underground railway system is extremely poorly adapted to wheelchair users. The development of the social model of disability was important because it highlighted the dangers of medicalizing the problems of those with disability and the importance of societal attitudes and structures to their experience of life. As a result of this model a distinction is often drawn between *impairment*—a reduction in physical, physiological, or psychological capacities relative to what is normal for the species (Bickenbach, Chatterji, et al. 1999; Buchanan, Brock, et al. 2000: 285), and *disability*—a reduction in function relating to impairment. Some have gone further, and defined disability explicitly as disadvantage arising from society's failure to take account of those with impairment. 'It is society which disables physically impaired people' (Oliver 1996). But this strong version of the social model of disability appears to go too far, and has been criticized, including by those from within the disability movement. This approach risks underestimating or ignoring the contribution of impairment or illness to the problems that those with disability face, and the potential benefits of medical interventions (Shakespeare 2008). It also appears to conflate disadvantage with discrimination and oppression. It is instructive to note that the quotation above talks specifically about physical impairment. It may be possible to overcome many of the disadvantages caused by physical impairment. However, cognitive impairment, particularly if severe, may lead to substantial challenges, even in societies that are well resourced and fully supportive of impaired individuals.

Is it discriminatory to withdraw life-sustaining treatment from an individual who is predicted to have severe disability? At first glance this does appear to be a form of discrimination. One test is whether the same decision would be made for a patient without that disability. Imagine that Baby Chloe's doctors and parents were weighing up whether or not she should receive cardiopulmonary resuscitation in the event of a sudden collapse or illness. If Chloe were predicted to have normal intelligence there is no question, of course resuscitation would be provided. So why isn't this discrimination? The answer is that not all discrimination is the same, and not all discrimination is problematic (Arneson 2006). When we are selecting which of a group of applicants to interview for a job it is appropriate to discriminate on the basis of the applicants' past experience, qualifications, and references. These are salient features to be taken into account in the decision since they are clearly related to how well the applicants would be able to perform in the job (they are morally relevant factors). But it would be *unjustly* discriminatory to choose which applicants to interview because they went to a particular school, or because they were of a particular racial background. Similarly the important question is whether disability is morally relevant to decisions about life-sustaining treatment or whether this is unjust discrimination. There are a couple of possible ways in which it could be relevant. Disability might affect the likelihood of treatment being successful (the quantity of life that treatment offers). It might also affect the benefits and burdens that the individual will experience during and after the provision of treatment. Sometimes disability will be relevant (sometimes it is highly relevant) for decisions about life-sustaining treatment. But it is important to recognize that it is not always relevant, and sometimes its importance may be exaggerated. The challenge is not to ignore the contribution of disability to the quality of life of the patient, but also to be sensitive to potential bias and overemphasis.

UK: Nuffield Report

a UK non-governmental ethics body, the Nuffield Council on Bioethics, published report in 2006 (Nuffield Council on Bioethics 2006). It covers a range of decisions both before and after birth for extremely premature and term newborn infants. The report, as with the RCPCH document, emphasises the primacy of the best interests of the child in determining whether or not to provide treatment. In another parallel with the Royal College guideline, it also draws on the concept of *intolerability*. According to this report:

It would not be in the baby's best interests to insist on the imposition or continuance of treatment to prolong the life of the baby when doing so imposes an intolerable burden upon him or her (Nuffield Council on Bioethics 2006: 12)

What sort of impairment would impose an 'intolerable burden'? The authors admit to some difficulty in defining this concept, noting that people may disagree both about what constitutes intolerability, and whether or not a particular infant's condition is intolerable. The report suggests that providing burdensome treatment to a child predicted to have a life 'bereft of those features that give meaning and purpose to human life' (Nuffield Council on Bioethics 2006: 12, para 2.13) may impose an intolerable existence. These features are not elaborated, but in a separate part of the report the authors discuss some of the potential benefits of treatment to be included in a 'best interests' determination: the capacity to establish relationships with others, the ability to experience pleasure, and independence from life support (Nuffield Council on Bioethics 2006: 161, para 9.33).

The authors of the Nuffield report discussed a couple of examples to put this in context. They did not believe that the future was 'intolerable' for a premature infant with predicted moderate motor impairment (spastic diplegia), but uncertain cognitive impairment (Nuffield Council on Bioethics 2006: 99–100). On the other hand the report judged that the future would be intolerable (and therefore that it was permissible to withdraw treatment) for a newborn predicted to have severe motor and cognitive impairment (Nuffield Council on Bioethics 2006: 101). Again, this appears to potentially exclude some of the cases described above (for example Cases 1 and 2) since they have lesser degrees of cognitive impairment.

The Nuffield report notes in several places the inherent uncertainty in prognosis for newborn infants. But the report is ambiguous about the role of uncertainty in decision-making. For extremely preterm infants of 23 weeks gestation the uncertainty of the prognosis is cited as justifying giving parental wishes precedence in determining resuscitation (Nuffield Council on Bioethics 2006: 82, 151). This appears to contradict, however, other parts of the report that suggest that for it to be in the best interests of the infant to die a 'high degree of certainty' would be required that the infant will suffer intolerably (Nuffield Council on Bioethics 2006: 16). One reason for this apparent contradiction is that the report distinguishes between what is in the best interests of the infant, and what decisions may be made. It differs from the Royal College guideline in that it explicitly embraces the idea that interests other than the child's might be taken into consideration. While the best interests of the child are a 'central' consideration in decisions about treatment, the interests of parents may also be relevant to take into account. The implication is that these other interests would permit treatment limitation in the face of uncertainty. But though the report is explicit in setting out examples of how this could be applied to resuscitation decisions for extremely preterm infants, it is less clear how this should be applied to withdrawal of treatment for infants with other conditions, and not clear at all about whether this could or should be extrapolated to older children.

Re J

J was an ex-premature infant with severe brain injury whose case appeared before the Family Court of England and Wales in October 1991 when he was 5 months old. (Re J 1991)

J had been born three months prematurely (at twenty-seven weeks gestation) weighing just over one kilogram. He had suffered brain injury at the time of birth, and was initially critically ill, but then improved and was weaned off respiratory support after one month. Subsequently J had repeated episodes of seizures and cyanosis (going blue), and was put back onto the breathing machine several times. He was briefly discharged home when he was three and a half months old, but was fairly quickly readmitted with further cyanotic episodes. Over the course of the next month doctors attempted repeatedly to take him off the breathing machine, and succeeded on their fourth attempt. At this point they approached the court asking it to approve a decision not to reinstitute breathing support if J required it again.

The vast majority of treatment withdrawal decisions in the UK and in other countries do not ever come before a court. But in J's case he had previously been made a ward of the court for reasons unrelated to the current issue of treatment. Although his parents agreed with doctors that treatment limitation would be appropriate, his legal status as a ward meant that the court was required to endorse the doctors' decision. The case was first heard by a local judge. This judge agreed with the doctors that it would not be in J's best interests to put him back on mechanical ventilation. J's case was then appealed by the Official Solicitor who claimed that it was never justified to withhold life-sustaining treatment from a child on the basis of their quality of life.

At the time of the case the main form of neuroimaging used in newborn intensive care was ultrasound of the brain. J's cerebral ultrasound showed large cystic areas within his brain relating to areas of brain tissue that had died and been replaced by fluid. The most optimistic of the doctors caring for J predicted that he would develop spastic quadriplegic cerebral palsy, be blind and deaf, and have severe cognitive impairment. It was believed that his life expectancy had been reduced—probably to teenage years, though he might not live that long.

The distinctive feature of J's case for the United Kingdom was that unlike previous cases there was clear acknowledgement that J was not terminally ill, and that with treatment he might survive into late childhood or adolescence. However, the court rejected the Official

Solicitor's argument; it held that it could be in the best interests of a child to withhold life-saving treatment even if survival was possible. In the summary of Re J, this decision was explicitly related to the concept of intolerability:

> where, viewed from... [his position], his future life might be regarded as intolerable to him the court acting solely on his behalf might properly choose a course of action which did not prevent his death. (Re J 1991: 34, para C)

US: American Academy of Pediatrics

Across the other side of the Atlantic there have been a number of influential guidelines and policy statements. In 1983 the President's Commission for the study of ethical problems published a report entitled 'Deciding to forego life-sustaining treatment' (President's Commission 1983). That report had a chapter relating to decision-making for newborn infants that set out the criteria for withdrawal of treatment from impaired newborn infants in their best interests.

> permanent handicaps justify a decision not to provide life-sustaining treatment only when they are so severe that continued existence would not be a net benefit to the infant. (President's Commission 1983: 28)

It also suggested that some cases were more difficult, particularly in the face of prognostic uncertainty. In the face of 'ambiguous' outcome the Commission suggested that parents' wishes be honoured.

Subsequently the American Academy of Pediatrics (AAP) has published two policy statements that are relevant—a guideline from 1995 on forgoing life-sustaining treatment, and a more recent guideline from 2007 on 'Non-initiation or withdrawal of intensive care for high risk newborns'.

The 1995 guideline does not provide specific criteria for forgoing treatment (AAP 1995). Like the President's Commission it specifies that for incompetent patients whose previous wishes are unknown (for example newborns or children), decisions should be guided by the best interests principle. It interprets this principle as involving a weighing up of the benefits and burdens of treatment (for life-sustaining treatment that specifically includes assessment of the benefits or burdens of ongoing life). The guideline refers to 'irremediable disability' in the lists of burdens, but there is no attempt to spell out what this means in practice. 'Irremediable' after all means only that disability cannot be cured, and does not specify the severity of impairment. It does not make clear the role of parents in decisions beyond a comment that for such serious questions decisions should usually conform to the family's wishes.

The later guideline also bases judgements on the best interests principle (AAP 2007: 401); it, too, is vague about how this should be interpreted in practice. The title refers both to withholding or withdrawal of treatment, though the guideline itself mostly refers to resuscitation decisions at birth, in particular for extremely premature newborns. It refers in several places to 'acceptable quality of life', though does not set out what this term means. It sets out a grey zone of permissibility where parental wishes should determine the treatment approach:

cases... in which the prognosis is uncertain but likely to be very poor and survival may be associated with a diminished quality of life for the child. (AAP 2007: 402)

The terms 'prognosis' and 'uncertain' here are ambiguous. In the penultimate paragraph, the AAP guideline expresses ambivalence about parents and their freedom to decide:

The important role of parents in decision-making must be respected. However... the physician must ensure that the chosen treatment, in his or her best medical judgement, is consistent with the best interests of the infant. (AAP 2007: 402)

Other Countries

Guidelines from other countries have generally been less detailed than the ones discussed above (McHaffie, Cuttini, et al. 1999). Most reports, including guidelines from Australia, Canada, Italy, France, and Malaysia relate treatment withdrawal to the best interests of the child or infant (McHaffie, Cuttini, et al. 1999; Baskett, Steen, et al. 2005; Hubert, Canoui, et al. 2005; NSW Health 2005; Royal Children's Hospital 2006; Giannini, Messeri, et al. 2008; Royal Australasian College of Physicians 2008). Like the documents mentioned above, a guideline from New South Wales supported limiting treatment if a child's condition would be intolerable to the child (NSW Health 2005). The Italian Society of Neonatal and Pediatric Anesthesia and Intensive Care recommendations are more cautious: 'parents and should exercise great prudence in considering the child's clinical ...ion and/or disability as "intolerable"' (Giannini, Messeri, et al. 2008: 591).

Charlotte Wyatt

A decade after the case of J the English courts were faced by a treatment question for another extremely premature infant with brain injury.

Charlotte Wyatt had been born at twenty-six weeks gestation (Portsmouth NHS Trust v Wyatt 2005a). Although she was only slightly more premature than J, Charlotte was significantly smaller weighing only 458 grams at birth. She required artificial ventilation for her first three months of life, and developed severe chronic lung disease, her lungs damaged as a side effect of her prematurity and the machines that had been keeping her alive. She was also believed to have profound brain damage and was described as being blind, deaf, and unable to make voluntary movements or to respond.

At the age of twelve months Charlotte remained in hospital, and had suffered a decline in her respiratory and neurological function. Like in J's case, her doctors sought court approval for a decision not to put her back on breathing support if she deteriorated further. At the time the most optimistic estimate was that she had a 25 per cent chance of surviving for a further year, though a more realistic estimate was said to be a 5 per cent chance of surviving a year. Her parents, who were devout Christians, wanted treatment to continue.

The High Court of England and Wales assessed Charlotte's best interests. Justice Hedley rejected the concept of intolerability:

the concept of 'intolerable to that child' should not be seen as a gloss on, much less a supplementary test to, best interests. (Portsmouth NHS Trust v Wyatt 2005a, para 24)

Instead Justice Headley placed emphasis on a weighing up of the benefits and burdens of treatment. He noted that

Charlotte has no sense of sight or sound and is (and will remain) effectively without volition. That substantially precludes physical or emotional response to another human. It is clear that she can experience pain as the nursing evidence clearly demonstrates. (Portsmouth NHS Trust v Wyatt 2005a, para 31)

The judge ruled that doctors could withhold treatment from Charlotte, but six months later Charlotte remained alive, and her parents appealed for a reversal of the earlier decision. At that point Charlotte's physical condition was more stable and she showed some limited response to her environment: her eyes would track the movement of a colourful toy and she was reported to occasionally smile. However, her head was noted not to have grown at all in the previous six months, a marker of the severity of her brain damage. She was diagnosed with spastic quadriplegic cerebral palsy with profound cognitive impairment. The doctors accepted that she was not in constant pain and that her life at that point was not intolerable. However, they argued that if she required mechanical ventilation there would be a significant chance of her being unable to be weaned off respiratory support, her condition would again become intolerable, and that it would prevent a peaceful and dignified death. The court confirmed its previous approach to assessing best interests:

The court must conduct a balancing exercise in which all the relevant factors are weighed, and a helpful way of undertaking this exercise is to draw up a balance sheet. (Portsmouth NHS Trust v Wyatt 2005b, para 87)

It held that doctors could withhold mechanical ventilation if Charlotte had a respiratory deterioration and required respiratory support again. At age two the parents had a partial victory when the court reviewed the treatment order again, and rescinded their previous order declaring that doctors could withhold treatment without consulting the parents or the court. Within a few months, however, when Charlotte had again deteriorated, it was reinstated. At age four Charlotte was still alive, and was out of hospital. In the meantime her parents had apparently separated and she had been placed in foster care (Dyer 2005; Rennie and Leigh 2008).

Putting Best Interests to the Test

UK and North American guidelines draw on the concept of the best interests of the infant for determining whether or not treatment may be withdrawn. There are two different approaches that emerge from these guidelines for determining the best interests of infants in relation to treatment withdrawal. Some of the guidelines draw on the concept of 'intolerability'; the key question is to determine whether future life would be intolerable—if so it would be in the best interests of the child to withdraw life-sustaining treatment. This is the approach favoured by the Royal College guideline and Nuffield Council report. Others emphasise a balancing of benefits and burdens: life-sustaining treatment is not in the best interests of the child and may be withdrawn if the burdens outweigh the benefits. This latter approach appears to be the one favoured by the North American guidelines, as well as by the UK courts in more recent judgements such as that of Charlotte Wyatt.

None of the guidelines or legal decisions referred to above mentioned the idea of a 'Life Worth Living' (LWL), a concept that I referred to in Chapter 1. Briefly though, one key difference between the 'intolerability' and the 'balance sheet' approaches is their respective ways of judging whether or not life is worth living. The intolerability test uses a *subjective* sense of a LWL: it looks to the viewpoint of the patient and their ability to tolerate continued treatment and life. Life is worth living if the patient would judge their life to be tolerable. The balance sheet approach is closer to what we might think of as an objective sense of a LWL: it reflects an attempt to impartially weigh up the positives and negatives of different courses of action.

We saw above that guidelines are not terribly specific about the severity of impairment that would make life intolerable or tip the balance against treatment. But could we use these different tests to yield an answer? Can we apply the intolerability test or the balance sheet approach to the outputs of the Carmentis machine?

Intolerability

Getting to Grips with the Concept

What does it mean to say that life is intolerable? The concept of intolerability is not defined in legal or ethical guidelines. Indeed, the Nuffield report and Royal College guidelines mentioned above go so far as to suggest that it cannot be defined.

In proposing 'intolerability' as a threshold to justify decisions not to insist on life-prolonging treatments, the Working Party acknowledges the fallibility of language and the uncertainty of interpretation of evidence. Reasonable people may disagree... about what constitutes 'intolerability'. (Nuffield Council on Bioethics 2006: 13)

A severe/intolerable disability is indefinable. (Royal College of Paediatrics and Child Health 2004: 25)

But if we cannot define intolerability how are we to apply it to the results of the Carmentis machine? One of the tools that philosophers use when analysing concepts is to try to break them down into their important elements. Even if there is no published definition of intolerability perhaps we can set one out? As a starting point, the *Oxford English Dictionary* defines 'intolerable' as something:

that cannot be tolerated, borne or put up with; unendurable, unbearable, insupportable, insufferable. a. physically. b. mentally or morally. c. in loose sense, as a strong intensive: Excessive, extreme, exceedingly great (cf. awful).

From here we might set out three different components that appear to be important:

i. First, there is the subjective nature of the judgement. It requires the perspective of the individual. In the case of J, Lord Justice Taylor wrote:

I consider the correct approach is for the court to judge the quality of life the child would have to endure if given the treatment and decide whether in all the circumstances such a life would be so afflicted as to be intolerable to that child. I say 'to that child' because the test should not be whether the life would be intolerable to the decider. The test must be whether the child in question, if capable of exercising sound judgment, would consider the life tolerable. (Re J 1991: 55F)

This description of intolerability has some similarity with the use of substituted judgement in decision-making for incompetent patients.

ii The second component of intolerability is the sense that it involves a *particularly negative* state of existence. Lord Justice Taylor referred to 'extreme' circumstances and the 'cruelty' of life (Re J 1991: 55). In an earlier English case (that of 'B') the judge referred to a life 'full of pain and suffering' (Re B 1981: 1424C). Similarly the Nuffield report refers to 'extreme suffering or impairment' (Nuffield Council on Bioethics 2006: 13). This relates to part c of the dictionary definition given above.

iii. A third conceptual element relates to the process of toleration. To tolerate something means putting up with or accepting the negative features of a situation. It requires awareness of those negative features (it makes no sense to tolerate something of which we are unaware or that causes no discomfort or annoyance). It also often involves a conscious weighing up of those negatives against some other goal, or benefit. For example, we might tolerate a toothache because we wish to continue our day's work, or because we hope that it will improve with time without the need to go to a dentist. The severity of pain that can be tolerated will depend in part on what else we need to do; even a severe toothache might be tolerated if we had an urgent work deadline or personal commitment. Conversely a toothache that is intolerable disrupts our daily activity and prevents us from working or taking part in planned activities.

These three elements might be combined into a formal definition

An *intolerable* condition is one that
1. From the perspective of the individual child
2. involves extreme suffering or adversity AND
3. is more than they are able or willing to endure.

As this is our first working definition of intolerability we will call it intolerability (1).

Can there be degrees of intolerability? The last condition here suggests that there may be. Some conditions may be literally intolerable, in the sense that there is no benefit that could persuade the individual to bear the condition. (Perhaps some forms of physical torture are literally intolerable in this sense?) Other conditions are relatively intolerable; they are sufficiently bad that the individual is not willing to endure them. However, it is possible that the patient would be physically or psychologically able to tolerate them if absolutely necessary or if they were sufficiently motivated to do so.

Although our first definition of intolerability appears plausible, there are problems in its application, as we will see shortly, and other versions are possible. The Royal College guideline suggests that the first condition above is optional.

Intolerable may mean 'that which cannot be borne' or 'that which people should not be asked to bear'. (RCPCH 2004: 25)

It is possible to envisage a level of disability that doctors believe to be intolerable, i.e. no reasonable person would want to live with it, and yet an individual sufferer may attach value to their existence. (RCPCH 2004: 26)

This version of intolerability then potentially adopts the perspective of a third party (i.e. not the patient), and introduces an additional dimension in suggesting that the patient *should not be asked* to endure it. So then the concept would be:

An *intolerable* condition is one that
1. From the perspective of a third party
2. involves such extreme suffering or hardship for the child that
3. they (the third party) would not be willing to endure it themselves.

We will call this second definition 'intolerability (2)'.

One question is why intolerability (2) is actually referred to as 'intolerable', since the guideline admits that individual patients may be able and willing to tolerate such conditions? It can't be literally intolerable. We might think of this as a judgement about probability: conditions that are intolerable (2) are probably, though not necessarily, intolerable in the first sense described above (i.e. for the patient). Another possibility is that it is intolerable *for the third party* that the child is in this condition:

An *intolerable* condition is one that
1. From the perspective of a reasonable third party
2. involves such extreme suffering or hardship that
3. they (the third party) are not able or willing for the child to endure it.

This third sense (intolerability (3)) could incorporate into an assessment of intolerability the fear or distress of parents or caregivers at the extremely unpleasant state that a child is facing.

Problems with Intolerability

1. How Could We Know? There are significant epistemic problems for the first two versions of intolerability. An epistemic problem is a philosophical term for a problem with acquiring knowledge and with getting to the facts of the matter. As noted above, intolerability (1) invokes a form of substituted judgement. But substituted judgement for patients who have never been competent (for example infants or young children) is difficult, since they have not been in a position to express preferences about treatment. It necessarily involves an attempt to imagine what the judgement of the individual would be.

Consider Phillip (Case 3), with predicted severe cognitive impairment and moderate physical impairment after his traumatic brain injury. There are different ways of arriving at a substituted judgement for a child like this (Archard 2008). The first way is to imagine that Phillip now were able to weigh up his condition and able to tell us whether his future life is tolerable to him. But since we are not likely to have knowledge of the six-year-old Phillip's views about significant future impairments it is difficult, if not impossible, to know what judgement Phillip would make. Would he want treatment to continue or to stop? It is highly unlikely that we will have a clear answer. (It would be even more difficult for the infants in Cases 1 and 4.) The second possibility is to imagine Phillip grown to maturity (with impairment), and to substitute his future retrospective judgement. In other words, we want to know whether he now (in this future hypothetical state) judges his life to have been intolerable, and whether he is glad or regrets his life having been saved. This possibility is somewhat more appealing since we have the evidence of adults with impairment, including those who have had head injuries, and their views about the quality of their lives. But the views of such individuals may not be representative of the future anticipated for Phillip. For example we have no way of knowing what the views of severely or profoundly cognitively impaired adults would be about their treatment in intensive care. They are unable to tell us what life was like or is like for them. These reports also represent only the views of those who have survived. Infants and children who died prior to reaching adulthood would be unrepresented. This may be a distinct possibility for children with serious impairments and illness. The third alternative is to imagine Phillip as a competent adult reflecting on treatments that may or may not be provided for him in childhood. This is also problematic, however, since it requires the judger to imagine lacking capacities that are essential to their identity and to their judgement. There is a worry that such forms of substituted judgment are inevitably prone to bias, because the prospect of losing capacities often appears overwhelming. Individuals tend to overestimate the impact of future negative life events, and underestimate their ability to adapt to changes (Ditto, Hawkins, et al. 2005). This may be why healthy individuals fairly consistently rate illnesses and impairments more negatively than those who have actually experienced those conditions (Ditto, Hawkins, et al. 2005). Our third definition of Intolerability avoids the difficulties of substituted judgement since it asks only whether a third party is able or willing to tolerate for Phillip to be in a severely impaired state.

2. The Tolerability Paradox When we try to apply the concept of intolerability in practice other problems emerge. Which predictions of the Carmentis machine are intolerable? Many of those who have invoked the concept of intolerability have cited conditions involving severe physical suffering. But they have also referred particularly to conditions involving severe or profound cognitive impairment. For example one of the judges that I have cited several times in relation to the case of J described

a child... so damaged as to have negligible use of its faculties and the only way of preserving its life was by the continuous administration of extremely painful treatment... or... sedated continuously as to have no conscious life at all. (Re J 1991: 55c)

The judge also listed as first amongst the factors justifying withholding treatment in J's case 'the severe lack of capacity of the child in all his faculties which even without any further complication would make his existence barely sentient'. In another case of treatment limitation for an infant with severe impairment Justice Ward referred to 'intellectual function as the hallmark of our humanity' (Re C 1990: 35C). The Royal College guideline argued that the lack of the capacity for meaningful communication would make life intolerable (Royal College of Paediatrics and Child Health 2004: 24), and the Nuffield report refers to lives lacking those features that give life meaning and purpose as an intolerable existence 'even in the absence of great pain or distress' (Nuffield Council on Bioethics 2006: 12, para 12.13).

But here is another potential problem for these accounts. There is a seemingly paradoxical improvement in tolerability with severe cognitive impairment (Wilkinson 2006). What we might call the tolerability paradox is the following: intuitively, if impairment can make life intolerable, it seems that this is most likely for severe or extreme forms of illness or impairment. There are some reasons, however, to think that beyond a certain point more severe degrees of cognitive impairment may make life more tolerable rather than less tolerable. This is illustrated schematically in Figure 2.1.

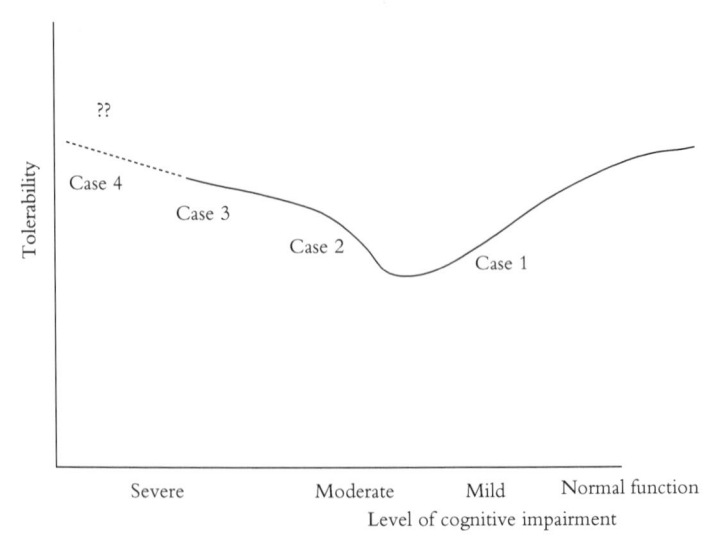

Figure 2.1 Tolerability and cognitive impairment.

There is a sense in which it could be better for an individual to be severely cognitively impaired than to be mildly impaired or cognitively normal. Why should this be the case? The first reason is that how difficult an individual finds life may be influenced by the severity of impairment. Individuals with mild intellectual impairment are often aware of their limitations and sometimes frustrated by them. They may be sensitive to the looks and attitudes of others, and be conscious of being treated differently. (Those with cognitive impairment are often subject to bullying (MENCAP 1999).) They may be distressed by difficulty in communicating and achieving their desires, by lack of opportunity, or by the socio-economic disadvantage that is often associated with impairment. There is some evidence that clinical depression is more common in those with cognitive impairment (McBrien 2003). But more severe cognitive disability may be less likely to cause this sort of distress. For example, in a large study of quality of life in children with cerebral palsy, those with an IQ <50 were *less* likely to have low ratings for mood, emotions, and self-perception than children with mild cognitive impairment or normal IQ (Arnaud, White-Koning, et al. 2008). A similar phenomenon is sometimes apparent at the other end of life. In patients with progressive cognitive decline associated with dementia, there is often an initially distressing phase when they are conscious of being unable to do things or remember things that they could previously. However, with further cognitive decline, there is sometimes some relief associated with the loss of insight, and an improvement in the patient's mood.

Consider Angelos (Case 2), the young child with severe muscle weakness who is dependent on a mechanical ventilator. The Carmentis machine predicts that he will have moderate cognitive impairment. This might make doctors and Angelos' parents concerned about whether ventilatory support should continue. However, his experience of life could be significantly worse if he were mildly impaired or cognitively normal and aware of his surroundings than if he were moderately or severely impaired and, to some degree, unaware (Nuffield Council on Bioethics 2006: 139). Those who care for such children sometimes worry that they will feel trapped or imprisoned by their bodies, unable to communicate their wishes or discomfort. Paradoxically life may be more tolerable for Phillip (Case 3) than for Amelia (Case 1), despite the much more severe cognitive impairment in the former's case.

Secondly, very severe forms of cognitive impairment may be incompatible with the second condition of all three versions of intolerability described above. Lord Justice Taylor described as example of an intolerable life where a child were continuously sedated and permanently unconscious. Yet in fact, such a life appears a paradigm example of a life that is able to be tolerated since it involves no negative experiences whatsoever. Similarly, since it would seem incoherent to describe anencephaly (a condition where there is absence of the cerebrum) as involving any suffering or hardship for the patient, it would not be intolerable on any of the definitions that we have developed.

What is more, at severe or profound degrees of cognitive impairment, the third element of intolerability may lose traction. As highlighted above, to tolerate implies a sense of trade-off, of enduring some experiences for the sake of others. It requires a minimum level of awareness and continuity of experience. But at very severe levels of cognitive impairment, such as that experienced by Baby Chloe (Case 4) the individual may not only be unable to communicate whether their life is tolerable, the concept of tolerance itself may not apply.

In summary, the problem with interpreting 'intolerability' when we are trying to make sense of the predictions of the Carmentis machine, is that there are substantial problems in determining the tolerability or intolerability of conditions for infants and young children—even where there is certainty about prognosis. Moreover it is difficult to take into account the apparent importance of severe cognitive impairment within a conventional analysis of intolerability.

Our third definition of intolerability (the 'third-person' form) may avoid some of these problems. We can determine the tolerability of a state simply by asking caregivers their views; we do not need to perform difficult feats of imagination to assess the child's view of life. A parent or doctor might find it intolerable for a child to be on life support in a persistent vegetative state for example, though that state involves little or no actual negative experiences and the perspective of the child himself is unknowable. Nevertheless, this version of intolerability is vulnerable to other objections. Firstly, the tolerance of a third party may depend on what they have been exposed to, or are accustomed to, or equally on their views about disability and impairment. In the past it was judged by many reasonable parents to be intolerable for a child to have Down syndrome, whereas now this is often cited as a paradigmatically tolerable condition. Can tolerability be so contingent on societal attitudes, and so subject to change? Secondly, there is a risk of circularity in the part of the definition that specifies that these must be the views of a 'reasonable' third party. Imagine, for example, that members of one society found trivial cosmetic impairments (e.g. cleft lip and palate) to be more than they were willing to bear for their children. We might well question whether or not this was the judgement of 'reasonable' people. But on what grounds is reasonableness to be judged? It cannot be on the basis that mild impairments like cleft lip are actually tolerable without going in a circle. We would be assuming what we are attempting to determine (this is what philosophers call 'begging the question'). Finally, if tolerability is related so fundamentally to the tolerance of a third party, why think that this is a test for the best interests of the patient? Lord Justice Taylor appeared to exclude intolerability (3) in his comments on Re J, when he noted that 'the test should not be whether the life would be intolerable to the decider' (1991: 55F). There may be reasons to take into account the wishes and views of parents (we will return to this in Chapter 7), but we should distinguish that question from the question of whether life with certain severe impairment is in the best interests of the child.

MB

MB was an infant with severe muscle weakness whose case was heard by the family division of the England and Wales High Court in 2006 (An NHS trust v MB 2006).

At the time of the court hearing MB was eighteen months old. He had a severe congenital neuromuscular disorder (type 1.1 spinal muscular atrophy), had been in hospital since seven weeks of age, and ventilator-dependent for six months. Spinal muscular atrophy is caused by a genetic mutation that leads to degeneration of the nerves running from the spinal cord to muscles. It varies in severity, and in the rate of degeneration. In MB's case, his condition led to progressive loss of muscle strength and tone, so that although he could initially cry audibly, smile, and move his limbs, by the time of the court hearing he could only move his eyes. He was essentially in a form of locked-in syndrome, though this description is not usually used for infants. Although MB had profound motor impairment he was not believed to be cognitively impaired. MB's doctors believed that continuing mechanical ventilation was 'cruel', and that it would be in his best interests to withdraw life-saving treatment and allow him to die. His parents, on the other hand, opposed the withdrawal of treatment.

The judge in the case, Justice Holman, sought to determine what would be in the 'objective' best interests of MB. He asked the advocates on either side to draw up a list of the benefits and burdens of continuing or discontinuing mechanical ventilation, and included the list provided by MB's legal guardian in his judgement. Justice Holman placed significant emphasis on the process of weighing up benefits and burdens, though noted huge difficulties in reliably appraising the benefits of treatment, deciding what weight to give to future burdens, and in arriving at an overall balance (An NHS Trust v MB 2006, para 62). The judge ruled that continued mechanical ventilation was in the best interests of MB. In reaching this decision the judge placed importance on the absence of cognitive and sensory impairment.

So far as I am aware, no court has yet been asked to approve that, against the will of the child's parents, life support may be withdrawn or discontinued, ... [from] a conscious child with sensory awareness and assumed normal cognition and no reliable evidence of any significant brain damage. (An NHS Trust v MB 2006, para 11)

As he can hear and see, I accept the evidence of his parents that he is attentive to TV, DVDs, CDs, stories and speech; and as all these things may give pleasure to other children of 18 months, I must and do assume they give pleasure to him. (An NHS Trust v MB 2006, para 65)

[MB's] life does in my view include within it the benefits that I have tried to describe... Within those benefits, and central to them, is my view that on the available evidence I must proceed on the basis that M has age appropriate cognition, and does continue to have a relationship of value to him with his family, and does continue to gain other pleasures from touch, sight and sound. (An NHS Trust v MB 2006, para 101)

The significance of this case for treatment decisions lies in several factors. The judge's decision endorsed the idea of using a balance sheet of benefits and burdens to determine best interests, he supported MB's parents against the unanimous opinion of medical experts, and he placed significant emphasis on the presence of normal cognition and sensory abilities.

Balance Sheet

As described above, the English case of MB was decided on the basis of a weighing up of the benefits and burdens of different treatment alternatives rather than on the basis of intolerability. The 'balance sheet' approach was described first by Lord Justice Thorpe (Re A 2000) and includes both the process of determining best interests, as well as a threshold for decision-making. Surrogate decision-makers are instructed to document the separate benefits and burdens of treatment. If the benefits of treatment outweigh the burdens, it is in the best interests of the patient to provide it. On the other hand, if the burdens outweigh the benefits, it is not in the best interests of the patient to provide treatment and it may be withheld or withdrawn.

This definition doesn't specify how much the burdens need to outweigh benefits for it to be in the best interests of the patient to withdraw life-sustaining treatment. Perhaps, like the probability threshold for civil legal cases (the so called 'balance of probabilities'), a small excess of negatives over positives would be sufficient? But Lord Justice Thorpe in the case of Re A appeared to require a higher standard:

Obviously, only if the account is in *relatively significant credit* will the judge conclude that the application is likely to advance the best interests of the claimant. (2000: 560; emphasis added)

The balance sheet has been favoured over intolerability in recent court judgements in the UK, and there are several potential reasons for this. One reason is that it appears to be more instructive. The concept of intolerability, as elaborated above, does not provide any guide for how to determine whether a condition is intolerable. (And, as noted above, there are formidable difficulties in doing so.)

Secondly, some have suggested that intolerability expresses a conclusion about best interests rather than a test for best interests (An NHS Trust v MB 2006, para 17). Although we have tried to set out the conceptual elements of intolerability in the above analysis there is a risk that its definition becomes a form of concealed tautology. The third condition (an intolerable condition is one that the patient or third party is 'unable or unwilling to endure') in each of the definitions provided could be thought equivalent to 'an intolerable condition is one that is intolerable' and consequently trivial.

A third reason that intolerability has been recently downplayed is that it relies on a form of substituted judgement (at least in forms (1) and (2) above). In the UK, the courts have tended to place less emphasis on substituted judgement than US courts; they prefer an 'objective best interests' test, with the patient's wishes comprising only one component of their best interests (British Medical Association 2007: 13). In another much cited British case the court held that a decision for an incompetent patient about the reinsertion of a feeding tube should be based on their best interests, rather than on what they would have chosen if capable (W Healthcare NHS trust v H 2005). It was accepted that the patient would not have wanted the feeding tube reinserted, but the judge held nevertheless that it was in the patient's best interests to do so. The balance sheet determination of best interests appears, at least at first glance, more objective than intolerability.

Is this approach to determining best interests able to provide an answer to the question of whether treatment should be provided in the face of certain impairment, such as that predicted by the Carmentis machine? We will consider the role of different impairments separately.

Physical Impairment

How would physical problems affect the balance of interests for a child? Physical impairment or illness may lead to burdens particularly where those impairments are associated with significant pain or suffering. For example, a congenital abnormality that will predictably require multiple surgical procedures would impose a definite burden. Angelos (Case 2) will likely require major spinal surgery for scoliosis in mid-childhood, and will have ongoing burdens relating to his ventilator dependence. He is likely to require insertion of suction tubes into his tracheostomy multiple times a day, a procedure that is acutely distressing and uncomfortable. These burdens will appear on the negative side of the balance sheet when weighing up life saving treatment. But here lies one problem for the balance sheet approach. Even if future impairment is known with certainty, the degree of pain or suffering associated with that impairment may not be predictable. For example, one child might have a relatively uncomplicated course and short hospital stay, while another child might develop a post-operative infection, require repeat surgery, and have a long hospital admission. Children also vary in their tolerance of pain, some are squeamish, some are stoic. Perhaps Angelos will not be bothered by suctioning of his trachea, perhaps he will be intensely and repeatedly upset by it. It is difficult to know in advance how adversely affected any individual child would be. We could potentially gauge the average burden of an impairment predicted by the Carmentis machine, but some uncertainty will remain.

Other impairments may cause limitations in activity without leading to physical suffering. They wouldn't necessarily lead to burdens for the child (though they could if the child were frustrated, depressed, or anxious as a result of the impairments) but might be included instead as relative reductions on the benefits side of the balance sheet. For example, there are some pleasures that Amelia with spastic quadriplegic cerebral palsy (Case 1) will be unable to experience because she is unable to walk or run and is confined to a wheelchair. She is not likely to be able to go rock-climbing, or bush walking, ride a bicycle, or go ice-skating. That does not mean that she will not enjoy other things just as much, if not more than she would have enjoyed these precluded activities. It is difficult to know how much weight to give to these absent pleasures. However, profound physical impairment, such as that affecting Angelos (Case 2) may substantially affect his access to many activities that others are able to enjoy. This seems relevant to the balance.

Another problem, however, with weighing future physical impairments is that the degree to which the individual is disabled by their impairment is contingent upon the society in which they live and the support that is provided to them. This is one component of the social model of disability discussed above. If there is little provision for wheelchairs in society, an individual may be very limited in their ability to take part in social activities. On the other hand, if society provides a high level of support the limitation attributable to their impairment may be much less. So an attempt to include physical impairment in a weighted balance of benefits and burdens will need to take into account both the current level of support provided by society and the anticipated future level of support. There is a further question here about whether the socially contingent features of a disability should even be included in a decision about life-sustaining treatment. Imagine that a child's disability will be much worse because their society has not made any effort to provide social support for the disabled. Some will find it highly troubling to take this into account when deciding about treatment. It seems to endorse or accept attitudes that should not be accepted. We do not need to settle that question here; rather we might merely note the added difficulty in the weighing equation.

The final point to note about weighing up the benefits and burdens of physical impairment is that some individuals appear able to realize high levels of personal achievement and well-being despite overwhelming physical impairments. Examples often cited include writers Christy Brown and Christopher Nolan with severe cerebral palsy, or physicist Stephen Hawking with amyotrophic lateral sclerosis (Doyal and Durbin 1998; Wyatt 2005). Christy Brown had severe spastic quadriplegic cerebral palsy, but he was able to write four novels and three poetry collections and was able to paint with a brush or pencil held between the first and second toes of his left foot. Perhaps the life of Baby Amelia (Case 1) will be like this?

The balance sheet approach does not rely on the subjective judgements of individuals with impairment, but the evidence of individuals like Christy Brown could be used to substantiate the potential balance of benefits and burdens. In the Charlotte Wyatt case, Justice Hedley noted that intolerability might provide a role of this sort:

the concept of 'intolerable to that child' should not be seen as a gloss on, much less a supplementary test to, best interests. It is a valuable guide in the search for best interests in this kind of case. (Portsmouth NHS Trust v Wyatt 2005, para 24)

On this basis the lives of Christy Brown or Stephen Hawking might lead us to question whether physical impairment alone would necessarily tip the balance against continued withdrawal of life support.

Sensory Impairment

How should other impairments be taken into account in the balance sheet? Sensory impairment might be thought to affect the balance in a similar way to some physical impairments. Blindness or deafness could reduce the benefits of life but would not necessarily lead to burdens for the individual. Single sensory impairments might be relatively easily overcome, but the combination of sensory impairments (for example blindness and deafness) or sensory impairment with other physical impairments would make it significantly harder for a child to communicate, to be independent, and to fulfil their goals. Again, this would be dependent on the amount of support provided to the child/adult. Sensory impairment would not necessarily preclude a life that was of net benefit.

Cognitive Impairment

But what about cognitive impairment? One point to note about the positive examples cited above of individuals overcoming severe physical impairment is that these people not only had normal cognitive function, they had significantly greater than normal cognitive function. One possibility is that it is only individuals with extraordinary abilities who are likely to achieve public attention. (The media stereotype of the high-achieving individual with very severe disability is sometimes labelled the 'super-cripple' (Barnes 1994).) But another possibility is that there is something important about the presence of cognitive function for achieving well-being despite physical obstacles. In the previous section, I outlined the tolerability paradox, and suggested that cognitive impairment would not necessarily increase the burdens experienced by the future child or adult (indeed it may reduce them). But the other possibility is that cognitive impairment may reduce the benefits of life for the child (Wilkinson 2006). By preventing or limiting the individual from accessing a number of those things that almost all of us would think are valuable and important features of life (for example deep personal relationships, the development and attainment of personal goals), severe cognitive impairment may make it easier for burdens to outweigh benefits. This is reflected in the judgements in the MB case and a similar legal case in the same year of 'K'. While in the former case the presence of normal cognition was felt to outweigh the burdens of extreme physical impairment, in the latter case the absence of the benefits afforded by normal intelligence tipped the balance in the other direction.

In this case K... has a developmental age of only 3 months. She has no accumulation of experiences and cognition comparable with that of MB. She is not, and with her short expectation of life is never likely to be, in a position to derive pleasure from DVDs or CDs and the only indication of real feelings of pleasure in her limited developmental state is enjoyment of a bath. (K (A Minor) 2006, para 57)

On the other hand, the balance sheet also has considerable problems. While we have seen that future physical and cognitive impairment may affect the balance of benefits and burdens for treatment, it is far more difficult to know to what degree, and whether the balance has been tipped in favour of or against discontinuing LST. Even if the Carmentis machine gave us certainty about the degree and nature of future impairments for a child, there is no straightforward way of deciding how much weight to give to different benefits or burdens, how they should be aggregated or combined, and how they should be weighed against each other. It is a more general problem for the best interests principle that it sometimes, perhaps often, is unclear which interest is the strongest, or which course will best promote interests overall. Often we are comparing apples with oranges, trading off values that simply can't be easily compared.

In the case of the paralysed infant Angelos (Case 2), how does the benefit of watching DVDs or the comfort of familiar voices weigh against the potential distress of being unable to move, the pain of suctioning breathing tubes, the sense of suffocation when secretions build up or breathing tubes become transiently blocked? What is more, there is no obvious way of arbitrating whether a particular threshold has been reached. It is not clear what the 'significant credit' level, mentioned above, would correspond to in practice.

The balance sheet approach is sometimes referred to as an 'objective' best interests test because it involves a weighing up of different interests and does not rely on the preference or choice of the individual. But the above analysis suggests that there is no truly objective way of determining the balance.

There are problems with both of the tests that have been proposed for determining best interests in infants and deciding about withdrawal of LST. Although uncertainty about prognosis is a major problem for decisions, when such uncertainty is removed, as in our thought experiment of the Carmentis Machine, the underlying conceptual problems are brought into sharp relief. Determining whether future life is intolerable, or whether the benefits outweigh the burdens is not only difficult to answer; for infants with significant cognitive impairment it is fundamentally unanswerable. And yet, ironically, it is for infants with this sort of impairment that there is the greatest consensus that treatment may be withdrawn. One of the reasons why guidelines and the courts have failed to provide specific guidance in this area may be that the tests that they have recommended for the task are simply inadequate.

The problem with using the best interests principle for helping with decisions about treatment is that in difficult cases it does not appear able to provide an answer. There is a separate problem, which we will return to in subsequent chapters, that it also appears to leave parents out in the cold with nothing to say about treatment. If treatment is in the best interests of the infant, then parents should have no say in whether or not it continues. Alternatively if treatment is not in the best interests of the child, then why should parents' wishes be relevant for whether or not treatment continues? This appears to conflict, then, with the major role of parents in decisions about life-sustaining treatment in most parts of the world.

What alternative principles might be used to develop more specific guidelines for prognostication and treatment withdrawal and to help us know what to do with the predictions of the Carmentis machine? In the next chapter we will go to the other extreme and examine the philosophical arguments that have been proposed to permit the withdrawal of LST from infants with mild or moderate impairment. Are newborn infants or children replaceable?

References

American Academy of Pediatrics Committee on Fetus and Newborn (1995). 'The initiation or withdrawal of treatment for high-risk newborns', *Pediatrics* 96(2 Pt 1): 362–3.

——(2007). 'Non-initiation or withdrawal of intensive care for high-risk newborns', *Pediatrics* 119(2): 401–3.

An NHS Trust v D. [2000] 2 FLR 677.
An NHS Trust v MB. [2006] 2 F.L.R. 319.
Archard, D. (2008). 'Children's Rights', *The Stanford Encyclopaedia of Philosophy*, <http://plato.stanford.edu/archives/win2008/entries/rights-children/> (accessed 23/09/2009).
Arnaud, C., M. White-Koning, et al. (2008). 'Parent-reported quality of life of children with cerebral palsy in Europe', *Pediatrics* 121(1): 54–64.
Arneson, R.J. (2006). 'What is wrongful discrimination?', *San Diego Law Review* 43: 775–807.
Barnes, C. (1994). 'Images of disability', in S. French (ed.), *On Equal Terms*. Oxford: Butterworth Heinemann, 35–46.
Baskett, P.J., P.A. Steen, et al. (2005). 'European Resuscitation Council guidelines for resuscitation 2005. Section 8. The ethics of resuscitation and end-of-life decisions', *Resuscitation* 67 Suppl 1: S171–80.
Bickenbach, J.E., S. Chatterji, et al. (1999). 'Models of disablement, universalism and the international classification of impairments, disabilities and handicaps', *Soc Sci Med* 48(9): 1173–87.
British Medical Association. (2007). *Withholding and Withdrawing Life-Prolonging Medical Treatment: Guidance for Decision Making*. Malden, MA; Oxford: Blackwell.
Brody, H. and W.G. Bartholome (1988). 'In the best interests of', *Hastings Cent Rep* 18(6): 37–40.
Buchanan, A.E., D.W. Brock, et al. (2000). *From Chance to Choice: Genetics and Justice*. Cambridge: Cambridge University Press.
Ditto, P., N. Hawkins, et al. (2005). 'Imagining the end of life: on the psychology of advance medical decision making', *Motivation and Emotion* 29(4): 475–96.
Doyal, L. and G. Durbin (1998). 'When life may become too precious: the severely damaged neonate', *Seminars in Neonatology* 3: 275–84.
Dyer, C. (2005). 'Judge over-rules earlier decision on Charlotte Wyatt', *BMJ* 331 (7523): 985.
Engelhardt, H.T. (1989). 'Taking the family seriously: beyond best interests', in L. M. Kopelman and J.C. Moskop (eds), *Children and Health Care: Moral and Social Issues*. Boston, Kluwer Academic, 231–7.
Giannini, A., A. Messeri, et al. (2008). 'End-of-life decisions in pediatric intensive care. Recommendations of the Italian Society of Neonatal and Pediatric Anesthesia and Intensive Care (SARNePI)', *Paediatr Anaesth* 18(11): 1089–95.
Hubert, P., P. Canoui, et al. (2005). 'Withholding or withdrawing life saving treatment in pediatric intensive care unit: GFRUP guidelines', *Arch Pediatr* 12(10): 1501–8.
K (A minor). [2006] 2 F.L.R. 883.

Kopelman, L.M. (1997). 'The best-interests standard as threshold, ideal, and standard of reasonableness', *J Med Philos* 22(3): 271–89.

Lockhart, T. (2000). *Moral Uncertainty and Its Consequences*. New York; Oxford: Oxford University Press.

McBrien, J. (2003). 'Assessment and diagnosis of depression in people with intellectual disability', *Journal of Intellectual Disability Research* 47(1): 1–13.

McHaffie, H.E., M. Cuttini, et al. (1999). 'Withholding/withdrawing treatment from neonates: legislation and official guidelines across Europe', *J Med Ethics* 25(6): 440–6.

MENCAP (1999). *Living in Fear: The Need to Combat Bullying of People with a Learning Disability*. London, MENCAP.

NSW Health. (2005). 'Guidelines for end-of-life care and decision-making', <http://www.health.nsw.gov.au/policies/gl/2005/GL2005_057.html> (accessed 18/07/2011).

Nuffield Council on Bioethics (2006). *Critical Care Decisions in Fetal and Neonatal Medicine: Ethical Issues*. London: Nuffield Council on Bioethics.

Oliver, M. (1996). *Understanding Disability: From Theory to Practice*. Basingstoke: Macmillan.

Portsmouth NHS Trust v Wyatta. [2005] 1 F.L.R. 21.

Portsmouth Hospitals NHS Trust v Wyattb. [2005] 1 W.L.R. 3995.

President's Commission (1983). *Deciding to forego life-sustaining treatment: a report on the ethical, medical and legal issues in treatment decisions/President's Commission for the Study of Ethical Problems in Medicine and Biomedical and Behavioral Research*. Washington: The Commission.

Re A (Mental Patient: Sterilisation). [2000] 1 F.L.R. 549.

Re B (a minor) (wardship: medical treatment). [1981] 1 WLR 1421.

Re C (a minor) (wardship: medical treatment) (No.1). [1990] Fam 26.

Re J (a minor) (wardship: medical treatment). [1991] Fam 33.

Re OT. [2009] EWHC 633 (Fam).

Rennie, J. and B. Leigh (2008). 'The legal framework for end-of-life decisions in the UK', *Seminars in Fetal and Neonatal Medicine* 13(5): 296–300.

Roth, A. (1976). 'The tender years presumption in child custody disputes', *J Fam Law* 15: 423–62.

Royal Australasian College of Physicians. (2008). 'Decision-Making at the End of Life in Infants, Children and Adolescents', <http://www.racp.edu.au/index.cfm?objectid=B5603385-D3A3-F3B4-7159013AE33D4697> (accessed 26/07/11).

Royal Children's Hospital. (2006). 'Withholding or withdrawal of life-sustaining treatment (Clinical Practice Guideline), <http://www.rch.org.au/clinical-guide/cpg.cfm?doc_id=12348> (accessed 18/07/2011).

Royal College of Paediatrics and Child Health (2004). *Withholding and Withdrawing Life-Saving Treatment in Children: A Framework for Practice.* London: Royal College of Paediatrics and Child Health.

Shakespeare, T. (2008). 'Debating disability', *J Med Ethics* 34(1): 11–14.

Street, K., R. Ashcroft, et al. (2000). 'The decision making process regarding the withdrawal or withholding of potential life-saving treatments in a children's hospital', *Journal of Medical Ethics* 26(5): 346–52.

Veatch, R.M. (1995). 'Abandoning informed consent', *Hastings Cent Rep* 25(2): 5–12.

W Healthcare NHS Trust v H [2005] 1 W.L.R. 834.

Wilkinson, D. (2006). 'Is it in the best interests of an intellectually disabled infant to die?', *J Med Ethics* 32(8): 454–9.

—— (2010). '"We don't have a crystal ball": neonatologists views on prognosis and decision-making in newborn infants with birth asphyxia', *Monash Bioethics Review* 29(1): 5.1–5.19.

Wyatt, J. (2005). 'Quality of Life', <http://www.cmf.org.uk/literature/content.asp?context=article&id=1702> (accessed 25/05/2009).

3

Starting Again

Case: Christine

Christine is born twelve weeks prematurely following a caesarean section. She has respiratory distress syndrome and requires breathing support from a mechanical ventilator. In the first days of life she is noticed to be having epileptic seizures and is treated with anticonvulsants. The Carmentis machine reveals a large left-sided cerebral infarction (stroke) involving the cerebral hemisphere, basal ganglia, and internal capsule. Christine's doctors tell her parents that she will have movement problems affecting her right side (a right hemiplegia) of moderate severity. She will have fairly significant problems using her right hand and will walk or run with a limp. She will have some shortening and tension in the muscles of her right leg, and will need splints and an operation in childhood to correct this. The machine also indicates that her cognitive function will be in the low normal range.

What significance is it that if Christine dies her parents could conceive another child, one who would not have impairments of this sort, or at least is much less likely to? Should this affect decisions in intensive care?

Sometimes in newborn intensive care, well-meaning doctors or nurses, friends or family members, wonder about the effort that is being exerted to save the life of a child like Christine who appears likely to be damaged or impaired in some way. They are usually (though not always) too tactful to express such thoughts to the parents, but they wonder whether it would be better to give up on this infant, to start again afresh (Kuhse and Singer 1985: 65). In a study of doctors working in a tertiary Indian neonatal unit, some of those interviewed suggested that they would avoid treating infants with a high chance of dying or of needing long-term medical attention because 'it is better for them to go for a new baby' (Miljeteig and Norheim 2006). Parents, too, sometimes admit to such thoughts. In her book, *The Long Dying of Baby Andrew*, Peggy Stinson wrote an honest, but critical, account of her experience of having a very premature newborn infant in intensive care. She wrote in her diary 'I keep thinking about the other baby—the one who won't be born' (Kuhse and Singer 1985).

This sort of question, about conceiving another child in the place of a current impaired child, is a strange one. It is possibly only voiced at the beginning of life. Something similar is occasionally mentioned when serious congenital abnormalities are discovered before birth, and there is the question of whether the pregnancy should continue. Perhaps it does cross people's minds too in relation to slightly older infants, though I have never heard it uttered in paediatric intensive care. But it would seem odd in the extreme to contemplate that an adult suffering from illness or disability might be replaced by another individual not yet born.

But the idea of 'replacing' an impaired infant is not simply a passing fancy. Several eminent philosophers, notably Australian utilitarian philosopher Peter Singer and English philosopher R.M. Hare, have defended it as being a relevant and important consideration for newborn treatment decisions. If that were the case, if it is not only legitimate, but morally important to replace impaired infants like Christine, our answer to the predictions of the Carmentis machine would be strikingly different. It might mean that we should be much more permissive in intensive care, at least for newborn infants. We would be justified in allowing infants to die whenever they are predicted to have even minor disabilities as long as parents were able and willing to have another child. What is more, this may cast into question the huge efforts and expense that are put into saving the lives of newborns, such as those born very prematurely. This would be in stark contrast to the answers that are usually given. In the previous chapter we discovered that in difficult cases, where infants are predicted to have very severe degrees of impairment, the best interests principle fails to provide a clear answer to treatment questions. In less severe cases, though, the best interests principle would have no trouble in providing an answer. For infants or children like Christine, who have only mild or moderate degrees of impairment, it is unquestionably in their best interests to keep them alive and we should do so if at all possible.

Where does the idea of replacement come from? What weight should we give to it in decisions about newborn infants or children? What is its significance for prognostication and the Carmentis machine? In this chapter we will spend some time trying to unravel these questions. In doing so we will venture into philosophically murky waters—into questions about existence and non-existence, benefits and harms. We will see that the significance of replacement lies not in future or possible people, but in the interests of those who already exist.

Key Terminology

Before we start it will be useful to be clear about some terms. Like the concept of 'intolerability' discussed in Chapter 2 some of these concepts are ones that often go undefined. But we should make sure that we are talking and thinking about the same thing. If this appears confusing or unnecessarily technical it will hopefully make more sense shortly once we put the terms in context.

Replacement: describes killing an individual (for example a newborn infant or fetus) or allowing them to die, so that a different individual can be brought into existence (Singer 1993: 185; McMahan 2002: 351). A critical feature is that the replacement child would not otherwise have been born.

Substitution: describes a related but different choice; it is the decision to bring one child into existence rather than another child (where neither already exists). Substitution thus relates to decisions about the timing of conception, or potentially to decisions about embryo implantation.

Causing an Individual to Exist: refers to the more usual decision, where bringing an individual into existence is not dependent on the death of an existing individual, nor does it prevent the coming into existence of another individual. I will use this phrase (or sometimes just 'Conception' for short) to refer to the standard decisions that parents make to have a child.

Well-Being: how well or how badly a life goes. This will include the amount of happiness or unhappiness in an individual's life, but it might also include whether or not the individual achieves desires or preferences, or might include the attainment of other goods such as friendship, knowledge, love, etc. There are various different philosophical theories about well-being (Parfit 1984: 493–502; Griffin 1986: 7–76), and we do not need to choose between them for present purposes.

The other term that we have referred to in the previous chapters is this one:

Life Worth Living (LWL): a life that contains or will contain overall more intrinsically good experiences than intrinsically bad ones (Broome 2004: 66–8). It is equivalent to a condition where the benefits outweigh the burdens using the balance sheet approach described in Chapter 2. A subjective measure of whether a life is worth living is whether the individual whose life it is prefers for his or her own sake to continue to live rather than to die.

In this chapter we will focus on cases of *moderate* impairment, for example, infants like Christine with hemiplegic or diplegic cerebral palsy, who require aids or assistance to walk, or infants with a predicted IQ in the range of 35–50, able to communicate and interact socially to at least some degree. Some of the conditions that have been cited as justifying replacement include Down syndrome (also known as trisomy 21) or haemophilia. The reason for focusing on impairments of this sort is that for more severe impairments we may have concern about whether life is worth living; whether, for their own sake, infants or children should be allowed to die. The distinctive feature of the replacement argument, however, is that it would potentially justify allowing to die or even killing infants who are predicted to have lives worth living (Singer 1993: 185; McMahan 2002: 345).

The Non-Identity Problem and the Argument for Replacement

The starting point for many discussions of replacement is via an analogy with *substitution*. A typical example is what we might call the *Teratogen Case*. A mother has a temporary condition that is likely to lead to moderate impairment in her child if she conceives now. For example, she might have been prescribed medication for epilepsy that is associated with birth defects. When mothers are taking these drugs they are usually advised to use contraceptives. If they decide that they would like to have a child there will often be an attempt to change the medication to one that is less likely to cause birth defects. If she hasn't had seizures for some time, there may be an attempt to try a period without anticonvulsants. In such a case we generally think that it would be a good thing for the mother to wait before trying to conceive. More than that, many believe that it would be *wrong* for the mother to fail to wait, knowing that in only a few months' (say six months) time there would be a much lower chance of birth defects. On the other hand, if we knew that it would not be possible for the mother to be weaned off her medication safely, the risk and severity of problems in the child are not so great that she should be prevented from conceiving at all.

But, as famously highlighted by philosopher Derek Parfit, such thoughts cannot be based upon the interests of the child that she conceives, nor on a conventional notion of harm. One of the usual ways of understanding what it means to be harmed is that we compare two different possible states. Someone is harmed if they are worse off after an event than they would have been if the event had not occurred (Feinberg 1986). (I am harmed if you steal my wallet, because I would otherwise have enough money to pay for dinner, and wouldn't have to cancel my credit cards.) But, crucially, the child that the mother would conceive now is *different* from the child she would conceive in six months time. It would be a different combination of sperm and egg. Assuming that she has a life worth living, the impaired child who is conceived now cannot complain about her mother's impatience. She has not been harmed by the mother's choice, since she would not otherwise exist. In fact, she should probably be grateful to the mother for not waiting to conceive—since she owes her existence to that decision.

Parfit described this situation as a *non-identity* problem; it arises from decisions that affect the identity of individuals who are yet to be conceived. The striking feature of such cases is that they take away a central feature of most morally significant choices. If someone is harmed and made worse off by a decision, that gives us a strong reason to avoid it. But on the other hand, if there is no one who is harmed by a choice, why shouldn't we do it? In Parfit's book *Reasons and Persons* he provides a number of examples of the non-identity problem (Parfit 1984). There are cases like the teratogenic medication cited above. Another example (adapted from Parfit) is of a medical programme that could potentially prevent birth defects. Imagine that we had a choice between two hypothetical programmes that would prevent congenital rubella (a virus infection during pregnancy that causes, among other features, deafness, intellectual impairment, and heart defects). Programme A would screen women who were planning to conceive, identify those women who were not immune to rubella, instruct them to delay conception, and immunize them. Programme B would screen pregnant women, identify those who are not currently immune to rubella, and prevent them from acquiring the infection and transmitting it to their developing fetuses. (At present there isn't a vaccine for rubella that is accepted as safe during pregnancy, but let us imagine that we had one.) If the two programmes are equally effective, i.e. they would prevent the same number of cases of congenital rubella, which should we choose? We may intuitively feel inclined to think that they are equivalent, but Parfit highlights that Programme A is affected by the non-identity problem. Because it delays conception, the children who are born are different from the ones who would have been affected by congenital rubella. It seems to be a good thing to prevent congenital rubella, but our reason for doing so cannot be for the sake of affected children. If Programme A is adopted they will never be born. In contrast, if Programme B is adopted, some children who would otherwise have been affected by congenital rubella will be prevented from developing deafness, heart defects, etc.

When we think about such cases Parfit and other philosophers suggest that there are two different reasons that might motivate us. There are what we might call *individual-affecting* reasons to do something (McMahan 2009), when a course of action will affect existing or future individuals for better or for worse. We have an individual-affecting reason to adopt Programme B because that would prevent some existing, though unborn children from being born with congenital rubella. They would be better off if Programme B is funded, harmed if it is not. But, Parfit argues, we may also have reasons to act where individuals are not made either better or worse. These are *non-individual affecting* also sometimes called *impersonal* reasons (Parfit 1982). It is good to choose to undertake Programme A because it is good when people are happy, bad when they are in pain or unhappy. It is better that healthy children are born than children affected by congenital illness or impairment.

To return to the teratogen case, although there is not an individual-affecting reason for the mother to wait a few months before conceiving, there is an impersonal reason to do so. I know of no published survey data, but most people do seem to intuitively think that there is a moral reason for the mother to delay getting pregnant in the teratogen case. This appears to provide support for the significance of impersonal considerations, at least in substitution cases. But perhaps it also supports similar considerations for replacement? Another analogy is often drawn between substitution decisions and pre-natal testing and abortion. Many parents choose to terminate their pregnancy after diagnoses of conditions in the fetus that are moderately serious, but that are consistent with lives worth living. This might be at least partly on the basis of the thought that if this fetus dies another could be conceived who will not be disabled.

In his books *Practical Ethics* and (co-authored with Helga Kuhse) *Should the Baby Live?* Peter Singer defends the replacement of newborn infants with moderate impairments on the basis of just this sort of impersonal consideration. He argues that newborn infants lack *moral status*; they should be treated differently to older children or adults. But he also argues that we should give weight to impersonal reasons. It is morally important to increase the total amount of well-being in the world, either by increasing the well-being of those already in existence or by making sure that those who come into existence have as happy a life as possible (Singer 1993: 103, 184–206). According to Singer, the fact that another child that parents could conceive would have greater well-being than a current impaired child would justify allowing the current child to die and replacing them.

Arguments Against Replacement

At this point a number of objections may be raised.

Disability Isn't (So) Bad

One objection relates to the well-being of children with impairment compared to unimpaired children. After all, being healthy does not guarantee happiness, and there are plenty of children and adults with very significant impairments or illness who have happy and fulfilling lives. But the question is not about whether a child with hemiplegia or Down syndrome *could* have a happy life. It is about whether in general, or on average, such impairments affect how well a life could go. The disability paradox, mentioned in Chapter 1, may make us wonder whether some impairments are really as bad as they appear, or as we fear. But it would be a mistake to conclude that there is no downside at all to having such impairments. If we held this view there would be no reason either to prevent them or to treat them. However, the reason that it is important to fund medical Programme B is that even mild or moderate degrees of impairment or illness *are* bad things to happen. Imagine, in a different case, that Christine's cerebral palsy were due to a medical mishap. Would it be an adequate defence for the doctor to argue that many children and adults with hemiplegia are able to live happy lives, and therefore she hasn't been harmed by his mistake?

Moral Status

A second significant objection relates to the difference between substitution and replacement. Even if we accept that there is a reason in the Teratogen Case for a mother to delay childbearing, there is a difference between this decision, and a decision to terminate a pregnancy or to allow a newborn infant to die. There is no individual-affecting reason to conceive another child. But there *is* an individual-affecting reason not to terminate a pregnancy or to allow a newborn infant to die. The infant or fetus who dies in order to make way for the replacement child is harmed by such a choice. This harm gives rise to the most common objection to replacement of newborn infants, based on the moral status of the infant.

If infants like Christine do have moral status such that they may not be killed, that would undermine Singer's argument for infanticide on the basis of the acceptability of substitution or prenatal testing and abortion (Uniacke and McCloskey 1992; Uniacke 1997). We will return to look in more detail at the question of the moral status in the next chapter. But here, as in most of this book, we are focusing on cases that involve allowing infants to die. It is widely accepted that in certain circumstances it is permissible to withdraw life-sustaining treatment from newborn infants. So we need to know why infants' moral status means that replacement shouldn't be a reason in favour of letting infants die.

Absurd Conclusions

Other objections to replacement include the suggestion that if we accepted replacement arguments these would have absurd and patently unacceptable consequences (Calef 1992; Uniacke 1997). For example, some have asked why, if newborn infants are replaceable, older infants or children or adults are not replaceable? The answer to that question will depend on whether there are any significant differences between fetuses or infants and older children or adults, and returns to the moral status question. If there are differences, the absurd conclusions may not follow. But all of these arguments accept as a starting point Singer's claim that there is a moral reason that underpins replacement. In the rest of this chapter we will look at whether this claim stands up. In fact, when we pay attention to the impersonal reason to replace, and when we think about it in relation to other decisions that are made about future children, the argument seems thin indeed.

The Insubstantial-Reason Argument Against Replacement

American philosopher Jeff McMahan has analysed in detail Singer's argument for replacement in his book *The Ethics of Killing* (McMahan 2002: 345–62). The reasons that Singer gives to have a child with more well-being are impersonal. It is good to make happy children and adults. Yet, if we have an impersonal moral reason to maximize the well-being of people who do not yet exist, this would seem to imply that there is a moral reason to conceive. This is a striking suggestion. It conflicts with many people's beliefs about reproductive decisions. Most people do not think that there is a moral reason to conceive a child, nor that someone does wrong by using contraception or deciding not to have children at all.

The idea that certain versions of utilitarianism have counterintuitive implications for the morality of conception is not new (Hursthouse 1987: 143–4; Glover 1990: 69–70). Some, for example the philosopher Stuart Rachels, have tried to get around the problem by suggesting that although there is a moral reason to cause an individual to exist it is weak and easily outweighed by other factors. This would have less major implications for the morality of conception decisions (Rachels 1998). McMahan argues, however, that accepting such a compromise has implications for the argument for replacement. The minor reasons that are usually taken as sufficient to justify not having a child (for example personal preference for number of children, the need to buy a larger car, a desire to travel) would be enough to justify allowing an impaired newborn infant to die and replacing them. This seems untenable.

McMahan's line of reasoning can be turned around, though, to answer a different question. How *strong* is the moral reason to replace? The impersonal reasons to replace and to conceive are related. But when we compare these two types of decision with each other, the impersonal value of replacement appears to be *less* than that of conceiving a child (where the alternative is not to have a child). This is illustrated in Figure 3.1. Imagine two different versions of Christine's parents. In one version, Christine has been born, and they are weighing up whether she should be allowed to die. There will likely be greater well-being in the life of the next child than in Christine. In the second version Christine's parents decided not to conceive seven months ago, but are now wondering whether or not to have a child or to have no more children. (We can assume that a child that they would conceive now would be unlikely to have Christine's problems, and would have average levels of happiness and well-being.) As shown in the Figure, the difference in well-being in version one is less than in version two. In version one, it is the difference between an average child and Christine. In version two, it is the difference between an average child and no child. Consequently, there is a weaker reason to replace an impaired newborn infant than to conceive. If we accept the general view that there is at best only a weak moral reason to bring a child into the world, the reason to replace is slender indeed. We could call this the *insubstantial-reason argument* against replacement.

Since this can all appear quite abstract, an analogy may help. Imagine that I plant an apple tree in my front garden. After I plant it I discover that the root-stock of the tree that I have planted is not particularly healthy. Although it will produce apples it will produce fewer apples than average. The apples that it produces will be tasty, but there will not be a large crop. I know that if I dig up the tree and replace it with a new tree it is likely that I will have a significantly larger crop of apples. Should I replace the apple tree? The answer is that it depends how important it is to have the extra

Replacement

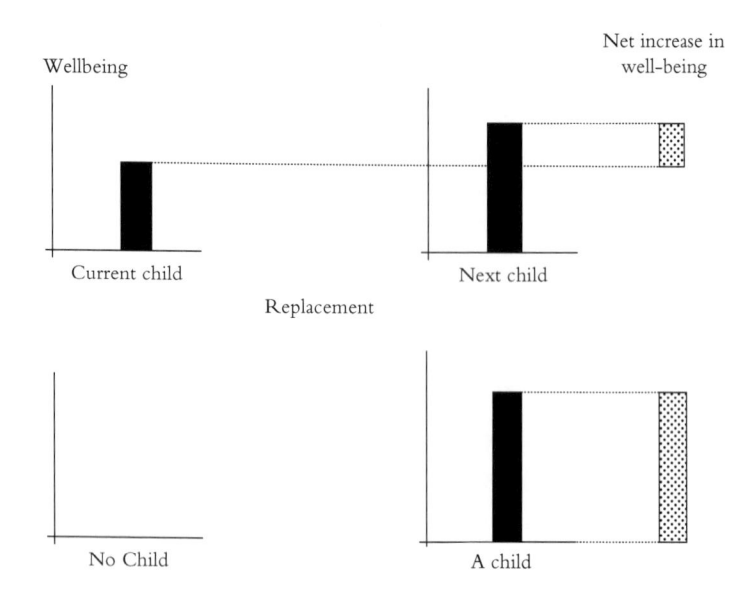

Wellbeing — Current child | Next child — Net increase in well-being

Causing an Individual to Exist

No Child | A child

Figure 3.1 Comparing a decision to replace with a decision to conceive

apples from a different tree. But, here the insubstantial-reason argument kicks in. If I do decide to replace the tree, the gain in apples will be less than the number of apples that I would have expected from planting a tree in the first place. The strength of the 'apple-reason' to replace the tree depends on how much it mattered to have a full crop of apples. If it was important to have a large number of apples (for example because they couldn't be bought elsewhere, or because I planned to sell them), then there might be a strong reason to replace the tree. But, like the situation facing a couple who might or might not decide to have a child, if there wasn't a strong reason to plant an apple tree in the first place (perhaps if I might easily have decided to plant a cherry tree or an ornamental tree or no tree), the reason to replace it must be even weaker.

To return to the question at hand: couples often decide not to have a child or not to have another child for a range of fairly minor reasons, for example the size of the family in which they were raised or the costs of raising a child, or perhaps that they already have one child of each gender. Are they doing something morally wrong by deciding not to bring another individual into existence? If we are convinced by Stuart Rachels' argument that factors like these are enough to justify not bringing a child into existence, then similar considerations (or weaker ones) would outweigh the impersonal reason to replace an infant such as Christine. There cannot be a strong impersonal reason for replacement.

At this point we might note one side-effect of the insubstantial-reason argument. Replacement and substitution decisions overlap in their dependence on impersonal reasons. But if the above argument reveals replacement to have weak foundations it may also undermine substitution; it may change our view about cases like the Teratogen Case. How strong is the reason to substitute? Contemplating decisions like that one, or decisions about genetic enhancement, Julian Savulescu has argued that where they have a choice there is a moral obligation for parents to bring into existence a child or children with the greatest predicted level of well-being. He refers to this obligation as the 'principle of procreative beneficence' (Savulescu 2001). This principle would explain why it would be wrong for parents to deliberately choose to implant an embryo predicted to have impairment or illness, when they have the choice of implanting an unaffected embryo. (For example, it would be wrong for parents to deliberately choose to implant an embryo with a gene for deafness.) It would also lead to the mother being obliged to wait to conceive in the Teratogen case.

On the basis of an argument that should now be familiar, however, there is less reason to substitute than there is to conceive a child. The types of reasons that would justify a couple choosing to limit family size or not to have children would also justify a decision to conceive a child with less than the best possible well-being. The mother taking teratogenic medication would relatively easily be able to justify a decision to conceive a child with moderate impairment rather than waiting and having a subsequent unimpaired child. Perhaps she doesn't want to wait, and is keen for a child now? On the other hand, we may not reach exactly the same conclusions about substitution and replacement decisions. One difference between substitution and replacement, is that there is often much less reason *not* to substitute. The insubstantial-reason argument does not mean that there is *no* obligation on parents to consider the well-being of the children that they could bring into existence, just that the prima facie reason is relatively weak. (A 'prima facie' reason is one factor among others to be weighed or taken into consideration; overall it may be outweighed by other duties or reasons.)

For parents who are already undergoing *in vitro* fertilization and who are choosing one embryo over another to implant there may be little or no moral reason not to follow the principle of procreative beneficence and choose the embryo with the best chances of happiness and health. In comparison, replacement decisions involve the death of the current fetus, newborn, or child. There may be considerable moral reasons pulling us in the opposite direction, towards keeping the infant alive.

The Next Child in the Queue

In his writings about replacement, philosopher R.M. Hare does not refer to impersonal reasons. He makes the argument vivid by imagining what he calls 'the next child in the queue', the child who would be conceived if the current infant dies. In a specific example, Hare compares the prospects for a fetus who will have a severe impairment if he is born (for example spina bifida), and the prospects for a possible child 'Andrew'. He imagines Andrew and his unnamed brother debating the relative merits of their lives in an imaginary other world, and weighing up which has the greater chance of a happy life (Hare 2006).

Both Hare and Singer refer to the interests of possible children:

I shall be arguing... that, where we have a choice between bringing someone into existence and not doing so, the interests of that possible person have to be considered. (Hare 1998: 279)

Putting the choice in these terms [of the conflict between the interests of the child and the family] overlooks someone, or a possible someone whose interests have been altogether neglected... The fetus and Andrew try to find a solution on the basis of equal consideration of both their interests in having a happy existence. (Kuhse and Singer 1985: 158)

Here, however, we must notice the other important interest... that of the next child in the queue. (Hare 2006: 331)

They also refer to the harm done to the possible child if they are not brought into existence; for example, in another article Hare notes:

But if it would have been a good for him to exist (because this made possible the goods that, once he existed, he was able to enjoy), surely it was a harm to him not to exist, and so not to be able to enjoy these goods. (Hare 1975: 221)

Some parents may think about future possible children in such concrete terms, perhaps even naming them in the way that Hare does. Peggy Stinson worried about her future child 'Jonathan' who was being prevented from existing by doctors who insisted that treatment continue for Stinson's sick premature infant. But does it make sense to talk about the interests of such children, or of them being harmed by decisions that lead to them not existing?

One reason that such thoughts lose coherence is that there is no single child who would be conceived if the current infant dies. There is no Andrew or Jonathan waiting in the wings for their chance. Rather there are a whole host of possible children, different combinations of sperms and eggs that could potentially be conceived. Should we worry about the interests of the innumerable possible individuals who could be brought into existence (but of whom the vast majority will never exist)?

Nor does it make any sense to talk about harming the interests of these possible children. If they are not brought into existence there is no entity, no individual who is harmed. We might think that Andrew or Jonathan would benefit if they are conceived. But, as noted above, the most plausible concept of harming someone involves the idea that they are worse off than they would otherwise have been. And Andrew or Jonathan cannot be worse off if they are not conceived; they cannot be anything since they do not and will not exist.

People sometimes think that it is worse to have something taken away from you than to be denied it. There is an apparent asymmetry between harms and benefits. Harms count for more. Some philosophers, and some philosophical outlooks, challenge this difference and suggest that this is partly or wholly illusory. If it is good for you to have $100, it is just as bad for someone to take $100 from you as it is for them to fail to give you $100 that you should rightly receive. However, even if we accept this argument there seems to be something special about the harm or benefit of coming into existence. If we conceive a child there is someone that we can identify who receives that benefit. But if we decide, for whatever reason, not to conceive them, they cannot be harmed—there is no 'they' at all.

Against the Insubstantial-Reason Argument

Having argued that replacement does not provide a strong argument in favour of allowing a newborn infant to die it will be worth considering the other side of the coin. There are a number of possible responses to the insubstantial-reason argument. Someone who wished to defend replacement may dispute one of the key components in the above argument. Perhaps they disagree with the general intuition and hold that there *is* a strong moral reason to bring a child into the world. If that were the case there would also potentially be a strong moral reason to replace (albeit less strong than the reason to conceive). However, although this is a possible response to the argument, it has some fairly unattractive implications for the morality of population policy, contraception, and abortion. One implication is that we may all be obliged to have as many children as we possibly can. It would be wrong for mothers to have an abortion, unless they plan to subsequently become pregnant again (Calef 1992). Many of our decisions about having children would be indefensible. I suspect that few would be willing to accept these implications.

Alternatively, the insubstantial-reason argument might be seen as a variation on a frequent criticism of certain moral theories (particularly utilitarianism) that they are too demanding (Williams 1973). There are many moral obligations that conflict with personal projects or common-sense morality, and this conflict does not in itself render implausible the idea of a strong moral reason to conceive. (It just makes it unattractive. As another example, a number of philosophers, including Peter Singer, have argued that those who are well-off in developed countries have an obligation to donate a significant proportion of their income to the poorest and most disadvantaged in the world. This makes many uncomfortable because it requires a degree of personal sacrifice from all of us in the West.) Nevertheless, the relationship between conception and replacement means that there is *more* reason on impersonal grounds to conceive additional children, than there is to replace. There is a stronger impersonal reason to advocate increased reproduction, and oppose contraception and abortion, than there is to advocate replacement of impaired newborn infants. That seems hard to accept.

STARTING AGAIN 97

Another objection arises from a common response to the suggestion that there is a moral reason to reproduce. Although bringing someone into existence who will have a life worth living is in principle a very good thing to do (there is a strong prima facie reason to conceive), there are other factors to consider, for example the resource and environmental costs of adding to the population. In fact there are multiple individual-affecting factors that weigh against the impersonal value of bringing someone into existence. In an overpopulated world with finite resources, once we take everything into account, there is not a strong moral reason to conceive (Glover 1990: 70; Rachels 1998). How does this affect replacement decisions? The insubstantial-reason argument would still apply; if the overall (taking everything into account) reason to conceive a child is not strong, there is an even weaker overall reason to replace (see Figure 3.2).

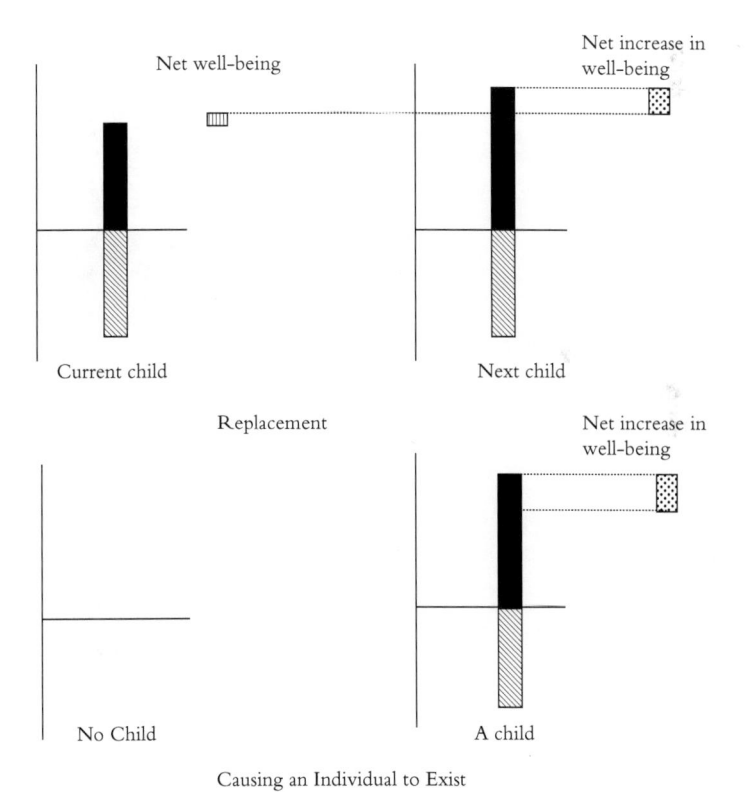

Figure 3.2 Comparing a decision to replace with a decision to conceive (all things considered)

One point to note is that the costs are not necessarily equal. There may be greater costs to Christine's family and to society if she lives than would be occasioned by a child without impairment. But unless those costs outweigh the impersonal value of bringing Christine into existence, there will still be greater reasons to conceive than to replace. In general we do not think that the costs of looking after a child with moderate cerebral palsy or haemophilia outweigh the value of that child's life. On the other hand, if the costs of keeping the current child alive *do* outweigh the impersonal value there would already be a decisive reason to let that infant die. There would be no need to justify the decision by invoking the well-being in another possible child.

Some philosophers have argued that coming into existence is always a harm (Benatar 2006: 18–57). Alternatively it might be argued that the costs of bringing even a healthy child into the world outweigh the impersonal value of their existence. If such views were true, then it would be better to replace than to conceive a child with average well-being. However, it would be better again not to have any children, or to let the current child die without having another child. There would be more reason to do so to replace them. Thus, this view does not provide a compelling argument for replacement in newborn intensive care.

Separating Replacement and Conception

In the insubstantial-reason argument we have compared replacement with decisions to cause an individual to exist. Some people would question this. It might be thought that the question of *which* child to conceive could be separated from the question of *whether* to conceive (McMahan 2002: 355). For example, some may believe that if parents are going to have a child it would be better for a healthy child to exist rather than a child with impairment like Christine's, but deny that this entails a moral obligation to bring children into the world. How would this be justified?

One reason to separate these judgements is on the basis of another distinction drawn by Derek Parfit. In substitution cases the same number of individuals exist in either option (they are what Parfit refers to as 'Same Number Cases'), while cases of causing an individual to exist involves adding an extra individual (it is a 'Different Number Case'). Different

Number cases raise perplexing questions for population policy that are hard to solve (Parfit 1984: 381–441). For example, if we think that it is good to increase the amount of well-being in the world, we could do so by having a world population that is extremely high. Even if everyone in this extremely crowded world had lives that were much worse than ours are now, the overall amount of happiness or well-being would be high. It would potentially be better to have a world containing a trillion people living lives that are only just worth living, than to have a world population that is much smaller with people living extremely contented lives. This surprising and highly counterintuitive result was coined by Parfit 'The Repugnant Conclusion'. Because impersonal reasons yield such unattractive conclusions in Different Number cases we might think that we should only take account of them in Same Number cases like the Medical Programme?

But there are problems with this line of argument. Replacement is also a Different Number case, so impersonal reasons would potentially not apply to it either. Although the same number of individuals exist after replacement as before, the total number of individuals who ever exist is different. In any case it seems ad hoc to apply impersonal considerations to one type of case but not the other. If it is morally important to increase overall well-being when that will not benefit any existing or future individual, it does not seem relevant whether that increase occurs by causing an additional individual to exist.

If the justification of replacement is impersonal, it must be related to decisions about conception. Once this relationship is clear, the reason to replace becomes weak and easily outweighed. But could the reasons in favour of replacement be *individual-affecting* rather than impersonal?

There are two ways in which replacement could provide a benefit to individuals. Firstly it might be thought that the benefit is to the replacement child. The idea of someone benefiting from being brought into existence is controversial (though we often think that individuals can be harmed by being brought into existence if they have a life that is not worth living). In this case the idea would be that both the current child and the replacement child benefit from their life—but since there is greater well-being in the life of the next child, that child will benefit more. Hare seemed to have something like this in mind when he wrote of the next child having a greater interest in coming into existence than the current child by virtue of the better life in store (Hare 2006). However, we should note that this isn't a comparative benefit—the child who comes into existence isn't better off than they would have been, since they would not otherwise have existed. So it isn't really 'individual-affecting', in the way that we described this above. In any case, if the benefit to the child of their future life is a relevant moral consideration in decisions about replacement or substitution, the same sort of benefit would apply to conception decisions. Any child with a life worth living that we bring into the world would benefit from being conceived. Once again, there would be a stronger reason to conceive a child than to replace.

The second potential way that replacement could benefit individuals would be its effect on *other* people who exist or who will exist, for example Christine's parents, other siblings, and other members of society. We could call this an *indirect* individual-affecting reason, since it does not relate to the individual whose existence will be affected by our decision. Parents' lives, and those of their other children, may go better if they have a healthy child rather than one with impairment. And it may be better for others in society who do not have to share the financial costs of Christine's treatment.

If replacement is justified in this way, indirectly, then the link between replacement decisions and conception breaks down. Although it is highly likely to be better for parents to have a healthy child rather than a child with impairment, it would not necessarily be better for them to have a healthy child than none at all. When parents conceive a healthy child, we may be unsure whether the effect of this on others will be positive or negative. The lives of parents may go better if they have a child, or they may go worse. Siblings may benefit from companionship, or they may suffer from competition. Others in society may benefit from the contributions of that child in the future, or may have to bear the costs of supporting them (if they are sick or unemployed, for example).

To return to the apple tree analogy, this would be like digging up the current tree not on the basis of the abstract benefit of the number of apples—but rather because I have a preference for more apples over fewer apples. I may not care particularly whether I have an apple tree or a cherry tree, but I may have a strong preference that if I do have an apple tree that it is heavily laden with fruit.

Reframed in this way, in the benefit or harm to others, both replacement and substitution have a much stronger basis. The principle of procreative beneficence would be supported by the effect on families and on others of conceiving a healthy child rather than one with impairment or illness. There would be a more tangible way of defending the intuition that the mother in the Teratogen Case should wait to conceive, and that parents should choose to implant a healthy embryo. It perhaps also helps to make sense about some judgements that take place when replacement *cannot* take place. Some infants in newborn intensive care are born to parents who have had considerable difficulty conceiving—they may have had multiple attempts at *in vitro* fertilization, with very little chance of being able to conceive another child. Or perhaps the mother has had a major complication of childbirth and had to have a hysterectomy. In such cases the child may be particularly precious to the parents, and there may be a greater reluctance to consider withdrawing treatment. It is the significance of the child *for the parents* given the lack of future children that makes the infant's survival particularly important.

But there are several points to note about this reconfigured argument for replacement.

Firstly, the way that some philosophers have referred to replacement has been to suggest that it provides a separate or additional reason to allow an infant to die. Thus R.M. Hare wrote

[T]here is the interest of the mother... [t]he other members of the family have a similar interest... [t]hen there are the interests which belong to those outside the family... and lastly there is another interest which is commonly ignored in these discussions, and which is so important that it often, I think, ought to tip the balance... that of the next child in the queue. (Hare 2006: 330)

But if replacement is primarily justified because it will be better for parents, family, and/or society, then in one sense it disappears as a separate factor in decisions about letting a newborn infant die. Doctors and parents already think about the interests of the child, the interests of the family, and perhaps the interests of others. Replacement is not an extra reason, though it may explain *how* the interests of others would be affected positively if the infant were allowed to die.

In addition, there is a generally accepted argument that the costs or benefits to society of a child's existence are not factors that should be considered when we are making decisions about life-sustaining treatment (Nuffield Council on Bioethics 2006: 21, 45). This is not to say that potential costs should have no role in decisions about newborn intensive care. Such costs might be relevantly considered by policy-makers (Wilkinson 2011). However, the costs of future treatment (or by extension the benefits to society) are not thought to be factors that should have any role in decisions about life-sustaining treatment in individual patients in intensive care. So the relevant reason for replacement comes down to the benefit to parents and siblings of having a different child instead of the current newborn.

Finally, we might note that this way of thinking about replacement is a different sort of justification than the one traditionally given. It is not about the abstract value of bringing happy people into existence. It is about the interests of parents and other family members. Whether it provides a decisive reason to let a newborn infant die will depend upon the reasons that we have not to let them die, and how the interests of parents and family should be weighed against those of the infant.

Conclusion

The question that we started with was this: if the Carmentis machine predicted a newborn infant or child to have mild or moderate levels of impairment would replacement justify the withdrawal of life-sustaining treatment? What difference would it make if the parents were able to have another child?

'Not much difference' is the answer if the reason to replace the infant is impersonal. The insubstantial-reason argument suggests that in impersonal terms the reasons to replace a newborn infant are weaker than the reasons to bring a child into existence. If we accept that there is a strong moral reason to conceive, there would remain a strong justification for replacement, but this has unpalatable implications. On the other hand if we believe that there is not a strong moral reason to conceive, then there is an even weaker impersonal reason to replace.

Alternatively, if the benefit of replacement were understood in individual-affecting terms, the answer would turn on the interests of others, and on the effect on other individuals' lives (principally parents and other siblings) if a healthy rather than an impaired child lives.

What does this mean for Christine, the premature infant with hemiplegia? Replacement would be relevant for our response to the results of the

Carmentis machine if her parents' lives would be better off with a different, unimpaired child. But their lives would also potentially go worse because of the loss of Christine. Most parents of critically ill infants are strongly emotionally connected to their child and experience a profound loss if the infant dies. In practice in newborn intensive care it is often difficult to persuade parents to let go and allow treatment to be withdrawn even when it appears to doctors highly unlikely that the infant will survive, or likely that if they do, they will have overwhelming impairment and illness. It does not seem likely that for many parents the potential improvement in their future life will outweigh the negatives of losing a loved and anticipated child. But what if the parents did want to allow Christine to die and to try again at conceiving? Would then replacement justify withdrawing treatment? It depends on how much weight we place on the impact of her survival (compared to an unimpaired child) on parents and other family members.

Investigating the idea of the replaceability of newborn infants has led into difficult waters, and to questions that can seem distant from the practical questions facing doctors and parents in intensive care. Discussion of impersonal and individual-affecting reasons and of the benefit or lack of benefit of conception may appear abstract and of questionable relevance to practice. Ultimately, however, we have seen that replacement turns on something familiar and more tangible, namely the relative weight that we give to the interests of the child and to the interests of parents.

This chapter has focused on newborn infants, since it is here, if anywhere, that the question of replacement appears to be significant. But should we treat newborn infants differently from older children? Should we give greater weight to the interests of parents in newborn intensive care than in paediatric intensive care? What are the relative interests at stake for the infant and for parents? That is where we will turn next.

References

Benatar, D. (2006). *Better Never to Have Been: The Harm of Coming into Existence*. Oxford: Clarendon.

Broome, J. (2004). *Weighing Lives*. Oxford: Oxford University Press.

Calef, S.W. (1992). 'The replaceability argument and abortion', *American Catholic Philosophical Quarterly* 66(4): 447–63.

Feinberg, J. (1986). 'Wrongful life and the counterfactual element in harming', *Soc Philos Policy* 4(1): 145–78.
Glover, J. (1990). *Causing Death and Saving Lives*. Harmondsworth: Penguin.
Griffin, J. (1986). *Well-Being: Its Meaning, Measurement and Moral Importance*. Oxford: Clarendon.
Hare, R. (1975). 'Abortion and the golden rule', *Philosophy and Public Affairs* 43(3): 201–22.
—— (1998). 'Possible people', *Bioethics* 2(4): 279–93.
—— (2006). 'The abnormal child: moral dilemmas of doctors and parents', in H. Kuhse and P. Singer (eds), *Bioethics: An Anthology*. Oxford and Malden, Blackwell, 329–33.
Hursthouse, R. (1987). *Beginning Lives*. Oxford, Blackwell.
Kuhse, H. and P. Singer (1985). *Should the Baby Live? The Problem of Handicapped Infants*. Oxford: Oxford University Press.
McMahan, J. (2002). *The Ethics of Killing: Problems at the Margins of Life*. New York: Oxford University Press.
—— (2009). 'Asymmetries in the morality of causing people to exist', in M. Roberts and D. Wasserman (eds), *Harming Future Persons: Ethics, Genetics and the Nonidentity Problem*. New York: Springer, 49–70.
Miljeteig, I. and O. F. Norheim (2006). 'My job is to keep him alive, but what about his brother and sister? How Indian doctors experience ethical dilemmas in neonatal medicine', *Dev World Bioeth* 6(1): 23–32.
Nuffield Council on Bioethics (2006). *Critical Care Decisions in Fetal and Neonatal Medicine: Ethical Issues*. London: Nuffield Council on Bioethics.
Parfit, D. (1982). 'Future Generations: Further Problems', *Philosophy and Public Affairs* 11(2): 113–72.
—— (1984). *Reasons and Persons*. Oxford: Oxford University Press.
Rachels, S. (1998). 'Is it good to make happy people?', *Bioethics* 12(2): 93–110.
Savulescu, J. (2001). 'Procreative beneficence: why we should select the best children', *Bioethics* 15(5–6): 413–26.
Singer, P. (1993). *Practical Ethics*. Cambridge: Cambridge University Press.
Uniacke, S. (1997). 'Replaceability and infanticide', *The Journal of Value Inquiry* 31: 153–66.
—— and H. McCloskey (1992). 'Peter Singer and non-voluntary "euthanasia": tripping down the slippery slope', *Journal of Applied Philosophy* 9(2): 203–19.
Wilkinson, D. (2011). 'Should we replace disabled newborn infants?' *Journal of Moral Philosophy* 8(3): 390–414.
Williams, B. (1973). 'A critique of utilitarianism', in J.J.C. Smart and B. Williams (eds), *Utilitarianism: For and Against*. Cambridge: Cambridge University Press, 77–150.

Exposure and Infanticide in Ancient Rome

There is ample evidence from literature, legal comment and, letters of the ancient Greek practice of 'exposing' unwanted newborn infants. The image of parents leaving their infants to die from dehydration or from the attack of wild animals is horrifying, and not all members of Roman society supported it. The early Christian writer Tertullian attacked the Romans for the cruelty of their treatment of children: 'you expose them to the cold and hunger, and to wild beasts, or else you get rid of them by the slower death of drowning' (Tertullian 1869, Ad Nationes Book 1, Ch. 15). But although it is clear that exposure of Roman infants sometimes took place, it is far from clear how often it took place, or what became of those infants who were exposed.

The English word 'exposure' conjures up both a sense of being subject to the elements (both extreme heat and cold would be perilous for newborn infants) as well as being vulnerable to danger. However, this may not have been the usual sense or implication of 'exposure' for Romans. The word 'expositio' in Latin, and its Greek equivalent, connoted instead a sense of 'offering up' or 'putting out'—perhaps closer to the modern word 'exposition' (Boswell 1984). There were places in Rome that were apparently well-known locations for leaving unwanted infants (much in the same way as there were foundling asylums with rotating doors in the Middle Ages). At least a proportion of those infants who were abandoned were adopted by childless families or saved to be raised as slaves or prostitutes (Westermann

1955: 86; Harris 1994). (This provided a second target for criticism on the part of early Christian writers. Tertullian noted that 'when you expose your infants to the mercy of others, or leave them for adoption to better parents than yourselves, do you forget what an opportunity for incest is furnished' (Tertullian 1869).) Most exposed infants were apparently clothed, and in some cases families left them with tokens or amulets that might allow them to be recognized or reclaimed later in life (Harris 1994). Stories of abandoned and adopted children later discovering their true identity filled numerous plays and myths, and there was a vigorous legal debate about the status of reclaimed children. In one notable literary instance of exposure, in Plautus' play *Cistellaria* (written about 200 BC) a servant abandons a newborn infant, conceived after a rape. American historian John Boswell noted that the mother's servant waits around the corner after abandoning the infant to see, not whether the infant would be rescued, but *who* would rescue the infant (Boswell 1984).

Some, but not all exposed infants died. How often did exposure happen? Two millenia after the fact it is impossible to know. There is some archaeological evidence; for example ninety-seven infant skeletons were found amongst Roman ruins at Hambleden in Buckinghamshire in the UK. It has been suggested that this is evidence of infanticide or exposure, perhaps at a brothel. However, such burial sites might be explained by the Roman practice of burying rather than cremating infants (Harris 1994; Scott 1999). Other historians have tried to argue that a high incidence of exposure or infanticide would contradict evidence of the stability of Roman population. However, there is so much uncertainty around the demographics of Rome and the different factors that could influence both live birth and death rates that it is impossible to reach any useful estimate (Harris 1994).

There were several reasons that might motivate Roman parents to abandon their children, including poverty, deformity, illegitimacy, and gender. Both abortion and contraception were available to Roman women, albeit considerably less reliable and more risky than today. One reason why Roman parents may have preferred exposure to contraception or abortion was because of the ability to choose the sex of their offspring (Harris 1994).

In contrast, infanticide appears much less often in Roman sources. Tertullian, writing around 200 AD, suggests that it was 'forbidden by the laws to slay new-born infants', though he goes on to claim that 'no laws are evaded with more impunity or greater safety' (Tertullian 1869, Ch. 15). If there was a legal distinction between infanticide and exposure that may, in part, explain why exposure appears to have occurred more frequently than the killing of infants. The other possible reason is that parents preferred to abandon their infants because of the possibility (as in Plautus' play) that the infant would be rescued. The Jewish writer Philo of Alexandria suggests as much: 'Others, again, carry them out into a desert place to expose them there, as they themselves say, in the hope that they may be saved by some one' (Philo, in Yonge 1855: 331). However, Philo, and later Christian writers such as the Roman jurist Paulus argued that exposure of infants were also acts of killing—and potentially more cruel to the infants concerned:

> Not only does a person who suffocates a child ... appear to kill, but also both a person who throws one away, a person who denies one nourishment, and the person who exposes one in a public place. (Paulus, quoted in Harris 1994: 11)

References

Boswell, J. (1984). 'Expositio and oblatio: the abandonment of children and the ancient and modern family', *The American Historical Review* 89(1): 10–33.

Harris, W.V. (1994). 'Child-Exposure in the Roman Empire', *Journal of Roman Studies* 84: 1–22.

Scott, E. (1999). 'The archaeology of infancy and infant death'. British Archaeological Reports. Oxford: Archaeopress.

Tertullian (1869). *The Writings of Tertullian*. Edinburgh: T & T Clark.

Westermann, W. (1955). *The Slave Systems of Greek and Roman Antiquity*. Philadelphia: American Philosophical Society.

Yonge, BA. (1855). *The Works of Philo Judaeus, the contemporary of Josephus*, translated from the Greek. *On Special Laws*, London: HG Bohn.

4

Competing Interests

In Chapter 2 we looked at the concept of the child's best interests as a way to decide what to do with predictions from the Carmentis machine. We saw that this principle fails to provide a clear answer in difficult cases. In the conclusion to that chapter I suggested a second problem with basing our decisions purely on the best interests of the infant—it appears to leave parents with no role in decisions about treatment. If we have decided that it is in the best interests of a child or infant for treatment to be provided or not provided there is nothing for parents to do or say except to go along with this. The best interests test gives no weight to the interests of parents or other family members.

Then, in Chapter 3, we looked at a different factor that might be relevant for treatment decisions based on the Carmentis machine—the interests or value of another child or other children who might be conceived if a current child dies. We saw that the significance of replacement lies largely in its effect on the interests of parents or other family members. If we were to take replacement seriously for decisions in newborn intensive care, this would require us to place a considerable weight on the interests of parents in decisions.

Both of these extremes seem to be the wrong answer. The crucial question is *how much weight* parents' interests should be given relative to the interests of the child? This chapter will focus on that central question for decision-making in paediatric and neonatal intensive care. There are two elements. We will look first at what is at stake for families, the nature of their interests, and the ways in which they are taken into account in treatment decisions. Then we will look at the interests of infants or children, and, in particular, at whether there is any difference between the interests of a newborn infant and those of an older child. That will determine whether decisions should be made in the same way, and on the same basis in newborn intensive care as in paediatric intensive care. As in previous chapters we will focus on decision-making in the face of certain prognosis, and the significance of these different interests for the Carmentis machine. Later, in Chapter 7, we will look at the interplay between uncertainty and the interests of parents, family, or the child interests.

Interests, Well-Being, and Moral Status

In ethics there is a lot of talk about 'interests'. But what does this term mean, and why is it important? In everyday language we use the word to refer to activities, hobbies, pastimes, areas of special knowledge or attention. It implies that I *take* an interest in that thing, I devote some time or energy or attention to it. However, the term 'interests' for philosophers is much broader. We *have* an interest in something if we stand to gain or lose depending on its nature or condition. Put more simply, we have an interest in something when we can be benefited or harmed by it.

When we think of it this way, having an interest is quite different from taking an interest. There are plenty of things that may benefit or harm me, but which I spend little or no time thinking about or actively caring about (for example, the sewerage system in my city). The opposite may also be true, at least to some degree. There are some things, perhaps the result of a sporting contest, or the fate of a character in a television drama, in which I take an interest, but which are neither in nor contrary to my interests (at least not in any important way).

Why do interests matter? They matter because, ultimately, much of ethics boils down to benefits and harms. If something is in an individual's interest it provides us with a reason to realize it or protect it. An individual's interests together contribute to their well-being—how well or badly their life overall is going. There are other ways of talking about ethics. For example we might ask what the rights of parents or the child are, or talk about the relevant duties or obligations, we might enquire about the attitudes or character of a good parent or doctor. But there is some reason to think that interests are primary; interests provide a fundamental starting point for analysis.

It is worth, briefly, mentioning a long-standing philosophical debate. Philosophers have argued for centuries about what it is that makes for a good life, and what, therefore, counts as benefiting or harming an individual. One way of dividing up existing theories about well-being is into three camps (Parfit 1984: 493–502; Griffin 1986: 7–74; DeGrazia 1995). In the first camp (hedonism) is the idea that interests are fundamentally based on pleasure and on pain. Hedonism is sometimes crudely caricatured as prescribing a selfish or slavish devotion to physical pleasure. However, there are sophisticated and subtle defenders of hedonism (Crisp 2006). The basic principle behind it is appealing—that things are important to us because and to the degree that they make us feel happiness or pleasure. There are of course other things that we value. However, ultimately (or so the hedonist claims), we value them because they make us feel good. A second group of well-being theories, sometimes referred to as desire or preference theories, holds that what makes our lives go well is to have our desires fulfilled. (Since we usually desire things that make us experience pleasure, and desire not to experience pain, desire theories will give similar answers to hedonism in many settings.) Desire theories have the advantage that certain things may appear to be good for us even if we do not experience them. For example, there is a common feeling that it would be bad for someone if their partner were unfaithful and lying to them, even if they never found out about this. A desire-based theory would capture this interest because most people prefer that their partners are faithful and truthful. The third group of theories of well-being are sometimes referred to as 'objective list' theories, and constitute a list of features of a life that could make it go well or badly irrespective of whether or not they are either perceived or preferred. For example, knowledge or friendship might count as constitutive of a good life, perhaps even if they do not lead to pleasure, or are not actively desired. Such lists are 'objective' because they point to something more than just the experience or preferences of the individual. However, they overlap with desire theories and hedonism, since experiencing pleasure and achieving desires are likely to be on any plausible list of objective values.

Interests are central to another philosophical concept, that of moral status (DeGrazia 2008). When we claim that some entity has moral status, what we mean is that they are worthy of moral consideration. It matters morally (for their sake) how we treat them. For example, there is debate about whether non-human animals have moral status. Does a mouse have moral status? We can rephrase this question as being about whether it matters how we treat a mouse. Is it wrong to cause a mouse pain? At least part of the answer is given by whether or not a mouse has interests. If a mouse can be benefited or harmed (by experiencing or not experiencing pain) that would ground a claim that a mouse has moral status. Conversely, if an entity (a rock for example) has no interests, it cannot have moral status. But there is a second question, the 'status' part of moral status, about how much it matters, and about whether it matters equally how we treat different entities. For example, does it matter equally whether we cause pain to a mouse or to a child?

There are two ways in which moral status could differ between different individuals. We could give their interests equal weight, but the interests themselves may be of different strength (we could refer to this as unequal strength of interests) (DeGrazia 2008). Alternatively two individuals could have similar interests, but they could differ in how much weight we give to their interests (unequal degrees of moral consideration). As another example, doctors in emergency departments often have to decide which patients are going to be treated first. If two patients arrive at the same time, but one is sicker, more in need of urgent attention, we think that it is justifiable for the sicker patient to be treated first. They have a stronger interest in receiving medical attention because they are in more pain, or at higher risk of dying if not treated immediately. It is not morally equivalent whether the doctor treats the sicker or the less sick patient first, but the reason for doing so is not because they are accorded a different level of consideration, rather it is because of unequal interests. But imagine a second example in which two individuals are injured in a car accident and are in equal amounts of pain with a non-life-threatening injury. However, one of the individuals is a child and one is a dog. If we decide to treat the child first it is not because the child's interest in having their pain alleviated is greater than the dog's. Instead we are judging that the child's interest matters more morally. There are a variety of ways in which we might justify such a preference, but if we do give greater weight to the child's interests than the dog's interests it implies unequal moral consideration between the child and dog.

In the discussion below we will be looking at the first type of moral difference, at the ways in which the interests of families may vary between different families and between different countries, at the ways in which the interests of a newborn or a child may vary, and at the ways in which interests may be affected by impairment. Where these interests vary in strength, this may justify different treatment decisions. But none of this discussion will be about different degrees of moral consideration.

Case RB

In late 2009 the UK Family court heard the sad case of RB. RB was a thirteen-month-old infant with an extremely rare disorder (congenital myasthenic syndrome, CMS) rendering him quadriplegic and permanently dependent on a ventilator to breathe. CMS is caused by a genetic problem in the connection between nerves and muscles. Although the nerves work, and the brain works, the signal between the two cannot get through. Severe forms of this problem affect infants from before birth, meaning that they develop joint contractures (their joints cannot move freely) from lack of movement and compression in the womb, and the infants require resuscitation and artificial ventilation as soon as they are born.

RB had been a patient in the intensive care unit since birth. He was not believed to have any cognitive impairment, but was unable to move his limbs, communicate, or even interact with those around him. He often would not open his eyes, though at other times would look around and watch things happening around him. He was described sometimes as wriggling with pleasure, and was able to move his hands enough to hold a drumstick. Although some forms of CMS respond to treatment, experimental treatments had failed to improve RB's condition. Long-term survival would be possible with a surgical tracheostomy and home ventilation treatment. However, RB's mother and doctors had come to the conclusion that it would not be in his interests to have this treatment; that, in fact, it would be best for him if his breathing support were to be withdrawn and he were allowed to die. The case came to court because RB's parents disagreed. His father believed that RB should have a tracheostomy performed and that life support should continue. Some doctors gave evidence that ongoing treatment would be in RB's interests. After several days of the court hearing, RB's father withdrew his objection to the medical treatment plan; RB was subsequently taken off the ventilator and died in his parents' arms.

The Interests of Families

What are the interests of families in decisions about life-sustaining treatment? In the real case of RB there was no Carmentis machine, but there was also no realistic doubt about his overall prognosis.

Cases of profound physical impairment like CMS or a similar condition known as 'spinal muscular atrophy' (SMA) raise questions about whether treatment is in the best interests of the child. But, in practice, if parents agree, the majority of infants with severe congenital neuromuscular disorders like CMS or SMA have life support withdrawn, usually within the first month or two of life after the diagnosis is able to be made with confidence.

The striking feature of RB's case was that his parents disagreed about whether treatment should continue. The reason that RB remained alive at 13 months of age was because, for a long time, both parents had opposed withdrawal of treatment. Had they both supported treatment withdrawal RB's case would never have come to the court and he would likely have died months earlier. If they had both wanted treatment to continue it is possible that it would have been provided. In some parts of the world there is increasing experience with providing long-term breathing support for infants with SMA or CMS (Sakakihara, Kubota et al., 2000; Bush, Fraser, et al. 2005). Whereas previously all such infants would have died, there are now a number of infants who survive into childhood, reflecting a willingness to contemplate providing long-term support (Geevasinga and Ryan 2007).

But why should parents have a say in such decisions? Why does it make a difference whether they support or oppose continued treatment? One possibility is that parents may help doctors to work out what is in the best interests of the child or infant, or perhaps they influence what would actually be best for the child. The two sets of interest may overlap. (We will return to this possibility in Chapter 7.) But the second possibility is that the interests of parents (and perhaps other family members) are also relevant to decisions about children and infants. The family's interests matter for our decisions.

How are parents affected by decisions in intensive care? There are benefits for many parents if an infant or child survives, even where the child's life is short or seriously compromised by impairment or illness. Some parents eloquently describe the ways in which their personal life, and those of other members of their family are enriched by the experience of caring for an impaired child (Yorgason 2003; Sheffield 2007; Wyn 2007). They may find fulfilment and purpose in their caring role; they may find that the challenges that the child faces put into perspective their own problems. Many parents also have a very strong desire that the child survive. This desire is perhaps sometimes stronger for parents who have had considerable difficulties conceiving, or who are unable or unlikely to be able to have further children. It is not that their love for their child is necessarily any greater, nor their grief at the child's death more profound. Rather, that if the child dies the parents may lose the possibility of being parents.

For cases like RB, the interests of parents, their fervent wish that the child does not die, and the significance of the child's survival for their own lives, is potentially a major reason why treatment is continued, though the normal course of events would be to allow the infant to die.

One Tattered Angel

In late 1988 writer Blaine Yorgason and his wife Kathy took over the foster care of a newborn infant with hydranencephaly. (Yorgason 2003) At the time they had six older children, and had fostered several other infants while an adoptive family was being found for them. However, there were no other families who wished to adopt Charity because of the severity of her underlying illness and her prognosis. The Yorgasons volunteered to care for Charity long-term, and adopted her into their family.

Hydranencephaly is a rare condition in which a very large part of the upper part of the brain, the cerebrum, is absent and replaced by fluid. The cause of the condition is not known, but it is suspected that it may be caused by a blockage to the blood supply to the brain while the fetus is developing. There may be small amounts of brain tissue remaining, but the main areas responsible for vision, hearing, and controlling movement are gone. In Charity's case her brain CT was described as showing 'severe brain loss in the supratentorial compartment. She has some occipital lobes bilaterally... She has essentially no visibly temporal, parietal or frontal brain.' The majority of affected infants die within a few weeks or months of birth; however, survival into late childhood (cAbee, Chan, et al. 2000) or even adulthood has been described (Bae, Jang, et al. 2008). Surviving children with hydranencephaly have been reported to be in a persistent vegetative state; some have been described responding to visual or auditory stimuli, smiling, and recognizing family members (Shewmon, Holmes, et al. 1999). The Yorgason's were told that Charity would not be able to see, hear, feel, taste, or smell, would neither experience nor be able to express emotions such as joy or love (Yorgason 2003: 26).

Charity was not expected to survive past infancy. However, her adopted parents quickly developed a very strong bond of love with her. They felt that they were meant to care for Charity, and that she did not wish to die. Charity clearly did appear to see and hear, she sometimes smiled and laughed, she was soothed by the singing of her parents. When she developed signs of pain and irritability because of a build-up of fluid in the cranium Charity had a ventriculo-peritoneal shunt inserted. However, she then developed a series of complications with the shunt including blockage, over-drainage, and infection. The shunt was replaced ten times over the next two years. At about eighteen months of age Charity developed an infection of her spinal fluid that was resistant to all treatment. Her doctors advised stopping all treatments except anti-epileptic agents and nutrition, and Charity was taken home to die. Within a few days, however, Charity spontaneously improved and recovered to her previous condition.

Charity's care imposed a major burden on the Yorgasons over a long period. Blaine Yorgason in his book *One Tattered Angel* described serious financial difficulties for the family over several years, complicated by his own difficulty in completing writing projects while

Charity was unwell. He described the enormous commitment made by his wife (who over a number of years also suffered from severe back pain). 'Never in my life had I imagined that an individual could so thoroughly sacrifice herself in behalf of another...Day after gruelling day, night after sleepless night, week in and week out for year after endless year I watched in awe as Kathy gave her every ounce of herself and then some to our tattered little daughter' (2003: 152). However, Blaine also described the enormous positive side of caring for Charity. 'She was like a sweet magnet drawing us all to her, and none of us could get enough of holding her, dancing with her, singing to her, and simply being with her' (2003: 73). 'Our family never stopped feeling overwhelmed by Charity's ability to give pure love—without asking or hoping for anything in return' (2003: 116).

Charity eventually died shortly before her eighth birthday. Although this had long been expected her family was overwhelmed by grief at her death. Yorgason eloquently describes the enormous sense of loss and emptiness that he and his wife felt in the months afterwards. Blaine Yorgason was also unequivocal that caring for Charity had enriched the lives of her parents and siblings. One of her siblings, Dan, wrote 'she helped us learn to love each other better...I can say without hesitation that Charity's coming into our lives is the single most important thing that has ever happened to our family' (2003: 132). Blaine wrote in the penultimate chapter: 'the more I ponder, the more overwhelmed with gratitude I feel...Through all eternity I will be thankful to God for bringing her into our lives and for allowing us to cherish her as our little angel daughter' (2003: 196).

On the other hand, other parents describe substantial negative consequences of the illness or impairment of their child. There are well-documented potential costs for families. Having a child with a serious illness or impairment increases the incidence of parents divorcing or living apart by 10–20 per cent (Corman and Kaestner 1992; Reichman, Corman, et al. 2004) and is associated with higher rates of psychological and physical ill health (Thyen, Kuhlthau, et al. 1999; Reichman, Corman, et al. 2004; Raina, O'Donnell, et al. 2005; Murphy, Christian, et al. 2007). Primary caregivers are at significant risk of clinical depression and abnormally low subjective quality of life (Cummins 2001). One study surveyed more than 200 Swedish families of children with autism and/or intellectual disability, and 200 control families. Almost half of the mothers of children with intellectual disability or autism had high depression scores (compared to 15–20 per cent in control mothers) (Olsson and Hwang 2001). The care needs of children with severe impairments do not diminish with age, and mothers are frequently unable to work outside the home (Thyen, Kuhlthau, et al. 1999; Curran, Sharples, et al. 2001); the impact on family income is compounded by a reduction in fathers' working hours (Reichman, Corman, et al. 2008). In the UK the financial demands of caring for a child with impairment are estimated to be more than three times the cost of bringing up a non-impaired child (Curran, Sharples, et al. 2001). Although state benefits supplement family income in countries like the UK, they do not bring that income up to the level of families without disabled children.

Many of these studies look at the average impacts of a range of degrees of disability. Norwegian researcher Berit Brinchmann interviewed a number of parents of very severely disabled children, all of whom had been involved in decisions about life-sustaining treatment in the past. Some of these parents described life as being like a prison, and dreamed of escape:

if only we could escape.... I'm aware that if I have one more sleepless night, more sickness and washing to do, I just can't cope.... There's a big sorrow inside us. It's there when we laugh and talk. It's there all the time, engraved independent of what's going on. The life of grief—or is it beyond grief? —that we live. (Brinchmann 1999)

When the Bough Breaks

In her book *When the Bough Breaks* writer and mother Julia Hollander describes her own experience of a traumatic birth and its consequences (Hollander 2008). Her second child Imogen developed hypoxic-ischaemic encephalopathy after a placental abruption, and sustained devastating brain injury. Hollander vividly evokes the emotional turmoil of the months following Imogen's birth.

In the early weeks and months Imogen was an extremely distressed and irritable infant. When she was awake she screamed inconsolably. Hollander and her partner struggled to cope with sleeplessness and disruption of daily life. She described shouting at her partner, at her older child, at the infant Imogen. A previously stable relationship started to show signs of wear. Her partner Jay chain smoked and ate alone; at one point he packed up his things to leave the family home (though subsequently he changed his mind). Imogen's older sister Elinor meanwhile became withdrawn, her behaviour out of character, and difficult to deal with. Elinor played at caring for an imaginary bed-bound mother. Hollander herself described dark fantasies in her diary:

> One night in the dark, with no moon and no candle, rocking Immie's angry little body back and forth, I feel myself swing just a little bit further. This is what it would feel like if I were to smash her head against the wall. It would be so simple... I must not tell anyone about my fantasy. It is too horrible, the ease with which I can truly imagine destroying my child.

Julia did not harm her child, though she wrote of being terrified by the possibility that she could. When she later spoke to other mothers of profoundly disabled children she found some consolation in the discovery that these sorts of illicit desires are actually not so unusual.

As Julia came to terms with the possibility of long-term impairment for her daughter she contemplated a future where she is identified as a carer rather than a mother, giving up on her career as a writer:

> I could picture my future, unable to afford a special needs carer, permanently holed up alone with miserable Immie whilst my sunny older child was farmed out to all the friends who wanted to help. (Hollander 2008: 162)

Imogen was admitted to hospital with seizures at a few months of age, and subsequently had a CT scan of her brain. It revealed severe global brain damage, with the majority of her brain tissue having been lost and replaced by fluid. Julia's partner withdrew further from Imogen, expressing an inability to care for a child 'without consciousness', who he feared would never even know him. In the book Julia is at turns angry, pessimistic, despondent, reckless, and close to suicidal.

After learning of Imogen's prognosis, Hollander researched the support services available for severely disabled children. She found precious little respite care available, and was advised that she was going to have to fight for support. She spoke to another mother of a severely disabled eleven-year-old child, and learned of her battle with social services to get her child admitted into residential care.

Ultimately, Hollander, at the end of her tether, despairing of the future years of caring for a severely disabled child, facing a family that was disintegrating around her, and the possibility of losing her partner, gave Imogen up for foster care.

Parents are not the only members of a family who are potentially impacted, positively or negatively, by decisions made in intensive care. Siblings may be significantly affected too. The impact of an impaired child on siblings' physical and psychological welfare has not been as well studied as that of parents. But siblings of children with intellectual impairment or chronic illness have been found to have more emotional and behavioural problems. In meta-analyses of more than seventy different studies siblings had higher levels of depression, loneliness, and anxiety, lower self-esteem and social functioning (Sharpe and Rossiter 2002). Siblings of impaired children report having to work around the home more than siblings of unimpaired children, and this has been suggested to affect the development of their self-identity. One study found children to be more socially isolated, and to spend more time in solitary pursuits than children without a disabled sibling. Again, the impact is not always negative. Siblings of children with Down syndrome have been reported to have no increase in psychological problems (O'Brian, Duffy, et al. 2009). Some reports have suggested that the presence of an impaired brother or sibling leads to greater psychological maturation (Findler and Vardi 2009), or may lead to greater empathy and appreciation of individuals with disability. Beyond the immediate family there are likely effects on grandparents and other members of the child's extended family. These have been even less studied.

Different Societies, Different Problems

There may be a significant impact on the interests of family members, perhaps in both directions. But one problem with taking these interests into consideration in decision-making, is that this impact varies between societies. It is, at least in part, dependent on the support that society provides for children with impairments and their families. The negative impact on parents and other family members of caring for children with impairment is likely to be significantly less in a society that provides ample publicly funded medical and social support services for disabled individuals and their carers than in a society that provides little or no such support. One of the factors that preyed on Julia Hollander's mind when she was contemplating a future as primary carer for her severely impaired daughter was the lack of available respite services and support. (Ironically, Hollander related that Imogen's foster carer was able to access more financial and practical support for Imogen's care than Hollander herself would have been eligible for had she continued to look after Imogen at home.)

Yet the United Kingdom, where Imogen was born, is a relatively wealthy country, with a comparatively large proportion of its gross domestic product spent on a public health care system and well-developed social care infrastructure. There are plenty of other countries where the financial and practical impact on families is likely to be substantially greater.

In a study of treatment limitation decisions in a public hospital in India Ingrid Miljeteig found that doctors worried about the impact of the survival of an impaired or ill child on families. Although treatment in this hospital was free of charge, ongoing medical costs and healthcare visits would be borne by the family. 'Who am I, a third person, to decide? His brother and sister might not go to school because of this. (Miljeteig and Norheim 2006: 28)' Treatment of a seriously ill infant might lead to economic ruin for the family or to the starvation of other children at home.

One problem with taking factors like these into account is that they might change. For example, a change in government or in government policy might lead to a substantial increase in respite care available for children like Imogen Hollander. Then part of her mother's concern about the future would be unwarranted. This is likely to lead to uncertainty about the interests of parents or other family members. But we may also feel that some of these factors *should* change. It is deeply troubling that parents like Julia Hollander should feel the need to pursue litigation against the hospital where Imogen was born merely in order to be able to afford to provide her ongoing basic care. It is unjust that parents of children with serious impairments face substantial out of pocket costs, and are financially penalized for care. It is disturbing that the only way that a parent like Hollander could access respite care was by convincing social services that her daughter was at risk if she continued to care for her. If part of the reason why the interests of parents and siblings are adversely affected by the survival of a severely impaired infant is an unjust and neglectful attitude towards disabled individuals, then we might worry about taking this into account in decision-making. Rather than allowing this impact to influence decisions about life-sustaining treatment, perhaps we should be agitating for greater support for parents of seriously ill or impaired children? There is a sense in which, if we allow social injustice to influence our decisions about treatment, we are participating in that very injustice. We are, to some degree complicit. We could call this the 'justice argument' against the inclusion of parental interests in end-of-life decisions.

One provocative related example is also mentioned in Miljeteig's study of decisions in an Indian neonatal unit. Many of the doctors that she interviewed described a concern about gender bias in decision-making. Although the doctors would not consider withdrawing treatment because of the gender of an infant they noted that parents were often more willing to agree to withdraw treatment if an infant was female, more likely to take an infant home against medical advice, and less willing to buy expensive medicines or attend follow-up appointments (Miljeteig, Sayeed, et al. 2009). Families were influenced by their lack of resources to take care of a daughter or other children, fear of having to pay high dowries later in the child's life, and fear of cultural stigma. These fears may be overstated or exaggerated by parents. But it appears that there was at least a perception by parents that their interests (and those of other siblings) were affected by the gender of an infant. But should we allow *this* factor to play a legitimate role in decisions in Indian neonatal units? Surely this sort of insidious discrimination should not be allowed? Even if it is true that there is a greater effect on the interests of parents and siblings for female infants, this factor ought not to be included in decision-making.

Is there a difference between taking into account the effect of disability on the interests of parents/siblings and taking into account the effect of gender? One difference is that even in an ideal world, in a perfectly just society with ample resources, there might be some negative effect of a seriously impaired infant on the interests of family members. Even if society provided a sufficiently generous support package for the caregivers of impaired children to prevent any impact on the career or finances of parents it is still possible that parents' well-being would be negatively affected by the survival of an infant or child with severe impairment. Parents might have ongoing grief for the lost opportunities that they had anticipated for their child, or for the activities that they had hoped to share with them. Even in this hypothetical just society parents may not feel able to conceive another child if the current infant survives. And it is hard to believe, even in this 'perfect' world, that parents would be able to devote as much time to other siblings as they would if the sibling were not impaired.

The first response to the justice argument is that even in a perfectly just society there is potentially some impact of an impaired child on parents' and siblings' interests. That is not the case for gender. In a just society it cannot make a difference for parents or siblings whether an infant or child who survives intensive care is male or female. But it is also the case that much of the effect on interests of impairment would be removed by the provision of generous support. So should we take this into account? There are two possibilities.

The *idealist's* response to the justice argument is to suggest that we should make our decisions as if we were in an ideal world. If we subtract from our deliberations those contingent and unjust features of our society, then it would reduce substantially the relevance of family interests for our decisions. But should we make decisions based on this ideal world standard? It seems unrealistic and unfair to apply this standard to decisions, for example, in low-resource countries where there is no prospect in the medium term that anything like this ideal level of support is going to be provided for families. Although we might regret the lack of support for families and for children with impairment in third-world settings we cannot ignore the fact that this is what families face through no fault of their own, and with no ability to change it. If we face the prospect, as the doctors in Miljeteig's study did, that the other children of a family will starve because of the cost of medical care for this child, or that they will be unable to go to school, is it right to refuse to allow this any role in decisions? One response would be to try to identify not only how much the effect on family interests would be in an ideal, just society, but also to try to identify how likely it is that injustice will be tackled within the lifespan of the child. The *pragmatist's* response to the discrimination argument is to identify as far as possible the impact on interests that the family is likely to face, and how much control they have over this. In this context it is instructive that some of the strongest evidence on the adverse effect of caring for a child with severe impairment comes from Scandinavian countries that are often held up as having the strongest and best funded social support systems (Brinchmann 1999; Olsson and Hwang 2001). It highlights just how difficult it is likely to be to eliminate negative effects on the interests of families. On the other hand, the pragmatist would potentially have a different response to gender discrimination. There are plenty of parts of the world where there is no impact for family interests of the gender of infants or children. There have been and there continues to be significant progress in reducing discrimination against women in developing countries. Many of the fears alluded to by the doctors in the Indian study could be reduced within a generation, and some are within the power of the family to control.

Finally, we should note that if we adopt the pragmatist's point of view and do take these factors into account that does not preclude us from identifying the status quo as unjust, nor from agitating to improve the level of resources available to care for impaired children. It is not contradictory to be influenced by the situation as it stands for our practical decisions, and simultaneously to seek to change that situation.

In practice how much do doctors take into account the interests of families in decisions in newborn and paediatric intensive care? This has changed over time, and differs between countries. In the US in the 1970s and early 1980s, when newborn intensive care was first developing, doctors placed a great deal of weight on the wishes of parents (Fost 1999). A survey in 1975 of American paediatricians and paediatric surgeons found that the majority would not perform surgery for a newborn infant with Down syndrome and a blocked intestine if parents refused consent (Shaw, Randolph, et al. 1977). But a decade later, following the very public controversy over Baby Doe, and the introduction by Ronald Reagan of the 'Baby Doe rules', the majority of Massachusetts paediatricians would seek a court order to perform surgery in the above situation if parents did not consent (Todres, Guillemin, et al. 1988). The shift in attitudes in the US away from the rights of parents towards the interests of the child reduced or eliminated the problem of undertreatment of mildly or moderately disabled newborn infants. However, by the 1990s in the US many were concerned that the pendulum had swung too far, and had led to a period of overtreatment (Fost 1999).

More recently it appears that doctors across a wide range of countries place some weight on the interests of families. In a survey of 1391 neonatal physicians in ten European countries, the majority of doctors in all of the countries surveyed believed that the burden on families was relevant when making end-of-life decisions for a child (Rebagliato, Cuttini, et al. 2000). In another survey of more than 300 physicians, this time in North America, and including doctors who worked in adult and paediatric as well as newborn intensive care units, over 90 per cent believed that family interests should have some role in medical decision-making for incompetent patients (Hardart and Truog 2003). Almost two-thirds of the surveyed doctors indicated that the interests of families should be considered even if those interests were not important interests of the patient.

To sum up our analysis so far, the interests of families may be affected in both positive and negative ways by decisions made for a critically ill newborn infant and child. The relationship between the desires of families and their wellbeing is not straightforward. For example parents' lives may predictably go worse overall if they have to care for a surviving child, and yet parents may have a very strong desire that the child does survive. It may often be the case that parents have interests both in the survival of the infant and in withdrawal of life-sustaining treatment. It is not clear how such competing interests should be weighed against each other.

It is, therefore, difficult to generalize about the strength of the interest that parents have in withdrawal of life support or in its continuation. But a couple of points appear reasonably plausible. Some families may have a strong desire and interest in treatment continuing for their child or infant. Other parents may have a strong interest in intensive care not being continued for their newborn infant. The strength of this latter interest is likely to be proportional to the severity of the child's impairment. This is because the greater the severity of impairment, the greater the demand that a child's care is likely to place on caregivers. Higher caregiving demands, in turn, are associated with lower physical and psychological well-being in caregivers and greater financial cost to families (Leonard, Brust, et al. 1992; Raina, O'Donnell, et al. 2005). Although some of the reason why families' interests are negatively affected is because of social injustice, and could, in theory, be reduced, it is nevertheless appropriate to take into account the way in which family interests are likely to be affected. It appears that in practice doctors in newborn and paediatric intensive care do take these interests into account.

But when should the interests of parents and siblings count, and does it make any difference whether we are dealing with a sick newborn infant or older child? To answer that question we need to know what it is that we have on the other side of the scales. What is the strength of the infant or child's interest?

The Interests of the Child

Although this chapter is focused on the potential conflict or competition between the interests of the family and those of the child it is worth noting that these interests will often coincide. There are, in fact, at least four possibilities. The most common situation in intensive care is that of an infant whose life will be worth living, and whose parents have a strong interest in the infant's survival. In such cases, obviously, there is no conflict or particular difficulty for decisions. Nor is there a problem when both the interests of the infant and the interests of parents lie in withdrawal of life support. These interests may also come apart, however. In the first sort of conflict the interests of the child, if taken on their own, would support withdrawal or withholding of life-sustaining treatment, but the family (the parents in particular) have an interest in treatment being provided (Death/Life conflict). In the second type of conflict the infant has an interest in continued life, but the family have an interest in withdrawal of the infant's life support (Life/Death conflict).

Death/Life

In the first type of conflict situation, the infant has an interest in life support not being provided. The strength of this interest will vary. We could imagine cases where future burdens just outweigh benefits, and there is a relatively small net interest in life support being withdrawn. But there will also be cases where future suffering vastly outweighs the benefits for the infant, and they have a strong interest at stake. Could the parents' interest justify providing treatment that is against the child's own interests? Is it permissible to, effectively, cause the child to suffer for the sake of their parents? Put this starkly, it seems difficult to justify such a course of action. If we were certain that the child were going to be significantly harmed by continuing treatment, we should surely not do so, even if it would distress his or her parents to stop treatment? In practice, however, there are a couple of reasons why we might adopt a course of action that respects the parents' wishes even if doctors do not believe that the treatment is in the child's interests. Firstly, we rarely, if ever, have that level of certainty about an infant's interests, so medical staff may not feel confident enough to override parents' wishes. Secondly, if our concern is about the infant or child suffering, there is usually something that can be done to ameliorate or eliminate that possibility. One situation that is not infrequently encountered in intensive care is where parents insist that intensive care continue despite an overwhelming likelihood that the child is going to die. This is often distressing to those involved in caring for the child, but in practice it is usually possible to provide sufficient sedation and analgesia to minimize the chance that the child is suffering. Then we may both respect parents' wishes and reduce or avoid the conflict with the child's. Thirdly, it seems at least theoretically possible that the parents' interests in treatment continuing might sometimes outweigh the child's interest in treatment stopping. If the child's interests were very weak, for example if they had only very brief, fragmentary episodes of consciousness, and only mild amounts of pain, perhaps the very strong desires of parents in treatment being provided would outweigh these interests of the child?

One question here is about which interest is greater, who has more at stake, the parent or the child? That is a difficult question, in part because we are comparing apples and oranges. There are different sorts of benefits and harms for the parent and child, and so it can be hard to stack one up against the other. There may well be cases where it isn't clear which interest is greater. But there will also be cases where it *is* clear that either families or the child have significantly more at stake. So then, the second question is what we do when there is an imbalance of interests. Do the child's interests dominate? If we think that it is never permissible to compromise the child's interests for the sake of parents or other family members, then in fact we would be giving no weight to the interests of the family. But that isn't the way that we think about other decisions that parents or families make. For example, it would often unquestionably be in the best interests of the child if parents were to purchase private education or private health insurance for the child. But parents are permitted to take into account the impact on themselves and on other family members of such decisions and to elect not to provide these significant benefits. Sometimes parents also make decisions that cause a certain amount of suffering for a child for the sake of their own interests. Perhaps they decide to move the family and child to another town, out of a school where they are happy and away from their friends, because the parent wants to pursue a different job. (Frequent house moves have been associated with significant long-term consequences on the well-being of children (Oishi and Schimmack 2010).) Perhaps a parent decides to spend a period of time pursuing a personal goal (for example to travel to Antarctica or climb Mount Everest), at the cost of causing a child a predictable amount of distress, fear, and anxiety. More controversially, parents are usually permitted to make medical decisions that potentially impose some risk on their children, for example electing not to have routine childhood immunizations (Dawson 2005). In each of these cases it appears that the parents' wishes and wellbeing appear to outweigh those of the child. One point that is worth making is that there is a difference between what parents should do, and what they should be allowed to do. We may feel, in the above examples, that it is wrong for a parent to fail to take out private health insurance, to move the family, to fail to immunize their child. But most of us would be willing to allow parents to make these sorts of potentially wrong decisions. There is considerable value in allowing parents to make decisions for their children and to bring them up as they see fit (within reason). A world in which the state interfered whenever parents failed to do the best possible for all of their children is not one that many would find terribly appealing. The second point is whether individuals *are* morally required to sacrifice all of their own interests once they become parents. Perhaps it is not wrong, where there is something very important at stake, for the parent to pursue their own interests at some cost to their children.

Is there any difference, in Death/Life conflicts, between newborn infants and older children? It is difficult to see how an infant's interest in not experiencing suffering would be any different from an older child's. One possibility is that the nature of that suffering would be different. An older child may be more aware of their condition. It is possible that because of this they would experience additional fear and distress at their physical state, and the prospect of continuing pain and discomfort. But it is also possible that their greater awareness would mean that they get greater consolation from the presence of family members and friends, or that they are able to understand the reason for medical procedures and anticipate that they will be over soon. In either case, we would include this in our assessment of the balance of benefits and burdens, and whether or not life is worth living for the child. Once we have done that, the principles should be the same across childhood. We should make similar decisions about continuing treatment (that doctors do not believe are in the interests of the child) for newborn infants and older children.

Life/Death

What about the other sort of conflict? Life/Death conflicts require more discussion since what is at stake for the child is an interest in future life. What is the nature and the strength of this interest? The answer is not straightforward.

It is generally thought that an individual's interest in continuing to live is one of the strongest interests that they hold. For adults and children we don't usually think that the lesser interests of others can outweigh the patient's interest in continued life. But are newborn infants the same? We will start by looking at two opposing suggestions.

No Interest? Peter Singer has controversially argued that infants have no interest in continued existence (Singer 1993: 97–8). If that were the case, then treatment withdrawal would potentially be justified whenever parent's interests were going to be adversely affected by the survival of an infant. Singer's argument is based on three claims. Firstly, he holds a desire-based view of well-being; it is necessary for individuals to have a desire for something for it to be in their interest (Singer 1993: 13, 94). Secondly, he claims that infants lack self-consciousness, and therefore they do not have a desire for continued life (Singer 1993: 169). Thirdly, Singer makes a controversial claim about personal identity: that infants are not the same person as the adult they subsequently develop into (Singer 1993: 97–8).

To make sense of this last claim, it is necessary to understand a little about what philosophers are talking about when they refer to 'personal identity'. If you compare yourself with a younger version, say yourself one year ago, there are going to be some physical differences. Perhaps you have a few extra grey hairs, have put on weight (or lost weight). You might have an extra scar, new freckles, a different hairstyle. On the microscopic level, all of the cells that would have made up the outer layer of your skin would have changed, as would all of your circulating red blood cells, and indeed many of your body's cells. You are obviously not physically identical with your younger self. But you are genetically identical with that younger individual, and there is good reason to think that (except in very unusual circumstances) you are the same person. When I reflect on what makes me distinctively 'me', what seems important is the combination of memories, likes, preferences, ways of thinking and acting in response to the world. Again, although there are going to be some differences, some new memories, some change in the things that I think are important, there is good reason to think that

I am the same person that I was a year ago. The Greek philosopher Heraclitus is quoted by Plato as saying that 'you cannot step into the same river twice' (Plato 2010), the implication being that when someone steps into a river for a second time both they and the river will have changed. Heraclitus was right of course, in that the water molecules that made up the river will have changed, and there will have been subtle changes in the edges of the river, in its flow, and in its contents. But there is another sense in which it *is* the same river that it was the first time. Likewise, in an important sense the person entering the river remains the same.

But what about when we think about ourselves much further back than one year? Peter Singer writes 'I am not the infant from whom I developed' (Singer 1993: 97) and, in another book, written with Helga Kuhse, 'When I think of myself as the person I now am, I realize that I did not come into existence until some time after my birth' (Kuhse and Singer 1985: 133). There are different levels of awareness. At the most basic level an individual is aware of their environment. Higher level of awareness involves perception of the self, and awareness of ongoing conscious experience. It is this higher level of self-consciousness that appears to develop in later infancy. The infant does not share central identity features of memory, desires, ways of thinking, with their older self. The implication of Singer's claim is that the toddler or young child who develops self-consciousness is a different individual from that same child at a slightly younger age. This claim is counterintuitive. Many will point to the physical continuity between infant and older child, or the genetic continuity, and reject out of hand any suggestion that the infant is not the same individual. But Singer's claim also risks being incoherent (McMahan 2002: 349). The problem is that at the moment that personal identity begins there must be a 'self' of which to become aware. But if personal identity only begins when that infant develops the higher-order awareness, then the lower-order conscious experience that they are starting to appreciate must belong to someone else? In any case, there are also reasons to think that there is some psychological continuity between the newborn and later fully self-conscious individual. Although few children or adults have any memory of early infancy (Hayne 2004), there are psychological ripples of unremembered events. For example, six-month-old infants who had been circumcised in the newborn period had a stronger pain response to routine vaccination at six months of age, an effect attenuated if local anaesthesia is provided for the procedure

(Taddio, Goldbach, et al. 1995). Two-year-old children have been demonstrated to retain non-verbal memories from events or training at six months of age (Hartshorn 2003; Bornstein, Arterberry, et al. 2004).

Singer might claim, in response, that the reason that the older child or adult is not the same person as the infant from whom they developed is because the infant is not a *person*. There are two different and competing concepts involved when we use the word 'person'. Person is often used synonymously with the term 'human being'. But there is a second meaning, particularly within ethical discourse. In a now famous paper on abortion written in the 1970s, philosopher Michael Tooley provided a definition of the morally relevant sense of 'person' (Tooley 1972). He argued that self-consciousness and self-awareness were the defining features of personhood. Tooley's account has significant overlaps with a much earlier account of the meaning of 'persons'; John Locke's famous 1690 *Essay Concerning Human Understanding* included a brief description of personal identity:

We must consider what person stands for—which I think is a thinking intelligent being, that has reason and reflection, and can consider itself as itself, the same thinking thing, in different times and places (Locke 2004, Chapter 27)

If newborn infants are not persons, then by definition they could not be the same person as an older child. But the psychological links between infant and child, and the gradual evolution of consciousness challenge this notion of personal identity beginning at some point in toddlerhood. It makes more sense to think of the development of personal identity as a gradual process, and of the newborn infant sharing at least some of the constituents of identity with their older self.

There are also reasons to cast doubt upon Singer's second claim, that infants lack self-consciousness. Newborn infants distinguish tape-recordings of their own cry from that of other infants; in one fascinating study infants stopped crying on hearing their own voice, while they continued to cry on hearing a recording of another infant (Martin and Clark 1982). In other studies, infants as early as an hour after birth have been shown to imitate adult facial gestures (Meltzoff and Moore 1977; Meltzoff and Moore 1983). But to imitate something requires awareness of the difference between self and other. The imitating behaviour of newborns appears to be non-reflexive, involves memory, and improves over time (Meltzoff and Moore 1994). These experiments, and others, suggest that infants have a degree of proprioceptive (i.e. non-visual) awareness of their own face (Gallagher 1996). They appear to have a form of primitive, non-conceptual self-consciousness (Bermudez 2001; Lagercrantz and Changeux 2009).

Still, even if newborn infants have some degree of self-consciousness, they do not appear to possess an explicit desire or preference for continued life. If Singer's first claim were true, about the importance of preferences for interests, then infants would still potentially lack an interest in living. They would not be harmed by their death, nor would they benefit from life-saving treatment in the newborn period. There is, however, a coherent and plausible sense in which a newborn is benefited by having their life saved in infancy. Compare two scenarios, John$_1$, where a newborn dies shortly after birth, and John$_2$, where the same infant lives to adulthood. John$_2$ experiences considerably more happiness than John$_1$, gets to have and fulfil more desires, hopefully establishes friendships, experiences love, achieves at least some of his hopes and goals. Few would doubt that John$_2$'s life is a better life than John$_1$'s. We have seen above that there are psychological links between John the newborn and his older self. Correspondingly the newborn infant John would benefit from experiencing the life of John$_2$; the infant has an interest in not dying in the newborn period (McMahan 2002: 352).

The above arguments provide reasons to reject Singer's claim; infants appear to be benefited by continuing to live as long as that future life would contain more intrinsically positive than negative experiences (i.e. they would have a life worth living). This interest in future well-being would be consistent with mental-state theories of well-being (i.e. hedonism), and is likely to be consistent with most objective-list theories. It would also be consistent with at least some versions of desire-based theories, those that admit informed desires or rational desires (Boonin 2002: 84). If infants were capable of having preferences and were given all appropriate information, they would want to continue to live.

This conclusion, that infants have an interest in continued existence, is not likely to be particularly striking for many. It fits with the widespread intuition that it is a bad thing for someone to die in infancy, a good thing to have their life saved. But how strong is that interest? The most widely held view is that newborn infants have a strong and overriding interest in continued life, equivalent to that of older children and adults (Kaposy 2007). Is that view right?

Strong and Overriding Interest? Most people have instinctively strong protective feelings towards newborn infants. Enormous efforts are made to save the lives of infants who are critically ill after birth. Parents and family members are usually devastated by the death of a newborn. It is believed to be a tragedy when this occurs—both for the parents and for the infant.

We have seen that death is a harm to infants because it deprives them of future happiness and well-being. But given that a newborn is typically deprived of significantly more years of life than a child or an adult, this loss appears greater for a newborn than for the child or adult who dies. This conflicts, however, with other widely held intuitions.

Consider the Transplant Choice:

> A six-year-old child with a severe cardiomyopathy is awaiting a heart transplant. She has had multiple admissions to hospital, and is becoming more unwell each time. It is feared that if she has to wait much longer she will either become ineligible to receive a transplant (because she will be too unwell), or will die. At the same hospital, a newborn infant is born with a rare congenital form of the same illness. He is critically ill and is put on a heart bypass machine. If he does not receive an urgent heart transplant he too will die.
>
> A heart becomes available that would suit either the older child or the infant. With transplantation the child and infant would have equal chances of surviving to early adulthood at least. Who should receive the transplant organ? (Whoever does not receive the heart is likely to die.)

The usual response to this dilemma is to refuse to choose between the children, perhaps to try to desperately find a way to treat both children. The dilemma is a variant of the terrible choice faced by a character in William Styron's book *Sophie's Choice*, who, at enormous personal psychological cost, must choose which of her children she will save from death in a concentration camp (Styron 1992). Clearly, if at all possible, we should try to save both children. But if forced to make a choice, most people choose the six-year-old (Ross 2007). In another survey, when doctors and non-doctors were asked to choose which of a series of children and adults of varying ages should be resuscitated first if they all needed emergency attention, greater priority was consistently given to resuscitating an older child than to resuscitating a newborn, even when the older child's prognosis was poorer (Janvier, Leblanc, et al. 2008a; Janvier, Leblanc, et al. 2008b).

These gut responses challenge the idea that newborn infants are viewed identically to older children. They suggest that for many people a newborn infant's interest in continuing life is not as strong as that of an older child.

Of course, even if such intuitions are widespread, it does not follow from this that newborns *should* be treated differently than other children. Our intuitions may be unjustified or unreliable. The authors of the second of the two surveys above have suggested that there is a bias against newborns, and premature infants in particular, and that such attitudes might have anthropological and evolutionary roots in the high neonatal mortality rates present throughout most of human history (Janvier, Leblanc, et al. 2008b). Given that half of all children born in ancient Rome did not make it to the age of 10, and that most of these deaths occurred in the first year of life, it would have made sense to save the life of an older child rather than a newborn. That older child was almost twice as likely to survive to support their parents (and pass on their genes). Others have suggested that the difference lies in the older child's lived experience, and the potentially greater grief for her parents (Ross 2007). If that is the case parents may have a stronger interest in saving the older child.

But neither of these accounts provides an adequate explanation for why it still seems worse for a six-year-old, or a 10-year-old child or a 20-year-old to die than a newborn. It seems worse *for* the individual to die after having lived a few years than to die very soon after birth. The evolutionary account might explain why parents would have greater attachment to an older than a younger child. But it does not explain why the death of a child who is genetically unrelated to us still seems worse than the death of a newborn.

A Reduced Interest Death is bad for a range of different reasons. It is bad because the experience of dying may be painful or unpleasant. It is also often bad because of the fear or anticipation that precedes death. But what if you were hit by a bus and killed instantly, would that be of no harm to you? If we think that it would be bad to die suddenly and painlessly, we need something else to explain the badness of death. There are two other factors that might help explain this. The first of these is, as noted above, that death deprives us of future life. The better and longer our life would have been, the greater the harm it is to us to die. But the second important element is that death is bad for us because it cuts short our desires, plans, and hopes for that future and severs the relationships that we have developed with those around us. The more of these that we have developed, the greater our psychological connection with that future and the more we have at stake. Where these connections are weak (for example in the presence of severe dementia, or at the very beginning of life), perhaps death would not be as bad?

In his book *The Ethics of Killing* American philosopher Jeff McMahan argues that the combination of these latter two elements helps to explain many of our intuitions about death (McMahan 2002). McMahan rejects Singer's arguments that it would be permissible to kill a healthy newborn infant because such infants lack an interest in continued life (McMahan 2002: 345–62). Newborn infants have some psychological links with their future selves. The future that they would lose if they died is their life. They have an interest in their future (McMahan 2002: 352). But this interest is not the same as that of an older child or adult. On McMahan's account, it is worse for a 20-year-old to die than a 40-year-old (because the 20-year-old would be deprived of more life). But it is also worse for a 6-year-old to die than a newborn because of the older child's greater awareness of herself, and richer psychological links with her future.

Time-Relative Interests

McMahan calls his view about the harm of death the 'time-relative interests' account. Interests are time-relative because they change in strength over time, but also, crucially, because they are affected by the nature and number of links that tie current and future selves. McMahan's time-relative interests account pays attention to the importance of how much an individual is psychologically invested in or connected to their future life (DeGrazia 2007). The time-relative interests account explains why the interest of a newborn in his future might be less than that of an older child. It also explains why the death of a newborn infant is worse (for the individual) than the death of a fetus, and why there is something worse about the death of a late fetus than a mid-gestation or very early fetus. This fits with many people's intuition that there is something more significant about a late abortion than an early abortion. The evolving neural connections in the second half of pregnancy mean that there is more at stake for the later fetus than the earlier fetus, and more again for the newborn.

(a) Deprivation Account

(b) Two-tiered Account

(c) Time-Relative Interests Account

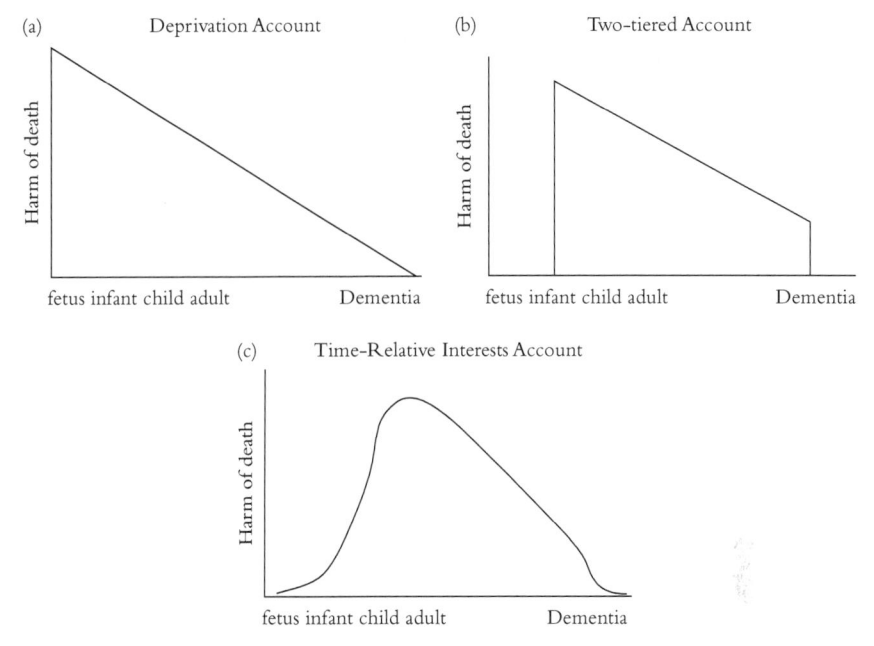

Figure 4.1 Three accounts of the harm of death.

But is this the right account of interests and death, and how does it compare with other ways of thinking about death? One approach to thinking about the harm of death focuses on the future life and happiness that death prevents an individual from experiencing. This is a 'deprivation' account of the harm of death (Bradley 2008). Figure 4.1a shows in schematic form the way that the harm of death changes over a lifetime from fetal life to death after a period of cognitive decline or dementia. The worst time to die is at the very beginning of life, when death deprives an individual of the most future life. Then, death progressively becomes less bad until, in old age, it is not very bad at all. But the striking thing about this theory is that it suggests that it is much worse to die as a fetus than as an infant or as a child or an adult. The worst death is that of an embryo or early fetus just after the start of their existence (McMahan 2002: 171). (Philosopher Don Marquis has famously claimed that abortion is immoral on the basis of just this sort of claim about the harm of death (Marquis 1989).) Deprivation accounts give the opposite answer in the Transplant Choice—the newborn should receive the heart because they are deprived of the most life.

A second way of thinking about the harm of death is the way that Peter Singer does, and that I have already described. This is a 'two-tiered' view of the harm of death. Death is not a harm at all for individuals who are not self-conscious. Figure 4.1b shows a dramatic change somewhere in early childhood when the infant becomes self-conscious. Suddenly, death is maximally harmful. Then, depending on the details of the theory, there may be a gradual reduction in the individual's interest in their future life—in a similar way to the deprivation account. At the other end of life there is another sudden change, when an individual with dementia loses their self-consciousness. In comparison, Figure 4.1c illustrates the potential changes in the harm of death on the time-relative interests account. The gradual increase in the harm of death early in life, and the gradual reduction at the other end of the lifespan, appears far more plausible than the sudden gain or loss on the two-tiered view.

The time-relative interest account appears to provide plausible answers to some problems. What does it yield for other ethical conundrums? McMahan defends his theory in considerable depth in *The Ethics of Killing*, and discusses a number of thought experiments and examples. It is beyond the scope of this chapter and this book to delve into these in any detail, but here is another area where this account yields answers that seem sensible. There is a famous thought experiment that involves a sinking lifeboat containing four adults and a dog. All will perish unless someone is thrown overboard. Is it permissible to throw the dog into the water (where he will certainly die) to save the humans? Even those who have advocated passionately for animal rights have argued that this would be permissible (Regan 1983). McMahan's theory provides a way to justify such a decision while still affording the dog equal moral consideration. While the dog has an interest in continuing life, he will be harmed less by death than would a human. He has less psychological unity, and is less invested and connected to his future than his human co-passengers (DeGrazia 2007).

Philosopher and economist John Broome has provided one counter-example to Jeff McMahan's time-relative interest account in his book *Weighing Lives* (Broome 2004: 250–1). He suggests the following problem, a variant of the Transplant Choice mentioned above: imagine that there is a choice between saving the life of a newborn infant A, and saving the life of a young adult, B. In Broome's example, both of these patients would, if their life were saved now, live for thirty years. If we were just to choose between the patients on the basis of the number of life years to be saved with treatment (or quality-adjusted life years), we would have a tie—both patients would have an equal claim to treatment. On McMahan's account, however, the newborn has a reduced interest in her future life, so we should save the young adult B rather than the infant A. But then Broome neatly turns the problem on its head. If we now think about the situation in thirty years, our newborn A would be a young adult, and the current adult would be at least middle-aged. Imagine that we have a new treatment for heart failure post-transplantation. At that point in time death for the younger patient would be worse, and if we could, we should save A rather than B. Broome claims that this swapping of preferences is incoherent.

The problem that Broome points to is one of 'dynamic choices' (Andreou 2008). What we have reason to do sometimes changes over time, and appears to contradict our previous choices. This problem can lead us into making choices that appear at the time to be rational, but lead us to a worse outcome overall.

However, in Broome's example the apparent inconsistency in the choices isn't really inconsistent. When we are making these difficult choices, we are trying to weigh up which patient has the stronger interest in treatment, and correspondingly stands to benefit more from receiving it. But it isn't a problem for that choice that in the future, the tables might be turned, and we would choose the second patient instead. We might think, on the contrary, that this shows us that we are not discriminating unfairly and that this is a virtue of our decision-making process. The same rules might benefit one individual on one occasion, but someone else on another occasion. Furthermore, because we are talking about life-saving treatment, there is no future time point at which we should save A rather than B. If we save B now, A will not live to be a young adult (and compete for treatment). If we save A now, B will not live.

Here is another example in which it is much clearer that preferences could change without that undermining our choice now. Imagine that we have two patients with different forms of cancer needing a bone marrow transplant. The patients are of identical ages, and if they have a successful transplant, have an identical life expectancy of five years. But while patient C has only a 10 per cent chance of going into remission with their transplant, patient D has a 90 per cent chance of going into remission. If we can only perform one transplant we should surely choose patient D over patient C? But there is an additional wrinkle to the problem. Although patient C has a low chance of remission with their first transplant, the nature of their cancer is such that if C needs a second transplant in the future, they have a high chance of going into remission again (say 90 per cent). But the situation for D is reversed. Their cancer is such that it is highly likely that they would go into remission now. But if they have a recurrence, and need a second transplant, their survival chance would be very low. Here, it does not seem to be a problem that when giving a first transplant we should choose D, but if we are faced with giving a second transplant we should choose C. Our allocation decisions should reflect the interests of those who currently stand to benefit from treatment. In any case, there is no paradox, since we cannot be faced with this choice twice.

Another apparent paradox for the time-relative interest account is provided by McMahan himself (McMahan 2002: 185–8). Imagine that we have a newborn infant currently dependent on life-sustaining treatment. Their condition is completely treatable, and they will be completely healthy throughout childhood and early adulthood, but they have an underlying condition that will cause them to die suddenly at age 35. On the time-relative interest account, it would be a much greater harm for the young person to die at age 35 than it would be to die now as a newborn infant. Therefore perhaps we should allow them to die now, to prevent this later, worse death? But that can't be right.

The key to solving this puzzle is the fact that our choices are not contemporaneous. We are choosing between death now for the newborn infant versus thirty-five years of healthy life and death later at age 35. The harm of later death is offset by the years of good life. Although it is certainly tragic for someone to die at age 35, we don't normally think that that makes their life to that point not worth living. The value of their life to them is greater than the harm of death. It is a worse death, but a better choice overall for the newborn to be saved now and die later. McMahan's response to the paradox is slightly different. Although the newborn's interest in continued life is currently weak, he nevertheless has an interest that we should respect now (McMahan 2002: 187). That interest will continue, and will grow stronger as the child ages. There is no point in time at which the individual's current interests will favour allowing him to die.

The last criticism that we will discuss of time-relative interests comes from philosopher Ben Bradley. Bradley dissects McMahan's time-relative interests account in an article titled 'The worst time to die' (Bradley 2008). He argues that it *is* worse for a 3-week-old baby to die than a 23-year-old student (if they had identically happy lives ahead of them, and died at age 80). Bradley contends that 'what is intrinsically good for someone does not change over time' (2008: 313). Although someone's attitudes towards death may change, Bradley argues that the overall value of death is unaffected.

One of the sources of the disagreement between Bradley and McMahan is a difference in their view about well-being, and therefore about what counts as being in an individual's interests. McMahan does not clearly state his own view about well-being, but Bradley points out that the time-relative-interest account is closely linked to a certain form of preference satisfaction or desire theory (2008: 310). Because McMahan's view specifically relates the harm of death to what an individual cares about, or has reason to care about, it is inextricably linked to the second group of well-being theories mentioned at the start of this chapter.

Bradley criticizes the specific assumptions about well-being that he sees as underpinning time-relative interests. In particular, he targets the way that McMahan restricts consideration to 'actual' interests. What does Bradley mean by 'actual interests'? In the examples that we have discussed above, the newborn has a relatively reduced interest in her future well-being. However, if she survives to become an older child or adult, she will then have a strong interest in her own continued life and well-being. If we choose to save the life of the newborn we should take those future interests into account. But those future strong interests don't get counted if, instead, the older patient receives the heart transplant. They never exist. Then, the only interests that count are the current weaker newborn interests. Bradley claims that the focus on those interests that actually exist is incoherent: it requires that we know in advance which patient we will save before we can work out which patient we should save (Bradley 2008: 312).

But while the time-relative interest account is complicated, it doesn't require us to know in advance which choice we will make. The 'actualist' assumption is based on a relatively simple and intuitively plausible principle—when we are evaluating a particular decision that will affect whether or not individuals exist, we should take into account the interests of all of those who currently exist as well as those who will actually exist if we make that decision. This means that we do not take into account the interests of people who will never exist if we make a particular decision.

There is an analogous version of this principle relating to interests—when we are evaluating a particular decision that will affect whether or not interests exist, we should take into account those interests that currently exist, as well as those interests that will exist if we make that decision.

If that all seems too complicated or obscure, here is an example that might make things clearer. (This example is a version of one suggested by Bradley.) My son does not currently support a football team. I know that if I encourage him (perhaps taking him along to football games, or buying him membership of a football club) he will likely develop a preference for a particular team, and in the future have a desire that that specific team (let's call them Philosophy United) win. He will be glad to support Philosophy United, and glad that I encouraged him in this. But if I do not encourage him, it is likely that he will, like his father, not develop a particular interest in football, and instead direct his attention and time to other things that he is already interested in. Should I

> Option a. encourage interest in the football team, or
> Option b. not actively encourage him?

When thinking about this I should certainly take into account how much potential pleasure he will gain from supporting football and seeing his team win. Against this I will factor in the potential pleasure involved in spending more time in other alternative pursuits. (He will have a future interest in experiencing pleasure regardless of which option I choose.) I might perhaps also factor in whether having this type of interest is good for him in other ways, perhaps by encouraging him to get more exercise, or by giving him something to talk about with friends. But let us assume that his other pursuits are equally pleasurable, and equally good for him in other ways. Should I then take into account his future preference for Philosophy United? This desire, and interest, will only come to exist if I encourage my son. We could count this future preference in favour of option a. If he develops an interest in football and Philosophy United wins in the future, my son's desire will be fulfilled. If they win more often than they lose, this might count overall as a positive for him. But we can't count this preference against option b. If I do not encourage him, he will never have an interest in Philosophy United. If Philosophy United win, but my son doesn't care about football it can't make his life go worse because he is not supporting them. Creation of a preference is, it seems, morally neutral (Singer 1993: 128).

Bradley suggests that the desire theory of well-being that lies beneath the surface of McMahan's account is implausible—but the above discussion and example show that it is not. He also claims that this is a very narrow theory of well-being that is supported by few people (Bradley 2008: 312). However, as noted at the start of the chapter, desire satisfaction is also likely to be a component of objective list theories. Then, the main theory of well-being that could not support time-relativity of interests is that of hedonism (Bradley's own preferred theory (Bradley 2009)). In fact, some forms of hedonism could accommodate the idea that well-being and interests are relative. Bradley asks 'how could it be the case that something actually fails to enhance my well-being, but would enhance my well-being if things had gone differently?' In the example above, if Philosophy United win the football finals next year, this would increase my son's well-being by causing him pleasure if I have encouraged him to support them—but it would not enhance his well-being if he remains uninterested in football. Next, some forms of hedonism accommodate preferences. So-called 'preference hedonism' embraces the idea that experiences are more pleasant if they are desired, and this is proportional to the degree that they are desired (Parfit 1984: 493–4). A strong desire for future pleasurable experiences could then ground a stronger interest in realizing them. Conversely, a weaker desire for those experiences (as seen in an infant), would yield a weaker interest.

Some may still not be convinced by the time-relative theory of interests, but may be attracted to the intuition that there is something worse, or more tragic about the death of a young adult than the death of a newborn infant. Both Bradley and McMahan note a number of different alternative justifications for this judgement (though Bradley does not himself endorse them). The first is the importance of investment (McMahan 2002: 176–83; Bradley 2008: 301). The young person has invested time and effort in certain pursuits and in directing their life in a particular way, while the infant has not. Peter Singer proposes a similar analogy. He imagines that someone decides to travel to Mount Everest. In the very early stages of his planning, he discovers, however, that this will not be possible. He will be disappointed, and we may be disappointed on his behalf—but nowhere nearly as much as he would if he had spent a long period of time preparing, planning, and spending, only to find at the last minute that he could not go (Singer 1993: 130–1). The second way of thinking about the difference between the young adult and the baby is in terms of the narrative of their life. The narrative of a young person's life takes on a particularly tragic shape when it is curtailed (McMahan 2002: 174–6; Bradley 2008: 301). In contrast, for an infant, the story of their life has barely started. If we think about the story or shape of an individual's life viewed as a whole, it seems that childhood or early adulthood may be the worst time to die.

The narrative account and the life-investment account are not competitors with the time-relative interests account. They are each arguably constituents of the strength of an individual's interest in continuing to live (McMahan 2002: 183).

I have argued, drawing on the time-relative interests account of the harm of death, that a newborn has a reduced interest in their future life compared to an older child. But the above argument does not establish just how strong the interest of a newborn is in their future. The difference between newborns and children might be sufficiently small that it only makes a difference in exceptional treatment dilemmas like the Transplant Choice described above. Alternatively, it might mean that treatment decisions for newborns are completely different from those in older children. Is there a way to define this further? One possibility would be to look at the relative importance of the different elements of interests. McMahan is not explicit about the relationship between future well-being and psychological connections. But one plausible way of expressing the relationship is that the strength of our time-relative interest in future life is directly proportional to both of these elements. They are equally important. We could express this in a mathematical way as

$$I \propto W \times P$$

(Where I is the strength of interests, W is the amount of future well-being, and P is the psychological connectedness of the individual with their future.)

But it is also possible that one of these is more important. Perhaps the amount of future well-being is the more important factor

$$I \propto W^2 \times P$$

or perhaps the psychological connectedness is more important

$$I \propto W \times P^2$$

It is not immediately clear which of these is the right way of understanding the relationship between the different elements of interests, nor whether some other possibility is the right one. It is also difficult to know how to quantify the degree of psychological connectedness. What would P be for a late-term fetus? Perhaps instead we could take a more indirect approach. We could examine our response to some further variants of the Transplant Case. In Transplant Case 2 the choice of a heart transplant is between

A. A six-year-old child who will live for twenty-five years if he receives a heart, and
B. A newborn infant who will live for fifty years if he receives a heart.

Who should receive the heart in this case? (Our intuitions here may be affected by a suspicion that it is impossible to be so sure about how long an infant or child will survive. But we should try to put those intuitions aside and assume that we are able to predict, perhaps with the Carmentis Machine, that the newborn will live twice as long.) If we still are tempted to give the heart to the six-year-old, what about Transplant Case 3 where we must choose between

A. A six-year-old child who will live for one year if he receives a heart, and
B. A newborn infant who will live for fifty years if he receives a heart?

If we still think that the six-year-old child should be prioritized in this third variant of the case, it implies that a newborn infant's interest in her future life is considerably less than that of an older child, perhaps less than a fiftieth that of an older child. That may mean that we are justified in giving substantially more relative weight to other competing interests, for example the interests of families. If we are willing to give the heart to the child in Case 2 but not Case 3, the newborn's interest appears to be less than half the strength of that of the six-year-old child, but more than a fiftieth. We could repeat the case with other variations to try to get closer still to the relative strength of this interest.

However, thought experiments like this can only take us so far. The aim of such experiments is to examine our intuitive responses to different cases, to put our moral judgements under scrutiny, to try to determine which are the important elements and which are less important. But the more unusual and specialized the thought experiment, the harder it is to generate a clear intuition about the right choice, and the less reliable those intuitions seem.

It is not clear what most people would answer to Transplant Case 3. It is also not clear whether we should determine our ethical principles through population thought experiments.

But even if we can't precisely determine the strength of an infant's interest in future life two points appear clear. Firstly, an infant's interest in her future is somewhat less than an older child's or adult's. Its strength is intermediate, between that of an adult and that of a fetus. Because of this it may be outweighed by other interests in situations where an older child's would not. Secondly, the strength of a child's or infant's interest depends on the amount of well-being in their future life. In Chapter 2 we looked at some of the challenges to determining the interests of an impaired child. It is difficult to know when the burdens outweigh benefits in an infant's or child's life. Nevertheless it was clear from that analysis that impairment can affect the interests of the child. Severe physical impairment is likely to increase the intrinsically negative features of future life. Severe cognitive impairment reduces the benefits of life. Both may thus reduce the strength of the child's interest in their future. Infants and children who are predicted to have such impairments, *particularly if combined*, have a comparatively weak interest in their future life.

Let us return to the question that we started with. For Life/Death conflicts when would families' interests outweigh those of a child or infant in continuing life? For an older child, as for an adult, it is going to be rare. But, as noted by paediatrician and ethicist Norman Fost, 'No patient is entitled to infinite resources from his or her family or from society' (Fost 1999: 2041). There must come a point where the benefit to the child is so small, and the cost to the family so great that it is unreasonable to demand it of them. In Chapter 8 we will draw on several different factors to try to generate more specific guidance for this level. However, as a starting point, this is conceivably the case where a child is predicted to live for only a very short period, or alternatively where they are predicted to live for a long period but in a state of very limited consciousness (for example in a minimally conscious state). The child would potentially benefit from life-sustaining treatment; they have an interest in continued life. But this benefit, this interest may compete against a very strong family interest in not providing or continuing treatment. Although there is a good reason to have a presumption in favour of the patient, and in favour of providing life-sustaining treatment, where there is a *substantial imbalance* in the interests at stake, family interests may legitimately lead to a decision not to provide treatment.

There are two central claims in this chapter. Firstly, that family interests count in treatment decisions, either in favour or against withdrawal of treatment. And secondly, that the interests of the child herself may vary depending on her age; the interests of a newborn in continued life are somewhat less than those of an older child. These two claims fit with the way that many paediatricians already think about treatment decisions. In the study mentioned above of US intensive care doctors, paediatric and neonatal intensive care specialists were significantly more likely than adult specialists to favour a model of decision-making that gave independent weight to the interests of families (Hardart and Truog 2003). Neonatal specialists were more likely than specialists caring for critically ill older children to think that the interests of the child and of the family should be given equal weight; in other words, they appeared to pay more attention to family interests for decisions in newborn infants. The above analysis suggests that this may be warranted, because the newborn's interests are not as strong.

Objections

What objections might there be to the claims in this chapter?

Interests Do Not Vary?

Some might still not be convinced that a newborn infant's interest in her future life is any less than an older child's or adult's. Philosopher Chris Kaposy has challenged Jeff McMahan's account and argued that an infant's interest in continuing life is not diminished by his or her lack of strong psychological connections to the future (Kaposy 2007). Kaposy accepts that the infant may not care about continuing to live in the way that you or I do. But Kaposy argues that this doesn't mean that a third party, for example the infant's parents or doctor, is justified in caring any less about that future. When we are making decisions on their behalf we reflect on what the infant should care about, if he or she were able to, not what they actually do care about. If a newborn infant dies in infancy they are deprived of a future life that (we expect) would be of overall benefit. According to Kaposy we should not discount this benefit because of the infant's developmental immaturity.

Kaposy is right to point out that parents and doctors do anticipate the future for an infant in a way that the infant himself is not able to. Much of the time this is a vitally important thing for us to do because the infant is likely to survive, and we need to make sure that we promote and protect the future interests that they will have. Imagine that we had a choice between two treatments for a newborn infant. One of them is marginally more effective than the other, but has a risk of causing childhood cancer. The time-relative interests account wouldn't justify us in ignoring this future cancer risk. Although the infant now may have a relatively weak interest in his future, he or she will, in the future, have a strong interest in not developing cancer (this is an 'actual interest'). It is that interest that we should be weighing up against the potential benefit of the riskier drug. But when we are trying to make decisions in intensive care about life-sustaining treatment those future interests are not certain, they are dependent on our decision. If we decide not to continue treatment the infant will never have those stronger interests. It is much less clear whether interests count where they may or may not come to fruition. This is the issue of future preferences discussed above in response to Ben Bradley's objections to the time-relative interests account. What we saw there was that it does not make sense to think about future possible interests in the same way as future actual interests. We cannot extrapolate infants' future interests (that they will have only if we continue treatment) to a decision about *whether* we continue treatment.

For Kaposy, the infant's interest in the future is based on the benefit that he will experience if he lives. But the other problem with this argument is that it runs up against some intuitions about the cases discussed earlier. Kaposy's view would imply that the infant has a stronger interest in her future than an older child or adult; we should give the heart to the newborn infant ahead of the six-year-old in the Transplant Choice. Perhaps even more significantly, if we imagine a slightly more far-fetched example where we were faced with a choice between saving the life of a fetus or that of a child, on Kaposy's account we should save the life of the fetus instead. It is possible that Kaposy would reject this conclusion of his argument, by pointing to the greater investment that the family has made to the six-year-old than to the newborn or fetus. Could family interests justify giving the heart to the child rather than the newborn? Although this is a possible response, the idea of taking family interests and investment into account in decisions about allocating organs for transplant would have some highly counterintuitive and controversial implications. It might mean that a family with only one child would get higher priority over a family, say, who had a number of other children. It would appear to mean that a twelve-year-old would get priority over the six-year-old, an eighteen-year-old over the twelve-year-old.

Kaposy makes a separate argument that may be relevant to the moral consideration that we give to human infants (as distinct from the strength of their interests). He argues that we have a special obligation to newborn infants because of our relationship to them and because of their dependency on us for survival. That is why it is worse to kill a newborn infant than to kill a non-human animal. Although Kaposy doesn't compare the treatment of infants and older children, his argument might be extended to imply that parents and doctors have a stronger obligation to newborn infants than to older children because of their special vulnerability and dependence on others for life. Again, there is something important to this argument. The fact that newborn human infants are particularly vulnerable is important. If we fail to care for them, feed them, keep them warm, they will die. That gives us strong reasons to make sure that they are cared for, fed, and clothed, stronger reasons than apply to adults or older children who might be able to look after themselves. But critically ill infants, children, and adults are all vulnerable and dependent. The patient in need of a heart transplant will die without one, no matter their age. So the vulnerability element doesn't help us when we are trying to make decisions in intensive care. In any case, although Kaposy is right that as parents we have important obligations to our children, these obligations are not limitless, and they may clash with other obligations, for example to other members of the family. The vulnerable patient is not entitled to 'infinite resources'.

Unlimited Treatment Withdrawal?

A second objection is that allowing parents' welfare interests to be taken into account in treatment decisions would lead to parents being given free rein in decisions about life-sustaining treatment. It would potentially lead to withdrawal of life-sustaining treatment from children or infants with only mild degrees of impairment, or on the basis of relatively trivial reasons.

There are several reasons, however, why this would not follow. The first is simply that the overwhelming majority of parents have a strong desire that their infants live—even if they will be impaired. In my experience, and in the experience of other neonatologists (Wilkinson 2010), it is very rare for parents to want to withdraw life-sustaining treatment in situations where doctors believe that survival without severe impairment is probable. It is not likely that allowing parental interests to be considered would lead to withdrawal of treatment from a large number of mildly impaired infants or children.

Secondly, and more significantly, the relative balance of interests is potentially quite different for an infant or child with mild or moderate impairment. As noted above, the strength of the family's potential interest in withdrawal of treatment is likely to be proportional to the severity of impairment. The impact on parents' lives is likely to be much less for an infant with mild or moderate impairment than for a more severely affected infant. It is much more likely (at least in countries that are well-resourced), that support from the community will mitigate or eliminate the negative effects of caring for the child. What is more, for infants with mild or moderate impairments the strength of their own interest in future life may not be substantially less than that of unimpaired infants. Children or adults with mild or moderate cognitive or physical impairment are usually able to enjoy a wide range of those things that are widely regarded as valuable in human life: developing friendships, attaining goals, achieving some measure of personal independence.

Finally, the third reason that the above arguments would not lead to withdrawal of life-sustaining treatment from mildly impaired infants or children is that there is the alternative of adoption or foster care, as evident in Imogen's case mentioned previously. For infants or children who will have a life worth living, adoption would respect the interests of parents to a similar degree as allowing the infant to die. Adoption would also be consistent with the child's interest in future life. It would be better to adopt the child or infant than to allow them to die.

On the other hand, adoption would not as easily resolve the conflict in interests for infants with predicted severe impairment. Permanent adoptive parents or foster placements are significantly harder to find for children with severe impairment than for unimpaired or less impaired children (Bain 1998; Local Government Association 2001). The impact on adoptive families is also likely to be great. Children who are unable to be placed and end up in institutional care, or those who have a succession of temporary foster placements, may experience additional emotional trauma. There is a risk that as a consequence such children are harmed by ongoing life. Finally, the supportive care of such children is very expensive. One estimate from over a decade ago suggested that it cost in excess of 50,000 Australian dollars per year to support a high-needs individual in a small group home (Bain 1998).

We noted above the difficulty in coming to a clear answer about the relative strength of a newborn infant's interests compared to those of an older child's. It wasn't clear when exactly a family's interest in treatment not continuing would outweigh that of the infant. Here we see a separate factor that provides a boundary to this consideration. The availability of adoption and foster care means that family interests are only going to count in the most severe cases. Beyond that point, if family interests are going to be significantly adversely affected by caring for the child we should seek an alternative home for them.

Unacceptable Implications for Pregnancy Decisions?

A quite different objection to the arguments in this chapter is that they would potentially have serious implications for pre-natal decision-making. If a newborn infant has an interest in their future because of the well-being that they have at stake if they die, then correspondingly so too would a fetus. A term newborn infant has at least a primitive degree of self-awareness and some psychological connections with their future. But so too might a near-term fetus. If parents' interests are to be given only limited weight in newborn decision-making, then perhaps this should also apply to decisions about pregnancy. This might have major implications for the morality of abortion or for decisions about the timing or mode of delivery. Perhaps mothers would not be allowed to choose a home birth, or to decline caesarean section if this would be contrary to the interests of the fetus?

There are several reasons why the view advanced in this chapter doesn't have this implication, however. Firstly, there are relevant differences between the fetus and newborn that would potentially warrant different treatment. There is an explosive phase of synaptic development in late gestation and especially in the period immediately following birth as the newborn responds to their environment (Bourgeois 2001). The infant rapidly adapts to her changing environment and starts to develop reciprocal relationships with those around her. Some have even argued that the primitive self-consciousness evident in newborns cannot be present in uterus because of the lack of interaction that is required to manifest phenomena such as the imitative features described above (Bermudez 1996). If that is right, the psychological connections in the fetus are substantially weaker than those of the newborn even of similar maturity, and there may be significant difference in the strength of interests between the near-term fetus and the ex-utero newborn. In any case, whether or not we are convinced by the arguments about lack of self-consciousness in near-term fetuses, there is no doubt that there are substantial differences in neurodevelopment between *early* fetuses and newborn infants. Prior to twenty-weeks gestation there are no cortical synapses in the fetus and no apparent capacity for consciousness (McMahan 2002: 267). This would justify the significant difference in treatment between first-trimester fetuses and newborn infants that is present in most societies.

Secondly, there are differences in the interests at stake when the fetus is in utero, compared to the ex-utero newborn. As famously argued by Judith Jarvis Thomson, even if the fetus has an interest in their future (or a right to life) as strong as that of an adult, there may be reasons to permit a mother to have an abortion (Thomson 1971). It is beyond the scope of this book to outline Thomson's argument in detail or the many responses to it. Nevertheless, the adoption alternative discussed in the previous section makes the situation for a newborn significantly different. We might require parents who do not wish to care for an infant with moderate or mild impairment to give the child up for adoption. This would not problematically conflict with the rights of parents in the way that prohibiting abortion or forcing mothers to have a caesarean section would.

Thirdly, the above arguments imply that parental interests may be taken into account in the face of severe predicted impairment for a newborn infant, a situation not radically different from the framework currently applied to late-term fetuses, at least in some jurisdictions. In the United Kingdom, for example, abortion is permitted in the later stages of pregnancy only if there is substantial risk of serious handicap, or if there is a grave risk to the life or health of the mother (Nuffield Council on Bioethics 2006: 55). The above arguments might have implications for abortion in jurisdictions that are more restrictive about third-trimester abortion.

Conclusions

In this chapter we have been grappling with questions that make treatment decisions for children and newborn infants distinctive. If we set aside uncertainty about prognosis using the Carmentis machine, how and when should we take into account interests other than those of the child? First we looked at the interests at stake for parents and siblings in treatment withdrawal decisions. These may be affected, both positively and negatively, by the survival of the child, and they may come into conflict with the interests of the child. The influence on families is likely to be greater for children than for adults, though it will not be so in all cases.

The way in which the interests of families are affected for the worse by the burden of caring for a child with severe impairment is, at least in part, dependent on the amount of support that a society provides. The impact is likely to be significantly greater on families in developing countries. Where this impact is the result of social injustice, we should seek social change. However, until that injustice is relieved it is legitimate and reasonable to give some weight to the likely impact on families of decisions about treatment.

Secondly, we have looked at the interests at stake for the child. For those situations where the child's interest would favour withdrawal of treatment, but the interests of the family would favour continuing treatment (Death/Life conflicts), the interests of the child will usually be the stronger and determine our decisions. Yet there may be situations where the child's interest is relatively weak and is outweighed by that of parents. When analysing the opposite situation, where the child's interest is in continued life and treatment, but the family's interest lies in treatment withdrawal (Life/Death conflicts), we need to assess the child's interest in continued life. Where there is a substantial imbalance in interests, such that the harm for the family is substantial, and the benefit for the child small, this may lead to a decision to withdraw or withhold treatment. When we focused on newborn infants we saw that infants have an interest in life, and in realizing their future. However, this interest is somewhat less than the interest of an older child or adult because of their developmental immaturity. It is easier for the interests of others, particularly those of parents and siblings, to outweigh the infant's interest. It is most likely that this will be the case for newborn infants with severe impairment.

The aim of the Carmentis machine thought experiment that has been behind the analysis in Part I of the book has been to try to focus on the central questions for treatment decisions. Uncertainty can cloud and complicate decisions, and it is helpful to know what we should do if we did not have the problem of uncertain prognosis. In Chapter 2, we saw that the best interests principle on its own is well meaning, but unable to help in difficult cases. It also appears to ignore other relevant considerations. In Chapter 3 we saw that the relevance of 'replacement' is almost entirely through its effect on parental interests. The two central conclusions of this fourth chapter are, first, that family interests should be taken into account in decisions in newborn and paediatric intensive care because they may sometimes outweigh the interests of the child, and second, that this is more likely to be the case for newborn infants than for older children. This difference in treatment between older and younger seems to imply a difference in moral status. But this difference is not because newborn infants are less valuable or valued, nor because they warrant a lesser degree of moral consideration. We have seen, rather, that the strength of their interest at stake, the harm to them if they die, is arguably less than that of an older individual.

It is time now to step back from the Carmentis machine. With a clearer idea of the relevant interests at stake we should now look at the role of uncertainty in decision-making. It may be some time before we have a machine that is able to provide a perfect prognosis for critically ill children and infants. Perhaps we will never have one. We need to assess how to make decisions in the face of uncertainty.

References

Andreou, C. (2008). 'Dynamic Choice', *The Stanford Encyclopedia of Philosophy*, ed. E. Zalta, <http://plato.stanford.edu/entries/dynamic-choice/>.

Bae, J., M. Jang, et al. (2008). 'Prolonged survival to adulthood of an individual with hydranencephaly', *Clinical neurology and neurosurgery* 110(3): 307–9.

Bain, K.J. (1998). 'Children with severe disabilities: options for residential care', *Med J Aust* 169(11–12): 598–600.

Bermudez, J.L. (1996). 'The moral significance of birth', *Ethics* 106(2): 378–403.

—— (2001). 'Nonconceptual self-consciousness and cognitive science', *Synthese* 129(1): 129–49.

Boonin, D. (2002). *In Defense of Abortion*. Cambridge: Cambridge University Press.

Bornstein, M., M. Arterberry, et al. (2004). 'Long term memory for an emotional interpersonal interaction occurring at 5 months of age', *Infancy* 6(3): 407–16.

Bourgeois, J.-P. (2001). 'Synaptogenesis in the neocortex of the newborn: the ultimate frontier for individuation?', in C. Nelson and M. Luciana (eds), *Handbook of Developmental Cognitive Neuroscience*. Cambridge, MA: MIT Press.

Bradley, B. (2008). 'The worst time to die', *Ethics* 118(2): 291–314.

—— (2009). *Well-Being and Death*. Oxford: Clarendon Press.

Brinchmann, B.S. (1999). 'When the home becomes a prison: living with a severely disabled child', *Nurs Ethics* 6(2): 137–43.

Broome, J. (2004). *Weighing Lives*. Oxford: Oxford University Press.

Bush, A., J. Fraser, et al. (2005). 'Respiratory management of the infant with type 1 spinal muscular atrophy', *Arch Dis Child* 90(7): 709–11.

Corman, H. and R. Kaestner (1992). 'The effects of child health on marital status and family structure', *Demography* 29(3): 389–408.

Crisp, R. (2006). 'Hedonism Reconsidered', *Philosophy and Phenomenological Research* 73(3): 619–45.

Cummins, R. (2001). 'The subjective well-being of people caring for a family member with a severe disability at home: a review', *Journal of Intellectual and Developmental Disability* 26(1): 83–100.

Curran, A.L., P.M. Sharples, et al. (2001). 'Time costs of caring for children with severe disabilities compared with caring for children without disabilities', *Dev Med Child Neurol* 43(8): 529–33.

Dawson, A. (2005). 'The determination of the best interests in relation to childhood immunisation', *Bioethics* 19(1): 72–89.

DeGrazia, D. (1995). 'Value theory and the best interests standard', *Bioethics* 9(1): 50–61.

—— (2007). 'The harm of death, time-relative interests and abortion', *Philosophical Forum* 38(1): 57–80.

—— (2008). 'Moral Status As a Matter of Degree?', *The Southern Journal of Philosophy* 46(2): 181–98.

Findler, L. and A. Vardi (2009). 'Psychological growth among siblings of children with and without intellectual disabilities', *Intellect Dev Disabil* 47(1): 1–12.

Fost, N. (1999). 'Decisions regarding treatment of seriously ill newborns', *JAMA* 281(21): 2041–3.

Gallagher, S. (1996). 'The moral significance of primitive self-consciousness: a response to Bermudez', *Ethics* 107(1): 129–40.

Geevasinga, N. and M.M. Ryan (2007). 'Physician attitudes towards ventilatory support for spinal muscular atrophy type 1 in Australasia', *J Paediatr Child Health* 43(12): 790–4.

Griffin, J. (1986). *Well-Being: Its Meaning, Measurement and Moral Importance.* Oxford: Clarendon.

Hardart, G.E. and R.D. Truog (2003). 'Attitudes and preferences of intensivists regarding the role of family interests in medical decision making for incompetent patients', *Crit Care Med* 31(7): 1895–900.

Hartshorn, K. (2003). 'Reinstatement maintains a memory in human infants for 1 (1/2) years', *Dev Psychobiol* 42(3): 269–82.

Hayne, H. (2004). 'Infant memory development: implications for childhood amnesia', *Developmental Review* 24: 33–73.

Hollander, J. (2008). *When the Bough Breaks: A Mother's Tale.* London: John Murray.

Janvier, A., I. Leblanc, et al. (2008a). 'The best-interest standard is not applied for neonatal resuscitation decisions', *Pediatrics* 121(5): 963–9.

―――― (2008b). 'Nobody likes premies: the relative value of patients' lives', *Journal of Perinatology* 28: 821–6.

Kaposy, C. (2007). 'Can infants have interests in continued life?', *Theor Med Bioeth* 28(4): 301–30.

Kuhse, H. and P. Singer (1985). *Should the Baby Live? The Problem of Handicapped Infants.* Oxford: Oxford University Press.

Lagercrantz, H. and J.P. Changeux (2009). 'The emergence of human consciousness: from fetal to neonatal life', *Pediatr Res* 65(3): 255–60.

Leonard, B., J.D. Brust, et al. (1992). 'Financial and time costs to parents of severely disabled children', *Public Health Rep* 107(3): 302–12.

Local Government Association (2001). Memorandum submitted by the Local Government Association. Adoption and Children Bill. Select Committee on Adoption and Children Bill.

Locke, J. (2004). *An Essay Concerning Human Understanding.* Adelaide: eBooks@-Adelaide.

Marquis, D. (1989). 'Why abortion is immoral', *Journal of Philosophy* 86: 183–202.

Martin, G. and R. Clark (1982). 'Distress crying in neonates: species and peer specificity', *Developmental Psychology* 18(1): 3–9.

McAbee, G.N., A. Chan, et al. (2000). 'Prolonged survival with hydranencephaly: report of two patients and literature review', *Pediatr Neurol* 23(1): 80–4.

McMahan, J. (2002). *The Ethics of Killing: Problems at the Margins of Life.* New York: Oxford University Press.

Meltzoff, A.N. and M.K. Moore (1977). 'Imitation of facial and manual gestures by human neonates', *Science* 198(4312): 74–8.

―― (1983). 'Newborn infants imitate adult facial gestures', *Child Dev* 54(3): 702–9.

—— —— (1994). 'Imitation, memory and the representation of persons', *Infant Behaviour and Development* 17: 83–99.
Miljeteig, I. and O.F. Norheim (2006). 'My job is to keep him alive, but what about his brother and sister? How Indian doctors experience ethical dilemmas in neonatal medicine', *Dev World Bioeth* 6(1): 23–32.
—— S.A. Sayeed, et al. (2009). 'Impact of ethics and economics on end-of-life decisions in an Indian neonatal unit', *Pediatrics* 124(2): e322–8.
Murphy, N.A., B. Christian, et al. (2007). 'The health of caregivers for children with disabilities: caregiver perspectives', *Child Care Health Dev* 33(2): 180–7.
Nuffield Council on Bioethics (2006). *Critical Care Decisions in Fetal and Neonatal Medicine: Ethical Issues*. London: Nuffield Council on Bioethics.
O'Brian, I., A. Duffy, et al. (2009). 'Impact of childhood chronic illnesses on siblings: a literature review', *British Journal of Nursing* 18(22): 1358–1365.
Oishi, S. and U. Schimmack (2010). 'Residential mobility, well-being, and mortality', *Journal of Personality and Social Psychology* 98(6): 980–94.
Olsson, M.B. and C.P. Hwang (2001). 'Depression in mothers and fathers of children with intellectual disability', *J Intellect Disabil Res* 45(Pt 6): 535–43.
Parfit, D. (1984). *Reasons and Persons*. Oxford: Oxford University Press.
Plato (2010). *Cratylus*. Boston: Actonian Press.
Raina, P., M. O'Donnell, et al. (2005). 'The health and well-being of caregivers of children with cerebral palsy', *Pediatrics* 115(6): e626–36.
Rebagliato, M., M. Cuttini, et al. (2000). 'Neonatal end-of-life decision making: Physicians' attitudes and relationship with self-reported practices in 10 European countries', *JAMA* 284(19): 2451–9.
Regan, T. (1983). *The Case for Animal Rights*. London: Routledge.
Reichman, N.E., H. Corman, et al. (2004). 'Effects of child health on parents' relationship status', *Demography* 41(3): 569–84.
—— —— —— (2008). 'Impact of child disability on the family', *Matern Child Health J* 12(6): 679–83.
Re RB (A Child) 2009 EWHC 3269 (Fam).
Ross, L.F. (2007). 'The moral status of the newborn and its implications for medical decision making', *Theor Med Bioeth* 28(5): 349–55.
Sakakihara, Y., M. Kubota, et al. (2000). 'Long-term ventilator support in patients with Werdnig-Hoffmann disease', *Pediatr Int* 42(4): 359–63.
Sharpe, D. and L. Rossiter (2002). 'Siblings of children with a chronic illness: a meta-analysis', *J Pediatr Psychol* 27(8): 699–710.
Shaw, A., J.G. Randolph, et al. (1977). 'Ethical issues in pediatric surgery: a national survey of pediatricians and pediatric surgeons', *Pediatrics* 60(4 Pt 2): 588–99.

Sheffield, K. (2007). 'Not compatible with life, a diary of keeping Daniel', <http://www.trisomyoz.bounce.com.au/#/danielsbook/4528173715>.

Shewmon, D.A., G.L. Holmes, et al. (1999). 'Consciousness in congenitally decorticate children: developmental vegetative state as self-fulfilling prophecy', *Dev Med Child Neurol* 41(6): 364–74.

Singer, P. (1993). *Practical Ethics*. Cambridge: Cambridge University Press.

Styron, W. (1992). *Sophie's Choice*. New York: Vintage International.

Taddio, A., M. Goldbach, et al. (1995). 'Effect of neonatal circumcision on pain responses during vaccination in boys', *Lancet* 345(8945): 291–2.

Thomson, J. (1971). 'A defense of abortion', *Philos Public Aff* 1(1): 47–66.

Thyen, U., K. Kuhlthau, et al. (1999). 'Employment, child care, and mental health of mothers caring for children assisted by technology', *Pediatrics* 103(6 Pt 1): 1235–42.

Todres, I.D., J. Guillemin, et al. (1988). 'Life-saving therapy for newborns: a questionnaire survey in the state of Massachusetts', *Pediatrics* 81(5): 643–9.

Tooley, M. (1972). 'Abortion and infanticide', *Philosophy and Public Affairs* 2(1): 37–65.

Wilkinson, D. (2010). '"We don't have a crystal ball": neonatologists views on prognosis and decision-making in newborn infants with birth asphyxia', *Monash Bioethics Review* 29(1): 5.1–5.19.

Wyn, N. (2007). *Blue Sky July*. Bridgend: Seren.

Yorgason, B. (2003). *One Tattered Angel: A Touching True Story of the Power of Love*. Salt Lake City: Shadow Mountain.

PART II

Predictions and Disability in Rome

Disability or deformity was one potential motivator for infanticide or exposure in Rome. The Greek-born physician Soranus, who wrote one of the earliest textbooks of gynecology/midwifery, and who lived in Rome for part of his life, provided a stringent list of characteristics for parents to take into account, when deciding whether or not to keep an infant alive. These included activity and vigour after birth, birth at full term, and absence of physical abnormalities.

How to recognise the newborn that is worth rearing:...By the fact that when put on the earth it immediately cries with proper vigor...also by the fact that it is perfect in all its parts, members and senses...that the natural functions of every <member> are neither sluggish nor weak...And by conditions contrary to those mentioned, the infant not worth rearing is recognised. (Soranus of Ephesus 1991: 79–80)

There may also have been a legal sanction against keeping deformed infants alive. The statute books of Rome have not survived, but one of the much cited laws of the Twelve Table apparently instructed parents to kill conspicuously deformed infants.

Deinde quom esset cito necatus tamquam ex XII tabulis insignis ad deformitatem puer, brevi tempore nescio IX quo pacto recreatus multoque taetrior et foedior natus est. (Cicero: Book 3, 19)

However, Cicero in this passage was not quoting the law directly, but was using it to complain about a law that established the power of plebeian tribunes. (He was suggesting by analogy that this particular law was deformed, and should be euthanized) (Coleman-Norton 1950).

Furthermore, there are various versions of Cicero's text, and there is some evidence that it was altered after he wrote it. Nevertheless it fits with other comments that deformed infants were killed after birth. How severe a physical abnormality would lead to such a decision? There is no clear answer from the texts. Cicero referred to 'insignis ad deformitatem puer' 'a boy notably deformed', while Seneca referred to 'si debiles monstrosique editi sunt' 'if they have been born weak and monstrous' (Rawson 2003).

Both suggest that it may have been particularly severe abnormalities that were treated in this way. However, there must also have been some discretion about these decisions, since there are descriptions of some adults who survived with disabilities, perhaps most notably the emperor Claudius, who is said to have had congenital talipes (clubfoot). Some historians have suggested that, contrary to the usual view, many disabled infants were allowed to live (Harris 1994).

Why did the Romans treat physically abnormal infants in this way? Soranus' features listed above may have been, like contemporary prognostic factors, useful in part because of their ability to predict the quantity of life. Severe physical malformations including imperforate anus, spina bifida, and perhaps even forms of cleft palate would have been likely to lead to death in early infancy or childhood even if infants were not actively killed or exposed. One potential reason why infanticide was chosen for deformed or disabled infants is that the infants would have been unlikely to have been adopted and survived exposure (Boswell 1984). But a second reason that was important to the Romans was that such physical abnormalities were often seen as very bad omens. Seneca claimed that families sometimes exposed infants in response to evil omens, and there is a story that the emperor Augustus' father had considered killing him in infancy because of an evil prophecy (Harris 1994).

References

Boswell, J. (1984). 'Expositio and oblatio: the abandonment of children and the ancient and modern family', *The American historical review* 89(1): 10–33.

Cicero, De legibus [On the laws], <http://www.thelatinlibrary.com/cicero/leg3.shtml>.

Coleman-Norton, P. (1950). 'Cicero's contribution to the text of the twelve tables', *The Classical Journal* 46(2): 51–60.

Harris, W.V. (1994). 'Child-Exposure in the Roman Empire', *Journal of Roman Studies* 84: 1–22.

Rawson, B. (2003). *Children and Childhood in Roman Italy*. Oxford, New York: Oxford University Press.

Soranus of Ephesus (1991). *Soranus' Gynecologyy*. Baltimore: Johns Hopkins University Press.

5

Sources of Uncertainty—Prognostic Research

> It's tough to make predictions, especially about the future. Yogi Berra[1]

Why is there uncertainty for critically ill infants and children? Why can't doctors determine with confidence whether or not a patient will survive, whether if they survive they will be impaired, and if so how? Doctors have been providing intensive care to sick children and newborn infants for more than forty years. It seems like it shouldn't be that hard to study a large cohort of patients, follow them up, and see what the outcome is, which ones do well, and which ones do poorly. And yet there remains considerable doubt. For many patients in intensive care the possible outcomes range from death, to survival with severe impairment, to survival without any long-term problems.

In this chapter we will look at some of the reasons why prognosis is uncertain. Some elements are unavoidable, and relate to intrinsic differences between patients in their response to an injury or illness. But other contributors to uncertainty are potentially avoidable, and relate to serious flaws in the way that researchers have performed prognostic research. We will look at the example of newborn birth asphyxia and the new technique of MRI. This will hopefully shed some light on why doctors have trouble with predictions. It will also reveal the value assumptions that undermine the usefulness of some of this research. In the second part of the chapter, we will investigate in some more detail a particular problem for outcome studies in

---

[1] Rabinstein, A.A. and J.C. Hemphill (2010). 'Prognosticating after severe acute brain disease: science, art, and biases', *Neurology* 74(14): 1086–7. Ironically, the provenance of this quotation is uncertain, and has also been attributed to Niels Bohr and Mark Twain, among others. *Economist*, 15 July 2007, 'The perils of prediction', <http://www.economist.com/blogs/theinbox/2007/07/the_perils_of_prediction_june>, <http://www.larry.denenberg.com/predictions.html>.

intensive care—that of self-fulfilling prophecies. Finally, since this is what is potentially most relevant for decisions we will also look a little at the evidence on quality of life for children and adults with severe impairment. We will examine evidence about the quality of life of individuals with severe cerebral palsy. Unfortunately this research is unable to answer the most difficult and important questions for treatment decisions.

Uncertainty in Prognosis

One difficulty for predicting outcome is that patients differ in the physical effect of similar insults. It appears that genetic differences may affect the amount of brain damage that a child suffers as a result of a given insult, but also the amount of recovery that they ultimately make. One example is the wide spectrum of illness in children who contract meningococcal infection. Some children are asymptomatic, others develop meningitis, inflammation of the external lining of the brain and spinal cord, others still develop septicaemia and multi-organ failure with disturbance of the body's clotting system. One study of more than 500 children with meningococcal infection in the UK found that a single variant in a gene that is involved in the normal coagulation process was associated with a doubling in the risk of death in children with meningococcal infection (Haralambous, Hibberd, et al. 2003). Animal models support the importance of genetic factors in the susceptibility to brain injury. Different strains of mice who all had identical mechanisms of brain injury (ligation of one of the main arteries supplying the brain) had significant variations in their risk of dying, and in the severity of brain damage (Sheldon, Sedik, et al. 1998). Human data is not as clear-cut, but, as an example, fairly commonplace genetic variations appear to affect the risk of developing cerebral palsy in very preterm infants (Nelson, Dambrosia, et al. 2005).

Apart from variations in physical susceptibility and recovery from injury there are also differences in psychological susceptibility, in the ability of individuals to adjust and cope with adversity. Different children have different degrees of resilience to injury or illness (Masten, Best, et al. 1990). Some cope extraordinarily well with major setbacks and challenges, others struggle with apparently less severe insults. Resilience is partly innate, and relates to differences in temperament and personality, but it is also significantly affected by the environment that children find themselves in, for example the amount of support provided by friends and family (Bradley, Whiteside, et al. 1994; Werner 2004).

A third factor that contributes to variations between individuals and to uncertainty in prognosis is neural plasticity. When areas of the central nervous system are injured there is a relatively limited amount of physical repair that is able to occur in damaged tissues. Unlike many other cells in the body, neurons in a mature individual have very little capacity to re-grow or regenerate. However, there is another possibility, that undamaged areas of the brain take over the functions that have been lost, or that pathways that would previously have traversed the area of damage detour around it instead (Johnston, Ishida, et al. 2009). This plasticity, the capacity of the brain to work around damaged areas of brain and restore function by developing alternative ways of performing tasks, is limited in adults but much greater in newborn infants or young children. The brain of a newborn infant is like a town or city whose streets have been marked out on the ground but not yet paved. It is much easier to accommodate unforeseen changes at that early stage than after the roads have been laid, rolled, and the tarmac is dry. That is the reason why a unilateral left-sided stroke in an adult, with the loss of blood supply to the area of the brain supplied by the middle cerebral artery, can lead to major physical impairment (severe weakness on one side of the body) and loss of the ability to use language. But the same lesion in a newborn infant usually leads to a much milder degree of long-term physical impairment (often none at all) and normal language and cognitive function (Ballantyne, Spilkin, et al. 2008). However, at this stage of our knowledge plasticity is hard to predict. Some individuals appear to manifest substantial plasticity, and have very little functional deficit from major injury. Others appear less able to remodel and are much more seriously affected.

As well as differences in genetic make-up there are also important differences in the environment in which children find themselves. These differences, in the amount of nurturing and support that a family provides, in the amount of stimulation that the child is exposed to, in the availability of therapies, tailored educational support, and rehabilitation, may be even more important than the innate differences within the child. The amount of external support may be predictable. For example a child may be fortunate to be born in a society with ample publicly funded medical and educational support for children with illness and impairment, and in a supportive and well-resourced family. However, there is always going to be some uncertainty about just how much time parents are going to devote to the child's needs and about the level of external services the child will receive. Other illnesses may also affect recovery. Infants with perinatal stroke who develop seizures have reduced functional plasticity (Ballantyne, Spilkin, et al. 2008). In addition, there is always the possibility that new types of services will be funded or developed, or that new treatments will become available. It is hard to predict how likely those currently unavailable or hypothetical treatments/interventions are to materialize, and how likely it is that they will change the outcome for the child.

Finally, it is worth noting a more general concern about prognosis, and the sort of inference that is required to make predictions. When we study a group of patients with a given problem and measure their outcome, we can assess the frequency of a particular outcome. Imagine that we have found that one-third of patients with illness X either die or are severely impaired. The number of patients that we have studied affects how confident we can be that if we repeated the study we would find the same or similar proportion of patients to have that outcome. If we have studied a very large number of patients, it is reasonably likely that one-third of future patients with the same illness and treated in the same way would die or be impaired. We are able to make an inference about the likely *frequency* of this outcome. But what we are really interested in, for prognosis, is not the frequency of that outcome in the population, but the *probability* of it occurring in an individual. We extrapolate from frequency data in cohort studies to estimate the probability of an outcome for an individual patient. However, that extrapolation may or may not be justified. Think about the next 100 children with condition X. Although we would expect thirty-three of them to die or be severely impaired, it isn't the case that each of those infants have a one-third chance of this outcome. Some may actually have only a very small chance of this outcome, while others may have a 100 per cent chance of being severely impaired if they survive. What parents want to know is the outcome for their infant, and the probability for their infant. Yet, there is a sense in which this information, the most important information, is simply not knowable.

This general concern about prognosis and inference from the general to the particular, from the global to the individual, might be taken too far. While it is true that we can't know the probability for individuals, information from population studies gives us the best way, probably the only way to estimate prognosis. The above factors (plasticity, genetic variation, environmental differences, etc.) give us reasons why the probability for an individual might deviate from that of a group, but the better the data, the closer that the patient resembles the studied group, the closer that the actual probability will be to this estimate.

Some of the above factors contributing to uncertainty differ between young infants and older individuals. We have already noted that newborns have a much greater degree of plasticity. One of the reasons why plasticity appears to vary between children is likely to be that the child's environment influences how well the brain is able to remodel. Because infancy and early childhood is a critical period for neurodevelopment, there is a much greater capacity for the infant to overcome their injury, but also a greater capacity for differences in the environment to influence that process. (The newborn period may also be a period of greater vulnerability to injury. In one study young children who had severe traumatic brain injury have worse long-term outcomes than older children with similar severity of brain injury (Anderson, Catroppa, et al. 2005).) Secondly, because of the length of time before adulthood, and the potential length of life ahead of infants and young children, there may be greater uncertainty about the possibility of novel, unheralded, treatments to improve their long-term function. And the third factor that potentially makes prognosis more difficult, and inherently more uncertain than in older children and adults, is a difference in clinical information available. Infants are more challenging to assess neurologically—their limited repertoire of skills means that neurological assessment is necessarily more broad-brush, and more uncertain. Furthermore, for infants for whom we have no information about prior function, we simply assume that they have the capacity to reach normal function unless there is evidence to the contrary. However, an older child or adult will have had time to demonstrate that they do or do not (prior to their acute illness) have certain capacities or functions. Although it is hard to predict how much worse off a patient is going to be following a critical illness, it is rare that a patient recovers to have *greater* function after their stay in intensive care than before.

Variations in innate susceptibility, resilience, plasticity, and environmental influences make prognosis one of the hardest tasks for a physician. Advances in technology and in knowledge may overcome some of these. For example, it may be possible in the future to identify some of the genetic determinants of variation. Combining this knowledge with detailed and accurate assessments of the severity of brain injury may give us a way to narrow our confidence intervals for predictions as imagined in the Carmentis machine. But what about current science? How close can we get with current technology to certainty?

Research in Prognosis—The Example of Birth Asphyxia

In Chapter 1 we looked at the use of magnetic resonance imaging (MRI) for prognosis in newborn infants with hypoxic-ischaemic encephalopathy (HIE). MRI is used by clinicians to help with decisions about treatment limitation for infants with HIE, and it is potentially one of the most important pieces of evidence prior to such decisions. How reliable is MRI or related technology at predicting outcome for infants with HIE? Which findings on MRI are the most useful?

There have been hundreds of research studies and papers published in the last twenty years relating to magnetic resonance imaging in this population. However, only a minority of these studies are really relevant to the question at hand. A recently published systematic review gathered together those studies that had performed an MRI or related test on newborn infants with HIE and looked at its relationship with the infants' outcome at one year of age or later. (This is probably the earliest point at which it is possible to get a reliable idea of the presence or severity of developmental problems in infants.)

Sudhin Thayyil and colleagues from University College London identified thirty-two studies including a total of 860 newborn infants with HIE (Thayyil, Chandrasekaran, et al. 2010). Their detailed analysis found MR spectroscopy (using MRI to assess the levels of different tissue metabolites) to be more accurate for predicting neurodevelopmental impairment than conventional imaging (MRI pictures of brain structure). In particular, they found that the ratio of two neurotransmitters in a deep part of the brain, the basal ganglia lactate/N-acetylaspartate peak/area ratio (Lac/NAA), was the most accurate prognostic marker for predicting adverse neurodevelopmental outcome. Abnormally high levels of this marker were present in 82 per cent of those infants who went on to have an adverse outcome (i.e. the test missed 18 per cent of infants with a bad outcome). Only 5 per cent of those infants with HIE who had elevated Lac/NAA did *not* have an adverse outcome measured at twelve months of age or later. In comparison, the presence of abnormal patterns on conventional MRI detected 91 per cent of infants with a later adverse outcome, but it had an almost 50 per cent false positive rate; half of the infants with abnormal patterns on MRI did not end up having a bad outcome.

The findings of this meta-analysis appear at first glance encouraging. At least some patterns on MRI appear to be pretty sensitive and highly specific for predicting an adverse outcome. In their review, Thayyil and colleagues suggested that abnormal Lac/NAA may be useful to help identify infants with the most severe brain injury, and help clinicians make 'objective decisions about the most appropriate clinical management' (Thayyil, Chandrasekaran, et al. 2010: e393). They do not explicitly discuss whether or not this includes decisions about the continuation or withdrawal of life-sustaining treatment. But this is arguably the most important management decision for infants with HIE. Do the results of the meta-analysis support the use of Lac/NAA to help decide about treatment withdrawal? Should the results of conventional MRI *not* be used in decision-making given their low specificity? When we look in more detail at the studies a number of problems become apparent.

Size

The first concern that we might have is about the size of the studies. The largest study that has looked at MRI and outcome in HIE studied 131 infants (it was part of a much larger randomized controlled trial) (Rutherford, Ramenghi, et al. 2010). However, half of the thirty-two studies included less than twenty-five infants. One of the strengths of meta-analysis is that it allows us to pool together small studies to have a larger sample size. But where most of the studies included in a meta-analysis are small, and there are few or no large studies (131 is still a fairly small sample) there is a greater risk that the results of the meta-analysis will be misleading (Egger and Smith 1995). Related to this concern, almost half of infants studied (in those studies that provided information about this) had either 'mild' or 'severe' encephalopathy (Sarnat stage 1 or 3). But infants with this level of HIE are not usually prognostically difficult. Those whose encephalopathy is classified as mild almost always have a very good long-term neurodevelopmental outcome; there is no question about whether or not intensive care should be continued. (Such infants usually do not need mechanical ventilation in any case.) Conversely, those with severe encephalopathy almost always have a very poor long-term outcome. If parents agree, clinicians would often be prepared to withdraw life support and allow such infants to die. It is the ones in between, infants with *moderate* HIE, where there is a genuine question about whether or not treatment should continue, and where MRI is potentially informative. The problem is that the inclusion of significant numbers of very mildly, or very severely, affected infants potentially distorts assessment of the usefulness of prognostic tests—it exaggerates the calculated sensitivity and specificity (measures of accuracy) of the test.

Selection Bias

Next, few of the studies cited by Thayyil and colleagues describe in any detail the population from which studied infants were drawn. This raises questions about how representative the samples are, and consequently how generalizable the results are. It potentially makes a big difference to our interpretation of the results if studies have come from specialized centres that are only referred the most severe, or most complex cases, or if most patients with the illness are excluded from study for one reason or another. In one MRI study (that did actually report the source population), out of 259 infants who met the inclusion criteria, only thirty-two had imaging and completed follow-up (Barkovich, Hajnal, et al. 1998). More than half of the parents of eligible infants declined to consent for the research, other infants were excluded because it was suspected that they had other medical conditions than just HIE, and others did not have follow-up data. Nine of the thirty-two studies in the meta-analysis included only surviving infants with HIE, making their results potentially less relevant to questions about withdrawal of intensive care.

Timing of Assessment

Studies of MRI in infants with HIE have varied in the timing of magnetic resonance imaging. Some of the studies in the meta-analysis performed scans in the first days of life, while others deferred imaging until after the first week. But the pattern of changes in brain imaging changes over time after a hypoxic brain injury, and the timing of imaging may be crucial if it is to be used in treatment limitation decisions. In infants with moderate or severe encephalopathy in recent trials, the majority of deaths relating to withdrawal of treatment occurred in the first three or four days of life (Gluckman, Wyatt, et al. 2005; Shankaran, Laptook, et al. 2005). Scans performed in non-ventilated infants in the second week of life are potentially much less relevant to treatment limitation decisions.

Self-Fulfilling Prophecies

Many of the studies of prognosis in HIE include death as an adverse outcome. But if treatment withdrawal decisions are influenced by prognostic tests, there is the potential for what are sometimes referred to as 'self-fulfilling prophecies'. This is a particular problem for assessing prognosis in conditions like HIE where a large proportion of deaths follow decisions to limit treatment. We will return to the general implications of this problem shortly. Interestingly, in only one of the studies included in the systematic review was there discussion of the potential relationship between MRI and treatment withdrawal decisions. That study acknowledged that MRI results were available to clinicians making such decisions, and potentially influenced withdrawal (Hunt, Neil, et al. 2004). The authors of the meta-analysis attempt to reduce the problem by considering outcomes of death or severe impairment together. This is only a partial solution since it depends upon the assumption that all infants who have treatment withdrawn would have survived with severe impairment. It also obscures for decision-makers a potentially relevant difference between death from multi-organ failure in the newborn period and survival with severe impairment.

Outcome Measurement

Importantly, studies of MRI in newborn infants have largely used vague and non-standardized means of assessing outcome. Only twelve of the thirty-two studies included in the systematic review reported blinding of outcome assessment to MRI results. (This raises the possibility that doctors who were aware of adverse findings on MRI looked harder for neurological abnormalities when they reviewed the infants in clinic, or rated them as more severe.) A particularly serious problem is that studies pooled a wide range of different outcomes together as abnormal. In many studies infants were classified as having an 'unfavourable outcome' if they had scores on developmental assessment that were more than one standard deviation below the mean. Other studies included infants in the unfavourable outcome category if they had any neurological abnormality. Infants with mild developmental delay or treatable epilepsy were considered together with infants with spastic quadriplegic cerebral palsy. On the basis of the published studies it appears that 95 per cent of infants who have high lactate levels in the basal ganglia will have an 'adverse outcome'. But the variability in classification of outcome between studies makes this information of questionable relevance for treatment withdrawal decisions. Are doctors and parents willing to withdraw intensive care from an infant who could survive with a mild form of physical impairment or mild developmental delay?

Testing in Isolation

Finally, there is a problem with many studies in that they consider a single test in isolation. So, for example, a study might report the relationship of MRI with outcome in infants with birth asphyxia, but not report the results of other important prognostic tests such as the infants' EEG or their clinical condition. The problem with this is that it makes it hard to assess how the test compares with other, existing, prognostic markers. The way that clinicians make decisions for newborn infants with birth asphyxia, or for other critically ill infants and children in intensive care, is to put together different pieces of evidence about prognosis. What would be most useful would be to know which combination of tests and clinical signs at a particular point in time is indicative of an unfavourable outcome.

Severe Disability

What does it mean to say that an individual is severely disabled? There are some standard definitions of severity. The World Health Organisation produced a classification system for disability in 2001 (the International Classification of Functioning, Disability and Health, ICF), to complement its widely used disease classification system (WHO 2001). The ICF distinguishes different elements to a disability. The severity of impairments of body function or structure, or the severity of impact on activities or participation, is related to the amount of time that the impairment is present, and the degree of disruption of day-to-day life.

A 'severe' impairment or difficulty is one that is present at least 50 per cent of the time and partially disruptive of the individual's day-to-day life. In comparison a 'complete' impairment or difficulty is present more than 95 per cent of the time and totally disrupts their day-to-day life. A 'moderate' impairment is present 25–50 per cent of the time, with sufficient intensity to interfere with day-to-day life.

The ICF allows (and encourages) disabilities to be graded in a multidimensional way, and distinguishes severe impairments of body function, from severe difficulties with activities or participation. So, for example, an individual might have a severe impairment of body function (for example they may be severely visually impaired), but have a moderate or mild difficulty in daily activities or social participation. Although the categories are vague, they are explicitly related to the impact on regular day-to-day activities, for example mobility, communication, self-care, learning, and applying knowledge.

There are other classification systems of specific types of impairment. For example, there is a standard classification system of intellectual impairment based on intelligence tests that relates severity to the normal distribution of intelligence and to ranges of intelligence quotient scores. For someone to be diagnosed with intellectual disability they must have a score on intelligence tests more than two standard deviations below the mean, with an accompanying difficulty in adaptive functioning. Severe cognitive impairment or intellectual disability refers to individuals with IQ approximately five standard deviations below the mean, or a score of 20–35 (Lin 2003). Individuals with severe impairment usually also have impairment of motor skills, and limited communication ability. Most require close supervision and care throughout life. Those with profound impairment (IQ <20) are only able to achieve even rudimentary self-care tasks with extensive training, and require total supervision and care (King, Hodapp, et al. 2000; Harris 2006). These categories overlap with the 'severe' and 'complete' categories of the ICF. By contrast, children and adults with moderate intellectual impairment (IQ range 35–50) are usually able to interact socially and able to carry out basic conversations. They usually require supported accommodation and employment, but may learn to travel independently.

What about other disabilities? Cerebral palsy is one of the most common and significant physically disabling conditions in children, and manifests in abnormal tone and muscle function. It is sometimes classified according to the number of limbs affected (monoplegia, diplegia, triplegia, or quadriplegia) and the type of abnormality of muscle tone or function (e.g. spastic, athetoid or dystonic, ataxic, and hypotonic). In more recent years a functional classification system has been developed, the Gross Motor Functional Classification System (GMFCS), that grades function from level 1 (walking without assistance) through level 3 (walking with assisted mobility devices) to level 5 (severely limited mobility) (Palisano, Rosenbaum, et al. 1997). 'Severe' cerebral palsy usually refers to those children who are unable to walk (GMFCS levels 4 and 5).

However, these categories of severity are not always applied consistently in outcome studies of infants or children. For example, in several large studies of infants with birth asphyxia (in the setting of randomized trials of a new treatment for asphyxia) 'severe' neurodisability was used for children with developmental scores (a proxy for later intelligence testing) of more than two standard deviations below the mean (<70), a GMFCS score of 3–5, blindness, or deafness (Ambalavanan, Carlo, et al. 2006; Rutherford, Ramenghi, et al. 2010). Similarly, a widely cited study of MRI in very preterm infants classified infants with developmental scores more than two standard deviations below the mean as having severe psychomotor delay (Woodward, Anderson, et al. 2006). A very large UK study of outcome for extremely preterm infants used a classification system of disability that classified children as severely disabled if they had a developmental score more than three standard deviations below the mean, were not able to sit or to walk without assistance, profound deafness despite a hearing aid, or blindness (Marlow, Wolke, et al. 2005).

There are several reasons why studies may have used a more generous definition of severe disability or impairment than the formal definitions provided above. One is that when children are assessed for their development at one or two years of age it may not be possible to clearly distinguish between very low levels of cognitive ability. In addition sensory impairments may make it difficult to apply standard developmental tests. A second reason is that for studies that are trying to develop treatments or improve outcome for critically ill infants or children it may be easier and require a smaller sample if a more inclusive definition is used. A third reason is that some of these definitions have focused on body function or structure rather than on functional impacts on activities and social participation. Again, these functional impacts may be more difficult to reliably distinguish at very young ages.

At one level it does not matter what terms we use. It is in a sense arbitrary whether we use 'severe' to refer to impairment that is two or three or four or five standard deviations from the normal range, or use it to refer to those who are wheelchair bound, or include all of those who need assistance with mobilizing (for example with a frame, or walker, or splints). But when we call something 'severe' there are particular connotations. The *Oxford English Dictionary* notes that a severe disease or illness is one that is 'attended with a maximum of pain or distress', and that, used as a descriptor of suffering or loss, it implies a 'grievous or extreme degree'. It is a 'thick' concept, one that simply by its use can carry connotations about what we ought to do. Other words that are used to describe certain outcomes from intensive care (e.g. 'poor', 'unfavourable', or 'adverse') also connote that such states are particularly negative. The language that we use to describe these states may be appropriate, but we should make sure that we do not prejudge the questions about what we should do by the language that we use.

What is most important is that doctors are consistent when they communicate with parents. If a particular prognostic factor or brain scan has been found to be associated with 'severe' disability, it is important to know what that refers to, and to communicate that specifically to parents. Severe disability may mean something quite different to the doctor and to the parent. Consistency is also important if we are to make guidelines about treatment decisions in intensive care. If, as is sometimes assumed, treatment withdrawal is permissible for infants or children with severe impairment we should make sure that we are clear about what we mean by this—and justify it.

Why aren't there more, and larger, studies of MRI and prognosis in birth asphyxia? Why haven't doctors been more explicit in discussing treatment limitation decisions, and why haven't they used appropriate and explicit outcome categories? Part of the answer to these questions relates to a problem with new technologies and research in clinical care. Magnetic resonance imaging involves some very sophisticated and expensive hardware, as well as complicated and advanced software to interpret the results, particularly where there is an attempt to make quantitative assessments (i.e. to put a number on different appearances). There have been enormous changes in that hardware and software over the two decades since it was first introduced. There have been changes in the power of the magnets used (recent studies use 3 Tesla magnets, compared to 1.5 or 0.5 Tesla magnets for earlier studies), in the computer power available to analyse results, and in the types of scans performed. It is not clear how well the results of early studies using MRI in birth asphyxia can be applied to current patients using a new generation of technology. This technological change also leads to a technological *imperative* in research. Researchers perform studies that use new protocols, or measure new markers, in part because they can, and in part because novel studies are more likely to be published in medical or scientific journals. Often the studies themselves involve only a relatively small number of patients, perhaps because there is some urgency to publish the results before a competing researcher does so. While many studies reveal a promising marker of prognosis, in relatively few cases is there then an attempt to repeat the study in a larger group of infants to validate that marker. These larger prognosis studies require significantly more funds to perform, take a relatively long time before they are complete, and may be harder to get published. There is also a risk that by the time they have been completed and published there will be new technology or imaging modalities available that may be superior. In a rapidly changing field there is a perverse disincentive to performing large, careful prognostic studies.

A second possible explanation is that studies of prognosis in birth asphyxia are less than ideal for informing treatment limitation decisions because they are focused on a different aim. We have concentrated up to this point on the use of prognostic information for making decisions about treatment withdrawal. However, in fact there are three distinct reasons why it may be useful to assess the prognosis of a critically ill child or infant.

1. Prognosis for treatment modification. One role of prognosis in intensive care is to identify subgroups of patients who may benefit from specific interventions to improve outcome. For example, it has recently emerged that cooling infants with HIE to about 34 degrees for seventy-two hours reduces their risk of death or significant impairment (Azzopardi, Brocklehurst, et al. 2008). Before such treatments start there is a need to determine whether infants are at risk of long-term complications, and consequently whether to institute cooling or other neuroprotective treatment. Some infants may be too severely, or too mildly, affected to benefit from these treatments.

2. Prognosis for anticipation. Prognostication may be used to identify infants or children with potentially abnormal neurodevelopment in order to inform parents. This may help parents to accept and to come to terms with the possibility of later disability. It may allow such infants or children to have careful follow-up with earlier detection of developmental or learning problems, and the provision of appropriate support.

3. Prognosis for treatment limitation/continuation. Prognosis is used to inform decisions about the continuation or withdrawal of intensive care support.

These purposes differ in their importance. The first aim depends on how much difference any interventions in intensive care make to long-term outcome. For example although neuroprotection with cooling for asphyxiated newborn infants is valuable, it has only a fairly modest effect on outcome (approximately 15 per cent reduction in the risk of death or significant impairment) (Jacobs, Hunt, et al. 2007). For a relatively low-risk treatment like cooling, it is sufficient to determine which infants have *some* risk of long-term impairment. There is no need to determine how high that risk is, nor the severity of impairment. If we had more risky treatments it might be far more important to have a very good idea about prognosis before applying them.

Prognosis for anticipation is also somewhat important. Parents are understandably anxious to know whether, and how significantly, their child might be impaired. But to date, there is no evidence that providing this information to parents or providing early developmental intervention is better for either parents or child than waiting until impairment becomes apparent (Evans 2007).

On the other hand, prognostication for treatment limitation/continuation decisions makes a huge difference to outcome. It obviously has the potential to lead to the death of an infant or to survival. Mistakes in prognosis for treatment limitation decisions have very serious ramifications for the infant and for parents. This third purpose of prognosis is arguably the most important, and the most important to get right.

It is possible that the studies reviewed above were deliberately designed to assist what I have called prognosis for anticipation rather than prognosis for treatment limitation/continuation. The above concerns about selection of patients, timing of imaging, self-fulfilling prophecies, and broad outcome categories may not matter if the study *is* designed for, and is used to help parents come to terms with the prognosis for their child. But if prognosis for treatment limitation is genuinely the more important prognostic question, it raises the question of why so much effort has been placed on prognosis for anticipation.

An alternative and more cynical explanation is that clinicians involved in research in birth asphyxia have been reluctant to openly discuss prognosis for treatment limitation because it is controversial. Few studies even mention treatment limitation preceding death in infants with HIE, though it seems highly likely that such decisions preceded death in most cases. There was explicit acknowledgement of the role of treatment limitation decisions in death (and consequently of the potential for self-fulfilling prophecies) in only one of the thirty-two studies in the systematic review by Thayyil and colleagues. The majority of studies provided no information at all about the cause of death. A number use euphemisms, stating that death was due to 'neurological problems', or was a 'direct consequence of their brain injury'.

Regardless of the cause of this undue focus, there are good reasons why future research should unambiguously focus on the most important prognostic question.

What about other conditions? We have focused on the example of newborn infants with birth asphyxia. But the problems listed above are not unique to newborn infants. Hypoxic-ischemic brain injury in children is uncommon, but raises similar ethical questions about prediction of outcome and continuation or discontinuation of intensive care. There have been only a small number of studies using magnetic resonance imaging to assess prognosis in affected children. A recent review noted that abnormalities in the basal ganglia, cortex, or brainstem are predictive of 'bad outcome' (Abend and Licht 2008). However, this conclusion was based on only two studies. The first of these studied forty children who had been admitted with hypoxic-ischemic brain injury and who had had MRI performed. The authors categorized as a 'bad neurologic evolution' children with mild or moderate cognitive or motor impairments, or epilepsy. More than half of the scans were performed more than one week after admission (Christophe, Fonteyne, et al. 2002). The second study looked at twenty-two children following near-drowning. All had imaging performed in the first six days after admission. It included categories of 'persistent vegetative state' or death as poor outcomes, though in fact children with 'severe cerebral disability' (dependent for daily support) were included with those who were vegetative, and very little detail is provided on the actual functional state of these children (Dubowitz, Bluml, et al. 1998). Neither study blinded outcome assessment to imaging, and neither documented whether or not treatment limitation preceded deaths, and if so, whether MRI results might have influenced treatment withdrawal decisions.

The Problem of Self-Fulfilling Prophecies

We noted above one difficulty for assessing the evidence for neuroimaging as a prognostic tool in infants with HIE—that prognosis is influenced by self-fulfilling prophecies. Sociologist Robert Merton famously introduced the idea of a self-fulfilling prophecy in the 1950s. Merton was interested in the nature of enquiry in the social sciences, and whether it is possible to get at the truth of the matter. Merton cited as an example the fictional Millingville bank. When a large number of customers are spotted queuing up in the bank, rumours of an imminent bank collapse develop (though in fact the reason for the surge in customers is pure chance); these rumours lead to a large number of people withdrawing their savings. This, in turn, leads to the actual collapse of the bank (Merton 1968: 476). The self-fulfilling prophecy raises the question of the overlap between prediction and predestination, echoed in mythology, literature, and in science fiction. Karl Popper, recalling the famous Greek myth, later referred to the same idea as 'the Oedipus prophecy' (Popper 2002: 139).

In medicine the problem of the self-fulfilling prophecy has been raised in many different contexts. Predictions may affect the mental state and behaviour of patients. For example giving patients the news that they have a short time to live may cause them to become depressed, to stop taking medicines, and may contribute to their early demise. Awareness of this problem has been argued to contribute to doctors' reluctance to make predictions about duration of survival (Christakis 2001). In intensive care the self-fulfilling prophecy is particularly apparent whenever decisions about withdrawal of life support are made on the basis of predicted high mortality. The concern is that if life support is withdrawn from patients who are predicted (if treatment were continued) to have a high risk of dying, this action then leads to a high mortality rate in that group of patients. This may occur whether or not the original prediction was correct. But since it is now true that the majority of patients with this condition die, subsequent similar patients are believed to have a high chance of dying and also have treatment withdrawn. It has been argued that the self-fulfilling prophecy contributes to mortality rates for extremely premature infants (McHaffie, Laing, et al. 2001; Mercurio 2005), infants with trisomy 13 or 18 (Embleton, Wyllie, et al. 1996; McGraw and Perlman 2008), as well as for adults with haemorrhagic stroke (Becker, Baxter, et al. 2001), hypoxic brain injury (Zandbergen, De Haan, et al. 1998), critical illness (Cook, Rocker, et al. 2003), and even brain death (Truog and Robinson 2003).

There are a number of ways in which predictions can affect outcome. They may generate an outcome that would not otherwise have occurred. They may increase the probability of an outcome occurring that had some chance of occurring otherwise. Alternatively, in some circumstances they may lead, by virtue of the prediction, to an outcome not taking place (Christakis 1999: 136).

Merton had in mind the first of these possibilities. He defined the self-fulfilling prophecy as a 'false prediction'; in his example Millingville bank would not have collapsed in the absence of the effect of rumours on consumer confidence (Merton 1968: 476). Yet the situation in intensive care is more like the second possibility. In almost all situations there is some significant chance of the patient dying even if no attempts at prognosis were made, and treatment were continued. We could think of the self-fulfilling prophecy in treatment limitation decisions as more of a self-*reinforcing* prophecy. The prophecy makes it more likely that death will occur.

Epistemic Problem of Self-Fulfilling Prophecies

The particular problem that I alluded to earlier in this chapter relating to the self-fulfilling prophecy is the difficulty that it creates in getting to the facts about prognosis (Bernat 2009). It is what philosophers refer to as an *epistemic* problem. Disentangling the prognosis for a group of patients from the effects of predictions can seem almost as intractable as the ancient conundrum of the chicken and the egg.

This epistemic problem, in turn, leads to two significant ethical problems for end-of-life decision-making. Self-fulfilling prophecies may compromise honest communication with families by causing doctors to mislead families about the patient's chance of survival. For example, parents anticipating the delivery of an extremely premature infant (say at twenty-two or twenty-three weeks gestation) may be told that all previous patients cared for at this gestation have died, or that the chance of survival in a published cohort of patients was very low or zero. However, the risk of death in both of these cited instances was likely influenced by treatment limitation decisions, and doctors may be wittingly or unwittingly deceiving families. Of course, it may be relevant to families to know that treatment is usually withdrawn in cases like this. But since the question is whether or not to continue life support, what families need to know is the chance of survival for the patient *if all supportive measures are provided*. Doctors may not be able to provide this probability because of the epistemic problems outlined above. Yet, sometimes at least, parents are misled into thinking that the answer they have been given is of this second sort, when in fact it is the former. The other problem for decision-making is that the self-fulfilling prophecy may affect the threshold for treatment withdrawal. Some doctors and families are unwilling to allow a patient to die unless the outcome is poor 'beyond reasonable doubt' (McIntosh 2002). However, the potential for a self-fulfilling prophecy may create sufficient uncertainty about outcome that it is felt to be impermissible to withdraw treatment—i.e. it may create reasonable doubt. Some have suggested that if the chance of survival with treatment is less than 1 per cent, a treatment may be judged 'futile', and withheld—even if the patient or their family requests it (Schneiderman, Jecker, et al. 1990). However, if we are basing our assessment of the chance of survival on studies or personal experience where at least some of the patients had treatment withdrawn or withheld it can be very difficult to know if the true chance of survival is this low or not.

The self-fulfilling prophecy is largely a problem for mortality rates in intensive care. Predictions of impairment are not likely to be affected by self-fulfilling prophecies in the same way. Treatment limitation doesn't directly affect impairment, so wouldn't be expected to cause quite the same problem. But there are three ways in which they could be affected. The first is that many studies of prognostic tests combine the outcomes of death and severe impairment (as in the meta-analysis discussed above), and physicians often use these combined statistics when talking to families. For example, the high probability of a poor outcome in children or newborn infants who have basal ganglia injury is based on a composite outcome of death or disability. Second, if a very large proportion of patients with a condition die following treatment withdrawal there will be relatively few survivors to provide data on impairment. This makes data on the severity of impairment less reliable. Third, in a small number of cases treatment limitation may actually increase impairment. For example, some infants who have life-sustaining treatment withdrawn survive because they are not in fact dependent on life support. However, they may have had a significant period of low oxygen levels or blood pressure after treatment withdrawal that could exacerbate future impairment.

Can we avoid self-fulfilling prophecies in prognostic research? One way to reduce the problem for new tests is to withhold the results of those tests from doctors in order to prevent them from influencing decisions. One careful study of somatosensory evoked potentials in children with brain injury took great care to make sure that the interpretation of the test was done by researchers who did not know clinical details of the patient, and that the results of testing were not available to medical staff, nursing staff, or parents (Carter and Butt 2005). But in many studies this is not done. Influential papers on cerebral blood flow velocity (measured on ultrasound) in HIE failed to mention whether there was a potential relationship between test results and decisions (Archer, Levene, et al. 1986; Levene, Fenton, et al. 1989; Ilves, Talvik, et al. 1998). Clinicians were blinded to test results in only six out of seventeen studies in a systematic review of prognostic tests for adults with anoxic coma (Zandbergen, De Haan, et al. 1998). The lack of blinding in many studies may be due to a blurring of the boundaries between research and clinical care, the simultaneous use of tests for several purposes, and ethical qualms about withholding or concealing results from patients and their families. This last is understandable given the emphasis that is placed in medical ethics upon truth telling and the provision of full information to patients. However, when the prognostic value of a given test result is not known or very uncertain, there may be little benefit from informing patients or families of those results, and there is a good case for not providing test results to caregivers. The problem is that once a certain amount of experience and information has accumulated about a test (as is the case now with MRIs), even if that information is imperfect, it becomes unethical to withhold the results of testing from doctors and families for the sake of future patients. It then becomes impossible to eliminate the possibility that test results will affect outcome.

A second way to obtain information about the validity of mortality predictions would be to deliberately avoid making any treatment limitation decisions in a cohort of patients, and to study their outcome. It is usually recommended that treatment is standardized for patients in prognostic factor studies (Simon and Altman 1994). But this is not as easy as it might sound. If we have literally no evidence about the risk of death in a group of patients, then it would be appropriate to continue life-sustaining treatment in all of them. It is far more common, however, that there is already some evidence that a high proportion of such patients die, and hence that withdrawal of treatment may be acceptable. Continuing life-sustaining treatment in order to determine the actual mortality rate risks prolonging the death of a number of patients, causing harm to them and to their families. Disregarding the wishes of patients and families in such a setting would be clearly unethical.

How else can the true validity of predictions be established? It may be possible to look at historical evidence of mortality in the first patients studied with a given illness, since self-fulfilling prophecies are least likely to have affected the management of such patients. But if treatment has changed since that early experience (as it is likely to have), that evidence will not be relevant. It will also be irrelevant to the assessment of recently developed prognostic tools.

Another possibility would be to try to determine statistically the impact of different prognostic factors upon outcome. In one study, researchers looked at a number of variables in a multivariate analysis of outcome in adults with intracerebral haemorrhage (Becker, Baxter, et al. 2001). Although commonly cited poor prognostic factors (the Glasgow Coma Score and size of haemorrhage) were associated with death, when decisions to withdraw treatment were added into the model no other factors remained statistically significant. The authors of the study claimed that this indicated a bias in decision-making, and that withdrawal of support was the most important determinant of outcome. But this conclusion is premature. All of the patients who had life-sustaining treatment withdrawn died. A combination of different prognostic factors, as well as the wishes of patients and family, are likely to have fed into treatment decisions (Rabinstein and Diringer 2007). Consequently, variables other than the decision to withdraw are individually unlikely to have as clear an association with death. It does not seem particularly striking that decisions to withdraw dominated the model of factors that contributed to death. An alternative technique is to use a statistical tool called propensity analysis. This technique attempts to take account of the different confounding variables that might be associated with a treatment decision. Propensity scores can be used to generate a matched cohort study that simulates a randomized trial. This has been used to look at the effect on mortality of decisions to withhold life-sustaining treatment (Chen, Connors, et al. 2008; (Shepardson, Youngner, et al. 1999). But one problem is that such models potentially ignore other prognostic factors that are difficult to quantify. Treatment limitation decisions may be a marker for mortality, rather than a cause of mortality (Sulmasy 1999). In any case, there may be other factors than mortality that influence decisions, including the probability of surviving with severe impairment. Such modelling may be useful but it is unlikely to provide a complete answer.

Finally, it may be possible to get an idea of the true mortality rate by looking at the outcome in patients predicted to have a poor outcome, but who nevertheless had intensive treatment provided. This might be a hospital or community that have a different philosophy about treatment withdrawal, or may be a group of patients whose family or surrogates refuse to permit treatment to be limited. For example, in a recent large study of outcome for extremely premature infants, researchers were able to distinguish the outcome for those infants who received mechanical ventilation (and hence were actively resuscitated) from those infants who died in the delivery room (Tyson, Parikh, et al. 2008). If all such patients die (or are severely impaired), we would then have good supporting evidence for the initial prediction. Conversely, a higher survival in this cohort may cause us to question the general assumption that prognosis is poor. There is a need for caution, however, in interpreting the outcome in the subgroup of patients who received intensive care or who had treatment continued. Firstly, they may not be representative of all patients who fit into a group predicted to have poor outcome. They may be younger, or fitter, from a different demographic or ethnic group. Any of those factors (or others less obvious) may impact both upon the doctors' decision to provide treatment or the family's willingness to withdraw life support, and on their chances of survival. In the study of premature infants mentioned above, those infants who were ventilated were heavier, less premature, and needed less resuscitation at birth (Tyson, Parikh, et al. 2008). Secondly, the presence of the previous prediction of extremely poor outcome may influence other management decisions. For example doctors may agree to continue intensive care for a patient with apparently very poor prognosis but negotiate with the family for non-resuscitation in the event of a cardiac arrest. Finally, it may be hard to systematically study this group of patients. Where families have disagreed with doctors about prognosis and continuation of life-sustaining treatment, there may be ongoing anger or distrust of medical staff. They may be reluctant to participate in research, or seek ongoing care elsewhere and be hard to follow up. Nevertheless, this is an extremely important cohort of patients to study since it may help in prognostication. The rate of favourable outcome in this group may help to estimate the maximum potential benefit of providing treatment.

Research in Quality of Life

The focus in this chapter has been on uncertainty in prognosis, and on the different factors that contribute to it. It is hard to predict the degree of impairment of a newborn or child with a brain injury, partly because of the way that research into prognosis has been carried out. But the importance of impairment for decisions about life-sustaining treatment is through its use to predict the quality of life of children. There is some research into the quality of life of children and adults with impairment. Does that research help with uncertainty in decision-making? I will concentrate particularly here on research that has looked at quality of life in children with cerebral palsy, and in survivors of newborn intensive care. Any limitations with this research are likely to be mirrored in research in other serious illnesses and impairments in childhood.

'Quality of life' is a term that is used in a fairly imprecise way by doctors and ethicists when they are discussing treatment decisions to refer to the experience of life for a patient if they survive. How good or bad would life be for them? In terms of the concepts that we referred to in Chapter 2, what are the future burdens and benefits going to be for a child, is life going to be tolerable? In particular, we might be interested in assessing whether the child's life would be, or could be, from their perspective a life not worth living.

When researchers attempt to measure and quantify quality of life the concept used is slightly different. In fact there are several different related concepts that are sometimes used interchangeably but are not actually the same. Some studies measure 'health status', assessing for the presence or absence and severity of problems in different domains of health. Others measure 'functional status', looking at the ability of an individual to perform a range of different day-to-day tasks. Still others attempt to gauge the patient's level of satisfaction with their life. The World Health Organisation definition of 'Quality of Life' encompasses this last sense: 'the individual's perception of their position in life in the context of culture and value systems in which they live and in relation to their goals, expectations, standards and concerns' (WHOQOL Group 1995: 1403). The idea is that 'quality of life' represents a subjective measure of overall well-being. One final concept worth distinguishing is that of 'health-related quality of life', which is an attempt to isolate the contribution of health to the individual's overall satisfaction and well-being.

It is difficult to compare levels of satisfaction between different people. If I rate my health as 'very good' is that the same as what you mean by 'very good'? There are a couple of ways that researchers have attempted to standardize measures of quality of life. One way is to ask the individual to compare their life with different alternative health states, and to use a standardized technique to assess how bad they feel their life currently is. For example, a patient might be asked to imagine that they have the option of treatment A, which will leave them in their current health state, or treatment B, which has a chance of recovery to full health, but also a chance that they will die. The probabilities are varied until the patient is ambivalent between treatment A and B. If the patient feels that the life that they are currently living is very good, it is unlikely that they would accept treatment B unless the chance of dying were very small. Alternatively, if they thought that their life were very bad currently, they might take treatment B even if the chance of dying were very high. This process is referred to as a 'standard gamble', and is a well-validated, though potentially quite complicated, way of generating a health 'utility' score from 1 (perfect health) to 0 death. (This 'utility' is not meant to represent 'usefulness', nor is it necessarily a reflection of 'utilitarianism' as an ethical or philosophical framework. Rather it is simply a way of generating a relative value (for the individual) of different health states.) Negative scores of health utility are also possible for states judged to be worse than death, though these require a different version of the standard gamble test (Patrick, Starks, et al. 1994). A slightly simpler way of getting to a similar score is to ask subjects to undertake a time trade-off. Instead of life with a fixed period (say twenty years) in their current health state, patients might be asked whether they would choose a treatment that would give them perfect health, but for a reduced period. The better the subjective judgement of current health, the less time that an individual would be willing to give up in order to achieve full health.

Because these comparisons are not straightforward to understand, an alternative way of generating utility scores for health states is to survey members of the population (without major illness or impairment) for the utility that they would assign to hypothetical health states. This is the only way to generate a utility score for conditions where the individual is unable to answer for themselves.

There is some evidence on the quality of life of children with cerebral palsy (from a range of causes). Unsurprisingly, health status and physical health is markedly reduced in children with cerebral palsy (Wake, Salmon, et al. 2003), more so in those with severe cerebral palsy (Venkateswaran and Shevell 2008). But researchers have also attempted to measure subjective reports of well-being. The largest published study (the SPARCLE study) reported subjective quality of life in 500 children aged 8–12 with cerebral palsy, who were identified randomly from cerebral palsy registries in six European countries. They did not report health utilities, but found that children with cerebral palsy experienced similar scores on a 'quality of life' (QoL) interview to other children (Dickinson, Parkinson, et al. 2007). This evidence has been drawn on to support the disability paradox that we referred to in Chapter 1, and to challenge the assumption that cerebral palsy leads to lives that are impoverished and of poor quality (Rosenbaum 2008).

However, this conclusion may not be warranted. Two-thirds of the responses in the above study were from children with mild forms of motor impairment (GMFCS 1 or 2), while only 14 per cent of respondents had severe motor impairment. Those children who did have severe physical impairment were much more likely to report lower physical well-being. In fact almost 40 per cent of the 818 children enrolled in the study were unable to answer questions about their quality of life. Most (93 per cent) of those children who were unable to self-report had significant cognitive impairment, but children who were unable to walk, or who had seizures were also less likely to answer the questions themselves (Dickinson, Parkinson, et al. 2006). In a separate part of the same study, parents reported on their perception of the QoL of their children (Arnaud, White-Koning, et al. 2008). While indices of QoL were not markedly different overall between children with cerebral palsy and those without, there were differences in QoL for children with severe cerebral palsy. Severe motor impairment was associated with reduced scores for physical well-being and autonomy, and a higher risk of psychological symptoms or social impairment (Parkes, White-Koning et al. 2008), while moderate or severe cognitive impairment was associated with reduction in the 'social support' domain of QoL (Arnaud, White-Koning, et al. 2008). We noted in Chapter 2 the 'tolerability paradox': that children with severe cognitive impairment were less likely to score low (by their parents) in those parts of the QoL tool that related to mood and self-perception. Interestingly, in another report from the SPARCLE study, severe cognitive impairment was associated with lower physical health status, while mild degrees of cognitive impairment were associated with worse psychosocial health status than either normal intelligence or severe impairment (Beckung, White-Koning, et al. 2008). Other studies have reported that children and adolescents with severe cerebral palsy are more likely to experience pain (Houlihan, O'Donnell, et al. 2004) and participate less in everyday activities (McManus, Corcoran, et al. 2008)

Does this evidence help? One problem with these studies is that, for the most part, they do not report separately on the quality of life of children with severe cerebral palsy. The SPARCLE study provides correlations between severity of cerebral palsy (GMFCS) and several domains of their QoL assessment. But it is not possible to compare directly the QoL scores of children with severe physical or cognitive impairment with those of other children. There is no way to use this information to give parents a genuine sense of what life might be like for their child if they survive. A second problem is a self-report bias: self-reported measures of QoL are much more likely in children with milder forms of impairment—potentially painting an overly positive picture of quality of life, and ignoring those children whose quality of life is potentially most relevant for treatment decisions. A third problem is that assessing the quality of life of surviving children in mid-childhood ignores the quality of life of children who died in infancy or early childhood. Children with the most severe forms of cerebral palsy have a significant risk of repeated hospitalization, and of death in early childhood (Strauss, Cable, et al. 1999; Hutton, Colver, et al. 2000). Furthermore, most children with cerebral palsy in these studies are likely never to have been critically ill in intensive care. What we need for decision-making in intensive care is a sense of the quality of life for children who survive intensive care, having been in a position where treatment withdrawal may have been a genuine alternative.

One study has looked specifically at quality of life of adolescents who were born prematurely and who had abnormal brain ultrasound appearances in the newborn period (Feingold, Sheir-Neiss, et al. 2002). Abnormal cerebral ultrasound is one of the most important tools that neonatologists currently use to prognosticate for very premature infants, and influences treatment decisions (Siperstein, Wolraich, et al. 1991). If we had good data on the quality of life of children who have had severely abnormal brain ultrasound appearances that would be potentially very useful for parents and doctors in newborn intensive care. The results of this study were surprising, in that teenagers who had more severe ultrasound abnormalities in the newborn period had higher rates of post-prematurity health complications, but rated their quality of life *more* favourably than teenagers without ultrasound abnormalities (or with mild abnormalities). This might again relate to the tolerability paradox. The authors of the study speculated that abnormal brain imaging in the newborn period led to reduced expectations on the part of parents or children, and consequently less stress in teenage years. However, there are problems in relating the results of this study to decisions in intensive care. There were relatively few teenagers included in the study with more severe ultrasound appearances. (There was only one participant with a grade 4 intraventricular haemorrhage, a pattern that is associated with the worst outcome and often used as a basis for treatment limitation.) The study provides no information on the presence or severity of physical or cognitive impairment in the children who were surveyed, so it is difficult to know in what ways children with abnormal ultrasound appearances were affected. Furthermore, given that quality of life measures were based on self-reports, it seems highly likely, as with the cerebral palsy studies, that any surviving children with moderate or greater degrees of cognitive impairment would have been excluded. Also, as with the cerebral palsy studies, there is no information provided on how many children with severely abnormal ultrasound appearances died in the neonatal period or in early childhood. Those children who survive to teenage years, and are able to answer a quality of life questionnaire, are likely to be a select cohort of less severely affected children.

Neonatologist Saroj Saigal at McMaster University in Canada has conducted a detailed and rigorous assessment of the health status, health utilities, and quality of life in ex-premature infants (born weighing less than 1kg) who were assessed in mid-childhood, adolescent years, and then in young adulthood. When assessed at age eight, health status was derived from clinical and psychological assessment of the children, and health utilities were derived from a separate group of parents of normal school-age children. Health utilities and health status were compared with a matched comparison group of non-premature children. The premature children were more likely to have functional limitations in one or more health areas than non-premature children, and these limitations were more likely to be severe and complex. The average health utility score for ex-premature children was lower than that for a reference group of non-premature children, though still fairly high (0.82 versus 0.95) (Saigal, Feeny, et al. 1994; Saigal, Rosenbaum, et al. 1994). When Saigal and colleagues reassessed these children at an older age, teenagers provided self-reports of their health status, and the majority were able to provide their own health utilities using a standard gamble technique. At this point, although ex-premature teenagers were more likely than their peers to have moderate or severe functional limitations (for example in cognition, vision/hearing, mobility, or self-care), their average health-related quality of life rating was only mildly lower than non-premature teenagers (0.87 versus 0.93). Approximately 70 per cent of both the ex-premature infants and the reference group rated their quality of life as more than 0.95

(i.e. very close to perfect health) (Saigal, Feeny, et al. 1996). In young adulthood (average age twenty-four), there was no longer any difference in the reports by individuals of their quality of life compared to the reference group. Furthermore, among the ex-premature young adults, there was no difference in self-reported quality of life scores between those who were impaired and those who weren't (Saigal, Stoskopf, et al. 2006).

One question raised by the latter piece of evidence is about the impact of impairment or disability on well-being. If young adults with impairment are just as satisfied with their life as those who do not have impairment, it appears to support the disability paradox, and undermines the idea that disabilities are even relevant for predictions about quality of life. However, there are a couple of reasons why that conclusion may be too hasty. There is now a considerable body of evidence about the phenomenon of 'hedonic adaptation' following illness or injury (Ubel and Loewenstein 2010). Research in a wide range of conditions suggests that following illness or injury there is an initial negative effect on an individual's mood and level of happiness. But this effect fades over time, and even if the illness or impairment remains patients often return to similar levels of happiness to those that they experienced prior to their illness and to those of other people without impairment. Patients who have become quadriplegic or who have had amputations after cancer have been reported to have similar affect and self-rated well-being to controls (Ubel and Loewenstein 2010). Another striking example is that of locked-in syndrome, a state of profound physical impairment, where the patient may be able to communicate only through eye movements. In one survey, 72 per cent of patients in a chronic locked-in syndrome rated their lives positively (Bruno, Bernheim, et al. 2011). The phenomenon of adaptation may be part of the explanation of the high levels of well-being in adolescents with impairment, though there may be an additional factor that is important. When someone acquires an impairment or illness part of their negative response is a reflection of the change in their experience, or in what they are able to do. However, when a child is impaired from birth or early childhood they do not have the same point of comparison. A child who is born visually impaired may not miss their sight because they have never experienced it.

How should we factor in hedonic adaptation into our assessment of the quality of life in different states? One reason to give us pause is this: if the subjective well-being of patients is unaffected by impairment, it would seem to imply that there is nothing bad for them in being impaired, and no reason to regret it. Nor would there be any reason to try to prevent such impairments. The most common impairment in the young adults in the McMaster study was visual impairment. This is likely to reflect the impact of retinopathy of prematurity—damage to the retina in premature infants, a fairly common problem at the time that these children were in newborn intensive care. Should we take this evidence to mean that we were wrong to invest considerable effort in trying to reduce the rate of retinopathy of prematurity? Secondly, our interpretation of quality of life evidence like that described above depends upon which theory of well-being we think is the right one. For example, patients who are on long-term renal dialysis report similar subjective levels of well-being to members of the general population (Evans, Manninen, et al. 1985). However, if they are asked a different question, namely whether they would prefer not to be on dialysis, patients give a different answer. Using the 'time-trade-off' technique, dialysis patients were willing to forego almost half of their remaining years in order to return to full health. Individuals' general levels of happiness are important on any plausible theory of well-being, but they are not necessarily the only thing that matters. On desire-based theories, or objective-list-based theories, there are other things that are important, namely whether their impairment prevents them from achieving what they would like to do, whether they would prefer not to be impaired, or whether it prevents or limits individuals from achieving objectively valuable features of life. In a different context the philosophers Amartya Sen (1993) and Martha Nussbaum (2000) have elaborated a list of 'capabilities' that are important for welfare independently of the individual's level of happiness. Sen and Nussbaum developed this list to take account of the phenomenon of adaptation in situations of considerable social injustice. (Those who are extremely poor and disenfranchised may not be unhappy, and may not have strong preferences that their situation change.) A similar capabilities approach to assessment of quality of life would potentially identify a number of serious impediments to well-being that are associated with severe physical or particularly cognitive impairment. This would support giving some weight to health status ratings as well as subjective markers of well-being.

How do the McMaster studies help with decision-making for very premature infants? Contrary to expectations, the subjective quality of life of these children and young adults appears fairly similar to that of children and young adults who did not need newborn intensive care. The first point to note is that this evidence relates to a cohort of extremely-low-birth-weight infants born weighing less than 1kg. So the principle relevance of the overall findings is for a decision about whether we should treat premature infants weighing less than 1kg. If we thought that the quality of life of premature infants born below this weight were so bad that we should not resuscitate or treat them, these studies should give us pause. But the real quality of life question for intensive care is not whether the average patient treated in intensive care has a good quality of life; rather it is whether there is a subgroup of children (those who have evidence of brain injury on ultrasound for example, or who are particularly premature and sick) who have substantial reductions in their quality of life. This sort of study and similar studies of survivors of paediatric intensive care (Taylor, Butt, et al. 2003; Conlon, Breatnach, et al. 2009) help us assess whether intensive treatment is generally or usually a good thing for groups of infants or children. It may indicate a subgroup with poor quality of life. However, existing studies do not help us determine how to predict which patients in intensive care will be in this state.

The McMaster studies are notable because they overcome some of the shortcomings and biases in other quality of life studies mentioned above. One helpful feature is that the researchers provide data on those children who did not make it to follow-up interviews and assessments. The premature infants who were studied were all born between 1977 and 1982. (This highlights a separate problem for quality of life studies arising from newborn intensive care similar to some of those noted above for new forms of neuroimaging. By the time that it is possible to get good data on the quality of life of survivors, so much time may have passed that the data is no longer relevant to current patients.) At that time in Ontario a fairly aggressive policy of treatment was followed; fifteen very premature infants did not receive intensive care, and eleven had life support withdrawn. Overall, 52 per cent of premature infants born under 1kg survived to discharge from hospital. Thirteen children died after discharge from the neonatal intensive care unit, six before the age of three, and seven later in childhood or adolescence. The researchers also provided proxy reports on quality of life for those children who were severely impaired and unable to self-report. In the study of teenagers, nine of the 150 survivors who were interviewed were in this group.

What is the quality of life of these severely impaired children? The McMaster studies don't provide separate scores for those children, though they were less than the average for the group as a whole. The problem is that although this is the group where 'quality of life' decisions are most often applied in intensive care, this is also the group where 'quality of life data'—i.e. the subjective reports of satisfaction and well-being—are unavailable. We are left with three options, though there are problems with each of these. The first is to use proxies (for example the quality of life scores that their parents or caregivers provide for them). In studies where quality of life has been reported simultaneously by both parents and children, parents tend to report lower quality of life and higher morbidity than the child. Other factors may influence parents' reports. For example high levels of parental stress are associated with lower scores for their child's quality of life (White-Koning, Arnaud, et al. 2007). On the other hand, parents' assessment of quality of life in some circumstances may also be biased in the other direction. For example, parents who have devoted large amounts of time and made substantial sacrifices in order to care for a child with severe illness or impairment may be predisposed to rate their child's quality of life positively, in part as a psychological defence mechanism or to avoid cognitive dissonance (Patrick, Danis, et al. 1988). The second option would be to draw on the preferences and utilities of other (usually healthy) individuals. However, third-party assessments of the quality of life in a severely impaired state may also be biased. There is a general problem (alluded to in Chapter 2) that when a healthy person imagines themselves in an impaired state they have to imagine losing capacities that they currently possess. In contrast, a child who is born in an impaired state never experiences this 'loss', and may view their state more positively. Specific groups may have biases in other ways. For example, health professionals reported lower utilities for severely impaired states than either parents or teenagers (Saigal, Stoskopf, et al. 1999). This could be because they have greater understanding or insight into these conditions. But doctors may also be more inclined to view such conditions negatively because their professional exposure tends to be especially with the negative consequences of impairment. (For example, doctors tend to see impaired children when they are sick or have problems.) Or they may have more negative views about certain types of impairment because their own professions place a very high value on cognitive performance. Finally, the third possibility is to just report functional state when we evaluate the quality of life of individuals who are unable to provide their own quality of life assessment. This would have the advantage of being less susceptible to bias; however, it then risks begging the question of the quality of life of severely impaired children and adults. How bad is it to be severely impaired?

There is no way around the most difficult questions relating to quality of life in severely impaired children and adults. The best that we can do is to be aware of the limitations of available evidence and to draw on information from a variety of sources, including proxies, and objective functional scores.

Conclusions

In this chapter we have looked at the different sources of uncertainty for prognostication in intensive care. Some uncertainty is intrinsic, and probably unavoidable. It relates to differences between patients in their susceptibility and potential to recover from acute illness or insult, and in the environment that they will be exposed to if they survive. Other uncertainty arises in part because of the ways in which research studies have been performed. Studies of prognosis and of prognostic tests have sometimes been undertaken in ways that may provide useful information for counselling parents of critically ill infants and children, but which have serious limitations when it comes to aiding decisions relating to continuation or withdrawal of intensive care. One pervasive problem is self-fulfilling prophecies relating to predicted risk of death, and the influence of treatment withdrawal decisions. There are ways around some of these problems, and if we are to reduce uncertainty in prognostication, if we are develop anything like the predictive powers of the Carmentis machine, a number of changes to prognostic research will be necessary (Table 5.1).

We also looked at some of the research data on quality of life for survivors of intensive care. Again, these studies have mostly been undertaken in ways that make it hard to apply to predictions of quality of life for particular patients. Future prognosis studies may be able to help reduce uncertainty about which prognostic factors are associated with reduced quality of life in survivors (Table 5.1) However, even if these studies provide more useful data, the hardest problem is going to remain. Those patients where assessments of quality of life are potentially the most important are also the ones where it is the most difficult. Empirical studies are not going to be able to

Table 5.1 Recommendations for improving prognostic research

1.	Studies of prognosis for critically ill children need to be large enough to assess for differences between groups and should be prospective rather than retrospective.
2.	They should measure multiple different prognostic factors so that these can be compared or combined.
3.	To be relevant to treatment decisions outcome studies should focus on those patients who were critically ill, and where treatment decisions may have been relevant.
4.	Cut-off points for continuous variables should be generated in a data-independent way (i.e. they shouldn't depend on the results of the study where they were measured).
5.	Follow-up should use validated, blinded outcome measures, present results in detail, and avoid overly inclusive outcome groups
6.	Research into new prognostic tests should ensure, where possible, that test results are not used to influence treatment limitation decisions.
7.	Where patients have died during or subsequent to their intensive care stay it is important to determine whether life-sustaining treatment was limited, and the basis for the limitation.
8.	Where tests may have influenced treatment decisions regression or propensity analysis should be used to try to determine the independent value of tests for prognostication.
9.	Patients whose treatment is continued despite a poor prognosis should be followed up, and reported separately.
10.	Quality of life should be measured in surviving children, using a combination of subjective and objective measures. Proxy reports and functional status should be recorded for children unable to self-report.

tell us what life is like for patients with moderate or severe cognitive impairment. Uncertainty about that is going to remain. We will need to decide how we should evaluate such health states.

How should we respond to uncertain predictions of impairment and quality of life? One way of reducing uncertainty in practice may be to defer prognostication and decision-making, and allow time to shed more light on the subject. What are the benefits and risks of such an approach? That is where we will turn next.

References

Abend, N.S. and D.J. Licht (2008). 'Predicting outcome in children with hypoxic ischemic encephalopathy', *Pediatr Crit Care Med* 9(1): 32–9.

Ambalavanan, N., W.A. Carlo, et al. (2006). 'Predicting outcomes of neonates diagnosed with hypoxemic-ischemic encephalopathy', *Pediatrics* 118(5): 2084–93.

Anderson, V., C. Catroppa, et al. (2005). 'Functional plasticity or vulnerability after early brain injury?', *Pediatrics* 116(6): 1374–82.

Archer, L.N., M.I. Levene, et al. (1986). 'Cerebral artery Doppler ultrasonography for prediction of outcome after perinatal asphyxia', *Lancet* 2(8516): 1116–18.

Arnaud, C., M. White-Koning, et al. (2008). 'Parent-reported quality of life of children with cerebral palsy in Europe', *Pediatrics* 121(1): 54–64.

Azzopardi, D., P. Brocklehurst, et al. (2008). 'The TOBY Study. Whole body hypothermia for the treatment of perinatal asphyxial encephalopathy: a randomised controlled trial', *BMC Pediatr* 8: 17.

Ballantyne, A.O., A.M. Spilkin, et al. (2008). 'Plasticity in the developing brain: intellectual, language and academic functions in children with ischaemic perinatal stroke', *Brain* 131(11): 2975–85.

Barkovich, A.J., B.L. Hajnal, et al. (1998). 'Prediction of neuromotor outcome in perinatal asphyxia: evaluation of MR scoring systems', *AJNR Am J Neuroradiol* 19(1): 143–9.

Becker, K.J., A.B. Baxter, et al. (2001). 'Withdrawal of support in intracerebral hemorrhage may lead to self-fulfilling prophecies', *Neurology* 56(6): 766–72.

Beckung, E., M. White-Koning, et al. (2008). 'Health status of children with cerebral palsy living in Europe: a multi-centre study', *Child Care Health Dev* 34(6): 806–14.

Bernat, J.L. (2009). 'Ethical issues in the treatment of severe brain injury: the impact of new technologies', *Ann N Y Acad Sci*.

Bradley, R.H., L. Whiteside, et al. (1994). 'Early indications of resilience and their relation to experiences in the home environments of low birthweight, premature children living in poverty', *Child Dev* 65(2 Spec No): 346–60.

Bruno, M.A., J.L. Bernheim, et al. (2011). 'A survey on self-assessed well-being in a cohort of chronic locked-in syndrome patients: happy majority, miserable minority', *BMJ Open* 2011; 1:e000039 doi:10.1136/bmjopen-2010-000039.

Carter, B.G. and W. Butt (2005). 'Are somatosensory evoked potentials the best predictor of outcome after severe brain injury? A systematic review', *Intensive Care Med* 31(6): 765–75.

Chen, Y.Y., A.F. Connors, Jr., et al. (2008). 'Effect of decisions to withhold life support on prolonged survival', *Chest* 133(6): 1312–18.

Christakis, N.A. (1999). *Death Foretold: Prophecy and Prognosis in Medical Care*. Chicago: University of Chicago.

—— (2001). 'Prognostication and bioethics', *Daedalus* 128(4): 197–214.

Christophe, C., C. Fonteyne, et al. (2002). 'Value of MR imaging of the brain in children with hypoxic coma', *AJNR Am J Neuroradiol* 23(4): 716–23.

Conlon, N.P., C. Breatnach, et al. (2009). 'Health-related quality of life after prolonged pediatric intensive care unit stay', *Pediatric Critical Care Medicine* 10(1): 41–4.

Cook, D., G. Rocker, et al. (2003). 'Withdrawal of mechanical ventilation in anticipation of death in the intensive care unit', *N Engl J Med* 349(12): 1123–32.

Dickinson, H., K. Parkinson, et al. (2006). 'Assessment of data quality in a multi-centre cross-sectional study of participation and quality of life of children with cerebral palsy', *BMC Public Health* 6: 273.

—— (2007). 'Self-reported quality of life of 8–12-year-old children with cerebral palsy: a cross-sectional European study', *Lancet* 369(9580): 2171–8.

Dubowitz, D.J., S. Bluml, et al. (1998). 'MR of hypoxic encephalopathy in children after near drowning: correlation with quantitative proton MR spectroscopy and clinical outcome', *AJNR Am J Neuroradiol* 19(9): 1617–27.

Egger, M. and G.D. Smith (1995). 'Misleading meta-analysis', *BMJ* 310(6982): 752–4.

Embleton, N.D., J.P. Wyllie, et al. (1996). 'Natural history of trisomy 18', *Arch Dis Child Fetal Neonatal Ed* **75**(1): F38–41.

Evans, N. (2007). 'Prognostic tests in babies: do they always help?', *Acta Paediatr* 96(3): 329–30.

Evans, R.W., D.L. Manninen, et al. (1985). 'The quality of life of patients with end-stage renal disease', *N Engl J Med* 312(9): 553–9.

Feingold, E., G. Sheir-Neiss, et al. (2002). 'HRQL and severity of brain ultrasound findings in a cohort of adolescents who were born preterm', *J Adolesc Health* 31(3): 234–9.

Gluckman, P.D., J.S. Wyatt, et al. (2005). 'Selective head cooling with mild systemic hypothermia after neonatal encephalopathy: multicentre randomised trial', *Lancet* 365(9460): 663–70.

Haralambous, E., M.L. Hibberd, et al. (2003). 'Role of functional plasminogen-activator-inhibitor-1 4G/5G promoter polymorphism in susceptibility, severity, and outcome of meningococcal disease in Caucasian children', *Crit Care Med* 31(12): 2788–93.

Harris, J.C. (2006). *Intellectual Disability: Understanding its Development, Causes, Classification, Evaluation, and Treatment*. Oxford: Oxford University Press.

Houlihan, C.M., M. O'Donnell, et al. (2004). 'Bodily pain and health-related quality of life in children with cerebral palsy', *Dev Med Child Neurol* 46(5): 305–10.

Hunt, R.W., J.J. Neil, et al. (2004). 'Apparent diffusion coefficient in the posterior limb of the internal capsule predicts outcome after perinatal asphyxia', *Pediatrics* 114(4): 999–1003.

Hutton, J.L., A.F. Colver, et al. (2000). 'Effect of severity of disability on survival in north east England cerebral palsy cohort', *Arch Dis Child* 83(6): 468–74.

Ilves, P., R. Talvik, et al. (1998). 'Changes in Doppler ultrasonography in asphyxiated term infants with hypoxic-ischaemic encephalopathy', *Acta Paediatr* 87(6): 680–4.

Jacobs, S., R. Hunt, et al. (2007). 'Cooling for newborns with hypoxic ischaemic encephalopathy', *Cochrane Database of Systematic Reviews* (online)(4): CD003311.

Johnston, M.V., A. Ishida, et al. (2009). 'Plasticity and injury in the developing brain', *Brain Dev* 31(1): 1–10.

King, B., R. Hodapp, et al. (2000). 'Mental Retardation', in B. Sadock and V. Sadock, *Kaplan & Sadock's Comprehensive Textbook of Psychiatry*. Philadelphia: Lippincott, Williams, and Wilkins, 2587–613.

Levene, M.I., A.C. Fenton, et al. (1989). 'Severe birth asphyxia and abnormal cerebral blood-flow velocity', *Dev Med Child Neurol* 31(4): 427–34.

Lin, J.-D. (2003). 'Intellectual disability: definition, diagnosis and classification', *J Med Sci* 23(2): 83–90.

Marlow, N., D. Wolke, et al. (2005). 'Neurologic and developmental disability at six years of age after extremely preterm birth', *N Engl J Med* 352(1): 9–19.

Masten, A.S., K.M. Best, et al. (1990). 'Resilience and development: contributions from the study of children who overcome adversity', *Development and Psychopathology* 2(04): 425–44.

McGraw, M.P. and J. Perlman (2008). 'Attitudes of neonatologists toward delivery room management of confirmed trisomy 18: potential factors influencing a changing dynamic', *Pediatrics* 121(6): 1106–10.

McHaffie, H.E., I.A. Laing, et al. (2001). 'Deciding for imperilled newborns: medical authority or parental autonomy?', *Journal of Medical Ethics* 27(2): 104.

McIntosh, N. (2002). 'Ethical issues in withdrawing life-sustaining treatment from handicapped neonates', in D. Dickensen (ed.), *Ethical Issues in Maternal-Fetal Medicine*. Cambridge: Cambridge University Press, 335–46.

McManus, V., P. Corcoran, et al. (2008). 'Participation in everyday activities and quality of life in pre-teenage children living with cerebral palsy in south west Ireland', *BMC Pediatr* 8: 50.

Mercurio, M.R. (2005). 'Physicians' refusal to resuscitate at borderline gestational age', *J Perinatol* 25(11): 685–9.

Merton, R.K. (1968). *Social Theory and Social Structure*. New York, London: Free Press; Collier-Macmillan.

Nelson, K.B., J.M. Dambrosia, et al. (2005). 'Genetic polymorphisms and cerebral palsy in very preterm infants', *Pediatr Res* 57(4): 494–9.

Nussbaum, M.C. (2000). *Women and Human Development: The Capabilities Approach*. Cambridge: Cambridge University Press.

Palisano, R., P. Rosenbaum, et al. (1997). 'Development and reliability of a system to classify gross motor function in children with cerebral palsy', *Dev Med Child Neurol* 39(4): 214–23.

Parkes, J., M. White-Koning, et al. (2008). 'Psychological problems in children with cerebral palsy: a cross-sectional European study', *J Child Psychol Psychiatry* 49(4): 405–13.

Patrick, D.L., M. Danis, et al. (1988). 'Quality of life following intensive care', *J Gen Intern Med* 3(3): 218–23.

—— H.E. Starks, et al. (1994). 'Measuring preferences for health states worse than death', *Med Decis Making* 14(1): 9–18.

Popper, K.R. (2002). *Unended Quest: An Intellectual Autobiography*. London: Routledge.

Rabinstein, A.A. and M.N. Diringer (2007). 'Withholding care in intracerebral hemorrhage: realistic compassion or self-fulfilling prophecy?', *Neurology* 68(20): 1647–8.

—— and J.C. Hemphill (2010). 'Prognosticating after severe acute brain disease: science, art, and biases', *Neurology* 74(14): 1086–7.

Rosenbaum, P. (2008). 'Children's quality of life: separating the person from the disorder', *Arch Dis Child* 93(2): 100–1.

Rutherford, M., L.A. Ramenghi, et al. (2010). 'Assessment of brain tissue injury after moderate hypothermia in neonates with hypoxic-ischaemic encephalopathy: a nested substudy of a randomised controlled trial', *Lancet Neurol* 9(1): 39–45.

Saigal, S., D. Feeny, et al. (1994). 'Comparison of the health-related quality of life of extremely low birth weight children and a reference group of children at age eight years', *J Pediatr* 125(3): 418–25.

—— —— (1996). 'Self-perceived health status and health-related quality of life of extremely low-birth-weight infants at adolescence', *JAMA* 276(6): 453–9.

—— P. Rosenbaum, et al. (1994). 'Comprehensive assessment of the health status of extremely low birth weight children at eight years of age: comparison with a reference group', *J Pediatr* 125(3): 411–17.

—— B. Stoskopf, et al. (1999). 'Differences in preferences for neonatal outcomes among health care professionals, parents, and adolescents', *JAMA* 281(21): 1991–7.

—— —— —— (2006). 'Self-perceived health-related quality of life of former extremely low birth weight infants at young adulthood', *Pediatrics* 118(3): 1140–8.

Schneiderman, L.J., N.S. Jecker, et al. (1990). 'Medical futility: its meaning and ethical implications', *Ann Intern Med* 112(12): 949–54.

Sen, A. (1993). 'Capability and Well-being', in M.C. Nussbaum and A. Sen (eds), *The Quality of Life*. New York: Oxford Clarendon Press, 30–53.

Shankaran, S., A.R. Laptook, et al. (2005). 'Whole-body hypothermia for neonates with hypoxic-ischemic encephalopathy', *N Engl J Med* 353(15): 1574–84.

Sheldon, R.A., C. Sedik, et al. (1998). 'Strain-related brain injury in neonatal mice subjected to hypoxia-ischemia', *Brain Res* 810(1–2): 114–22.

Shepardson, L.B., S.J. Youngner, et al. (1999). 'Increased risk of death in patients with do-not-resuscitate orders' *Med Care* 37(8): 727–37.

Simon, R. and D.G. Altman (1994). 'Statistical aspects of prognostic factor studies in oncology', *Br J Cancer* 69(6): 979–85.

Siperstein, G.N., M.L. Wolraich, et al. (1991). 'Physicians' prognoses about the quality of life for infants with intraventricular hemorrhage', *J Dev Behav Pediatr* 12(3): 148–53.

Strauss, D., W. Cable, et al. (1999). 'Causes of excess mortality in cerebral palsy', *Dev Med Child Neurol* 41(9): 580–5.

Sulmasy, D.P. (1999). 'Do patients die because they have DNR orders, or do they have DNR orders because they are going to die?', *Med Care* 37(8): 719–21.

Taylor, A., W. Butt, et al. (2003). 'The functional outcome and quality of life of children after admission to an intensive care unit', *Intensive Care Med* 29(5): 795–800.

Thayyil, S., M. Chandrasekaran, et al. (2010). 'Cerebral magnetic resonance biomarkers for predicting neurodevelopmental outcome following neonatal encephalopathy: a meta-analysis', *Pediatrics* 125(2): e382–95.

Truog, R. and W. Robinson (2003). 'Role of brain death and the dead-donor rule in the ethics of organ transplantation', *Crit Care Med* 31(9): 2391–6.

Tyson, J.E., N.A. Parikh, et al. (2008). 'Intensive care for extreme prematurity—moving beyond gestational age', *N Engl J Med* 358(16): 1672–81.

Ubel, P.A. and G. Loewenstein (2010). 'Pain and suffering awards: they shouldn't be (just) about pain and suffering', *The Journal of Legal Studies* 37(2): s195–s216.

Venkateswaran, S. and M.I. Shevell (2008). 'Comorbidities and clinical determinants of outcome in children with spastic quadriplegic cerebral palsy', *Dev Med Child Neurol* 50(3): 216–22.

Wake, M., L. Salmon, et al. (2003). 'Health status of Australian children with mild to severe cerebral palsy: cross-sectional survey using the Child Health Questionnaire', *Dev Med Child Neurol* 45(3): 194–9.

Werner, E.E. (2004). 'Journeys from childhood to midlife: risk, resilience, and recovery', *Pediatrics* 114(2): 492.

White-Koning, M., C. Arnaud, et al. (2007). 'Determinants of child-parent agreement in quality-of-life reports: a European study of children with cerebral palsy', *Pediatrics* 120(4): e804–14.

WHO (2001). *International Classification of Functioning, Disability and Health (ICF)*. Geneva: World Health Organisation.

The WHOQOL Group (1995). The World Health Organization Quality of Life assessment (WHOQOL): position paper from the World Health Organization, *Social Science & Medicine* 41(10): 1403–9.

Woodward, L.J., P.J. Anderson, et al. (2006). 'Neonatal MRI to predict neurodevelopmental outcomes in preterm infants', *N Engl J Med* 355(7): 685–94.

Zandbergen, E., R. De Haan, et al. (1998). 'Systematic review of early prediction of poor outcome in anoxic ischaemic coma', *The Lancet* 352(9143): 1808–12.

6
Managing Uncertainty

Uncertainty makes decisions difficult in intensive care. But there is a solution available, of a sort. We could continue treatment until things become clearer, until we are able to get a good picture of the likely outcome for the child. At that point, if the outcome is sufficiently poor, treatment could be withdrawn. Is this the best approach to dealing with uncertainty?

The 'treat until certainty' option has been adopted in some parts of the world as the default for treatment of extremely premature infants at the margins of viability (Lantos and Meadow 2006: 92; Kipnis 2007). Infants of twenty-three weeks gestation have approximately a 50 per cent survival rate if resuscitated, and a 20 per cent risk of severe impairment if they survive (Tyson, Parikh et al. 2008). At the time of resuscitation, however, it is not possible to determine which infants are going to live, and which will be impaired. In the 'treat until certainty' strategy, infants are resuscitated if the attending physician believes that they have a chance of survival. If they respond to resuscitation they are admitted to intensive care, and treatment is provided until there is very clear evidence of impending death, or of very severe brain injury. This may mean continuing treatment for a few days, or it may mean continuing treatment for weeks or months.

A similar approach is sometimes applied for newborns or children with hypoxic brain injury. In this illness early clinical or radiological markers of outcome may be misleading. In Chapter 1 we saw the various tools that can assist with prognosis in newborn birth asphyxia including clinical examination, electrophysiological investigations, or imaging of the brain. Most of these tools face the same problem—that early predictions are more fallible than late predictions. In one study, neurological examination performed in the first four days of life had a false positive rate of 45 per cent, but this fell to less than 1 per cent when performed at the end of the third week (Mercuri, Guzzetta, et al. 1999). In some cases assessment can be overly pessimistic, as for example might be the case in an infant or child who has needed high doses of sedation or anticonvulsants. At other times early assessment can be overly optimistic. There is a second phase of cellular injury that sometimes occurs 24–48 hours after a hypoxic-ischemic event. This secondary injury can lead to a significant worsening of a child's condition and to an extension of the original area of brain injury. Clinical or radiological assessment before this point may underestimate the extent and severity of damage. By a week or more after the injury though, it is usually possible to make a better clinical assessment of children or infants. At this stage, multi-organ failure has often resolved or is resolving, and sedation or muscle relaxants are able to be weaned or stopped, allowing meaningful assessment of neurological responses. Imaging may be easier to interpret because areas of the brain that have suffered permanent damage are likely to be more demarcated, and brain swelling will probably have settled.

A waiting strategy is sometimes also applied where particular diagnoses can only be made after a period of time has elapsed. A diagnosis of a 'persistent' vegetative state is made twelve months after a traumatic brain injury, or three to six months after hypoxic or other brain injuries (The Multi-Society Task Force on PVS 1994). Before this period has elapsed, recovery is possible. Some children and adults may appear to be in a vegetative state for months after a traumatic brain injury and then start to show signs of responding to their environment. After this point if the diagnosis of a vegetative state has been made on the basis of robust and careful assessment, recovery is rare. Similarly, diagnoses of severe cerebral palsy, or severe developmental delay/cognitive impairment cannot be made with confidence in early infancy. Because newborn infants are yet to learn to sit, roll, and walk we can't test their skills in those areas. As time passes and they fail to achieve developmental milestones and behave in the way that their peers are behaving, it is possible to diagnose impairment and delay. Decisions about life-sustaining treatment might be deferred until the child's neurological state were clear.

The advantage of waiting is that it avoids making a particular type of mistake because of uncertainty. If we treat until certainty we reduce the chance that we withhold resuscitation from an extremely premature infant who would, if treated, survive without impairment; we make it likely that all those children with hypoxic brain injury who could survive without severe impairment do survive, and we reduce the risk of stopping treatment in children or infants who wouldn't end up severely developmentally delayed, or in a persistent vegetative state. But there are also costs of the waiting strategy.

One of the costs is that we risk prolonging suffering for a group of infants or children who end up dying in intensive care or after discharge from intensive care. One study looked at treatment over time for the most premature newborn infants in a region of Northern England (Swamy, Mohapatra, et al. 2010). Over a fifteen-year period there was minimal change in the overall survival for infants born at twenty-two or twenty-three weeks gestation. However, the duration of intensive care for infants who died increased significantly. The median survival had risen from 11 hours to 3.7 days by the mid 2000s. There was an apparent increase in the number of infants who were treated for several weeks before dying, and several infants died after fifty days or more of intensive care in the most recent period of the survey. Similarly, if we wait for months or years until we are confident of diagnoses of severe impairment or persistent vegetative state before making a decision to limit treatment, it is inevitable that some children will have a long period of invasive and potentially painful treatment and still die.

The other cost of waiting is that doctors and parents may miss the 'window of opportunity' for withdrawing treatment.

The Window of Opportunity

Doctors in intensive care often refer to a 'window of opportunity' for stopping treatment (Kon 2009; Wilkinson 2011), though it does not usually appear in ethics or intensive care textbooks. The term was introduced into popular discourse during the 1980s (it was used initially in relation to the nuclear arms race). In medicine it refers to a particular concern that if decisions are deferred or delayed, the patient may no longer be physiologically dependent on intensive care treatments. At that stage, even if decisions are made by family members to limit further intensive care there is a risk that the patient will survive with very severe degrees of impairment.

This problem is particularly apparent for acute severe brain injuries, for example adults or children with head injury, stroke, or hypoxic brain injury (Cochrane 2009). It also applies to decisions for very premature newborn infants. In these illnesses acute insults lead to multi-organ failure in the first part of their illness, though in many cases there is improvement within a short period. These changes influence treatment withdrawal decisions. During the first couple of days if mechanical ventilation is withdrawn the patient will die quickly in most instances. By contrast, if the decision is deferred by even a few days, infants and children have often resumed breathing and are less acutely unwell. Ironically, the use of specialized prognostic tests such as MRI can compound the problem of the window of opportunity. Obtaining an MRI can lead to delays in decision-making due to the difficulty in organizing an available time in the scanner, arranging transport for the child or infant, and then waiting for the scan to be reported by someone with appropriate experience (Filan, Inder, et al. 2007).

Does the window of opportunity impact on practice? In my interviews with UK neonatologists it was clear that this was an important consideration for at least some doctors caring for infants with asphyxia.

There is a 'window of opportunity' to withdraw with dignity for the child and for the family and if you don't withdraw during that window of opportunity, the child then may start to respond, may then start to breathe, may come off the ventilator and may survive and is profoundly handicapped.

Another clinician noted the potential impact of this on decisions:

there is some urgency... on the one hand you don't want to push parents, you specifically say you don't want them to rush to a decision about anything, on the other hand they need to be aware that there probably is a much greater chance of the child to survive without the ventilator the longer you delay.

However, two neonatologists expressed a degree of ambivalence about the idea of a window of opportunity.

I am not sure I quite buy into that personally... The fact that the baby might survive doesn't mean to say that you have made the wrong decision.

But whether it truly is used in decision making I'm uncertain. I'm not so sure that I use it.

So, the timing of decisions about withdrawal of life support in intensive care is important. It also makes parents' and doctors' decisions very difficult. The challenge is that there is an apparent trade-off between a number of values at stake, for example, between certainty in prognosis, and the risk of survival in

Table 6.1 Competing values in the timing of withdrawal of life-sustaining treatment.

Early withdrawal of treatment	Later withdrawal of treatment
More uncertainty about prognosis.	Less uncertainty about prognosis.
Lower risk of survival with severe disability because patient is more physiologically unstable.	Higher risk of survival with severe disability because patient is less dependent on life support.
Less time for caregivers to decide; risk of rushed decisions and later regret.	More time for surrogates to come to terms with prognosis and decide about treatment.
Withdrawal of life support easier, with prolonged death and patient suffering less likely.	May require consideration of withdrawal of artificial nutrition—more controversial, and may lead to prolonged dying.

a state of severe impairment (Table 6.1). We can manage uncertainty in decision-making by our choices about timing of predictions and decisions. If we make a decision early we potentially reduce the risk of an infant surviving with very severe impairment. If we defer decision-making, we can reduce the risk of an infant dying who would have survived without impairment.

There are two different ethical questions that are raised by this way of managing uncertainty that will be the focus for the rest of this chapter. Firstly, is it ethical for doctors and parents to take the 'window' into account in their decisions and withdraw early? Secondly, if decisions are made to delay decision-making, and an infant or child is no longer dependent on intensive care, is it ethical to withdraw other, less intensive, treatments? In particular we will look at the issue of withdrawal of artificial feeding, and whether it provides an acceptable solution to the problem of uncertainty.

The Ethics of Opportunity in Treatment Withdrawal

The reason to withdraw treatment early (or at least to offer this as an option to parents) is that delaying decisions risks infants or children surviving intensive care in a severely impaired state. But are there reasons to *avoid* considering the window of opportunity?

One general concern relates to quality of life judgements. As noted in Chapter 1, some clinicians, ethicists, and disability rights advocates contend that a diminished quality of life is not sufficient grounds for withdrawing life-sustaining treatment (Wyatt 2005; Ouellette 2006). If it is only permissible to withdraw treatment when death is inevitable, then a window of opportunity cannot arise. But this is not a distinct objection to decisions made to withdraw treatment early in the face of uncertainty. On this basis it would also be wrong to withdraw treatment later in the face of absolute certainty about outcome. In any case, as noted in Chapter 1, both professional guidelines and legal cases have supported the relevance of quality of life considerations in treatment decisions, and there are strong ethical arguments for allowing quality of life, at least sometimes, to justify withdrawing or withholding treatment.

Specific objections to the window of opportunity include discomfort with the term itself, uncertainty and the burdensomeness of treatment, and the doctrine of double effect.

Terminology

The term 'window of opportunity' could be one reason for the disquiet of some of the clinicians that I interviewed. The phrase potentially connotes that the death of the patient is 'opportune', while for families (and for the infant) death represents a terrible misfortune. It might be thought insensitive to raise or even to contemplate the 'opportunity' of death. But we could, if we wished, invent a different term to refer to this phenomenon, perhaps referring to the 'critical decision phase' for brain-injured patients. In any case, in some instances it may be a greater misfortune if the child survives.

Uncertainty

A second reason relates to avoidance of prognostic uncertainty. If we may only withdraw treatment when prognosis is certain, then early decisions to limit treatment would be precluded. Yet, as we noted in Chapter 5, uncertainty is virtually inevitable for predictions in intensive care. The important question is not *whether* there is uncertainty, but rather whether there is *sufficient* uncertainty that treatment must continue. Attempting to reduce uncertainty may have costs, and whether that is worthwhile depends on how those costs are weighed against the benefits of avoiding uncertainty. A related argument might be that uncertainty is a bad thing in decisions about life-sustaining treatment, so we should try to minimize it. If it is possible to improve certainty (by waiting) we should do so. However, again, it depends on which uncertainty we are talking about, and what the costs are of increased certainty. Waiting potentially increases uncertainty about another factor—whether or not a severely impaired infant or child will die. If it is sometimes appropriate to withdraw treatment in the face of less than complete certainty about outcome, there must be some cases where earlier decisions would be an option, even though later ones would be more certain.

Burdens of Short Treatment

A third possible objection is that the window of opportunity is not a relevant consideration for treatment decisions because we may not withdraw treatment from infants or children who only need short periods of life support. It might be thought that recovery of respiratory drive portends a good outcome, or a sufficiently good outcome that treatment withdrawal should not be countenanced. On this view, the most severely affected children will not become independent from a ventilator, or, if they do, will rapidly develop airway obstruction or aspiration. To my knowledge, however, there is no published evidence on the return of spontaneous breathing and prognosis for infants with HIE, extremely premature infants, or brain-injured children. Although it may well be the case that those who *remain* ventilator-dependent are a subset with worse prognosis, it is not necessarily the case that their prognosis is worse. (For example, children with a combination of lung disease and brain injury may remain on the ventilator for several weeks because their lungs are slower to recover— without this being any reflection on the severity of their brain injury (Conlon, Breatnach, et al. 2009).) Furthermore, some of those with poor prognosis do not remain dependent on intensive care. Some infants with HIE maintain or recover respiratory drive despite very severe patterns of brain injury (Miraie 1988; Paris and O'Connell 1991). It would have been permissible to allow these infants to die if they had still been ventilator-dependent.

A different version of this objection relates to the burdensomeness of treatment. If a child will only require a short period of respiratory support, the burden of treatment is relatively minor. It is unpleasant for the child to have a breathing tube in place, but sedation and analgesia can be provided to reduce any discomfort. On some accounts of treatment withdrawal decisions, it is only permissible to withdraw or withhold treatment when the burdens of *treatment* outweigh the benefits, and this may not be the case for a short period of life support. But in the face of severe predicted impairment there are other treatments that we feel it is reasonable to withhold that are even less burdensome than a short period of respiratory support. For example, in such infants or children it is sometimes felt to be acceptable (if the parents choose) to withhold antibiotics for a respiratory infection. Yet the discomfort and burden associated with a course of antibiotics is minimal. If it is permissible to withhold antibiotics it must be permissible to withdraw mechanical ventilation—even where that would only be required for a short period.

It may help to distinguish between different subgroups of quality of life treatment withdrawal decisions (Table 6.2). In one group of infants or children, the reason not to provide treatment, or not to continue treatment, is because the treatment itself is a bad thing and weighs heavily in the balance ('Burdens of treatment'). As an example, some children with severe muscle weakness reach a point where it becomes apparent that they are unlikely to be able to manage without permanent mechanical ventilation via a tracheostomy. Because the burden of this is so substantial for the child, it is often felt acceptable to withhold or withdraw treatment and allow the child to die. However, we would not withhold or withdraw life saving treatments from the same child, if they were not dependent on a breathing machine. Other very burdensome treatments that are sometimes treated as optional in this way include renal dialysis, extra-corporeal membrane oxygenation (ECMO), very complicated cardiac surgery, or perhaps bone marrow transplantation. But there are two other groups of infants and children where the treatment itself plays a minor or trivial role in the balance. The major negatives for these children arise from their underlying illness or impairment ('Burden of life'), or life itself may not provide a benefit to

Table 6.2 Three different groups of quality of life treatment decisions.

1. Burdens of treatment (e.g. prolonged mechanical ventilation, chemotherapy).
2. Burden of life (e.g. severe osteogenesis imperfecta, epidermolysis bullosa).
3. Lack of benefit (e.g. persistent vegetative state).

them because of profound cognitive impairment or depressed consciousness ('Lack of benefit'). It would be ethical to withdraw mechanical ventilation from children in these latter two groups. But even minor interventions to prolong life in these children may not be in their interests, and consequently appropriate to withhold. In such patients it may be appropriate to withhold treatments of little burden, including antibiotics, blood transfusions, or brief periods of mechanical ventilation. (We will look shortly at the specific questions relating to withdrawal of artificial nutrition.)

A more significant concern is that consideration of the window of opportunity potentially conflicts with the doctrine of double effect (DDE). It will be worthwhile addressing this concern in more detail, as the doctrine has a broader relevance for treatment limitation decisions in intensive care.

The Doctrine of Double Effect

The DDE is a rule that is often cited as providing a boundary for permissible actions in end-of-life decisions, and has its origins in Catholic moral theology (Nuffield Council on Bioethics 2006; Racine and Shevell 2009; Mason, Laurie, et al. 2011). It governs actions that have potential effects that are both good and bad. According to the DDE (or at least according to one part of the doctrine) it is not permissible to *intend* to hasten the death of the patient, but it is permissible to perform acts that unintentionally (or as a side effect) hasten death. For example, the doctrine is often drawn on to sanction the common practice of giving opioids to a terminally ill patient to relieve their pain, even though it is suspected that this may slow their breathing and lead to them dying sooner than they otherwise would have (see below).

Morphine and the Doctrine of Double Effect

The classic example used in discussions about the doctrine of double effect in end-of-life care is the use of morphine for terminally ill patients. This example has featured in numerous textbooks, and has been supported by the courts in a number of cases (Mason, Laurie, et al. 2011). For example Lord Goff, in the Tony Bland case, noted that it was established law that a doctor who is caring for a patient dying of cancer may 'lawfully administer painkilling drugs despite the fact that he knows that an incidental effect... will be to abbreviate the patient's life' (Airedale NHS Trust v Bland 1993:12).

Recently, though, a number of palliative care specialists have challenged whether morphine does actually hasten death when provided as an analgesic, and consequently whether the doctrine of double effect is relevant for decisions of this sort. There is no randomized controlled trial evidence (for fairly obvious reasons), but a large number of studies have looked at the timing of death in patients who did or did not receive opioids, or at the relationship between the timing of death and the dose of opioids received. In a number of studies of palliative care patients, sedative or morphine use was not associated with length of survival (Thorns and Sykes 2000; Morita, Tsunoda, et al. 2001; George and Regnard 2007). Indeed there is evidence that, paradoxically, higher doses of opioids and sedatives were associated with *longer* survival after extubation in the intensive care unit (Mazer, Alligood, et al. 2011; Edwards 2006). In other studies the opposite result was found: in one large study of hospice patients, higher morphine dosing was associated with shorter time until death; however, it appeared to be only a minor determinant of survival (Portenoy, Sibirceva, et al. 2006).

How should we interpret this evidence? If morphine does not shorten time until death, then physicians' concern about hastening death may be misplaced. We may not need to worry about the doctrine of double effect in much end-of-life care. But it remains possible that opioids could hasten death in some patients (for example those with chronic obstructive airway disease), or that other actions (or omissions) would predictably hasten death, and consequently that the DDE would be needed to justify them. One example is the use of high doses of sedation to induce unconsciousness in patients who are dying and continuing to experience pain or distress (so-called 'terminal sedation') (McIntyre 2004).

The problem for the window of opportunity is that if the timing of treatment withdrawal is influenced by whether or not the infant will die (when extubated) it may appear that death is either intended, or is, at least in part, one of the direct goals of extubation. Can the window of opportunity influence treatment decisions without conflicting with the DDE? For that to be the case, the intention of treatment withdrawal must be something other than death. There are a couple of possibilities. One option is that the primary goal of the doctor is to respect the interests of the child. It could be in the best interests of a child to have treatment withdrawn earlier rather than later, if later withdrawal will lead to survival in a state of severe impairment or to a slow death. But the problem with this solution is that it risks conflicting with a different part of the DDE.

In its full form the doctrine of double effect actually has four separate conditions:

1. The act itself must be one that is allowed.
2. The intention is to achieve the good effect, though the bad effect may be foreseen.
3. The good effect does not come about through the bad effect.
4. The good achieved by the act is enough to allow the bad side effect to occur (Frey 2005a).

Treatment withdrawal on the basis of the infant's or child's best interests would meet the first and second conditions. And clearly if we think that the seriousness of the child's condition warrants withdrawing treatment (even if they die), then the fourth condition will also be satisfied. However, the problem with the 'best interests' defence is that if it is in the best interests of the child to die, and it is those interests that are the goal of treatment withdrawal, the third condition of the doctrine would be violated. The good (interests) comes via the bad (death). In a different setting, the DDE rules that a doctor may not prescribe barbiturates to a patient in order to serve the best interests of the patient (where the death of the patient is believed to be in their best interests). The doctor may, however, permissibly give barbiturates in order to treat seizures (a different goal) even if this could conceivably hasten the death of the patient.

A second possible defence is that the doctor's goal in withdrawing treatment is not to hasten the child's death, but to respect the parents' request that treatment be withdrawn. If parents are justified in a belief that continuing treatment would not be in the child's best interests, we would usually think that their wishes should be respected. Then the child's death would be neither intended, nor a means of achieving the goal (respecting parents' wishes). This would potentially avoid clashing with the DDE. Yet one residual concern is that the reason that parents have chosen earlier withdrawal of treatment may be at least partly in order to avoid the infant's survival with severe impairment. So there might still be the possibility that the child's death is the means to achieving the aim of satisfying parents' wishes, again clashing with the third condition of the DDE. We might also wonder whether the DDE applies to parental requests as well as to doctors' actions. Even if they are not the ones withdrawing treatment, their request for treatment withdrawal leads to the child's death, and we might worry about whether this is intended or is the means of achieving an alternative aim.

A third possibility is that the doctor's (and parents') goal in withdrawing treatment is to alleviate or reduce suffering. This is perhaps the way that doctors most often rationalize treatment withdrawal decisions; it is certainly the way that they sometimes couch decisions when they are talking to parents. Is this the answer? Where the treatment itself contributes significantly to suffering for the child, then it does seem possible for us to decide to withhold or withdraw that treatment to prevent suffering without intending the child's death. This option is most plausible in the first group of quality of life decisions discussed above—those where the treatment is a major reason for judging the child's quality of life to be poor. It is more problematic in the second group, where we are contemplating not providing treatment that is of little burden (antibiotics, or a short period of ventilation for example). But in both cases there is a separate problem. Although it isn't included in the list of conditions above, there is another factor that is sometimes included in descriptions of the DDE: that if it is possible to avoid or reduce the bad side effect of the action this should be done (McIntyre 2004). This is, in a sense, a way of proving that the doctor's intention is not really to achieve the bad effect. On this condition, if there were another way of achieving the desired end (reducing suffering) without producing the side effect (leading to death), we should do so. However, there *are* often ways of alleviating or eliminating the suffering caused by medical treatment that do not lead to death. For example, a patient who is on a ventilator can receive high doses of sedatives and analgesics to ensure that they do not suffer. The reason that doctors don't always take this option is that there are other reasons to think that this is not a good solution; it might mean that a patient is consigned to long periods of intensive care without any capacity for conscious experience or any ability to wean off the ventilator. But the possibility of other ways of achieving the aim of reducing suffering without hastening death raises questions about whether we can avoid conflicts with the DDE in this way.

In fact, although we have focused on early withdrawal of treatment here, all of the above arguments (and problems) might also apply to later decisions to withdraw life-sustaining treatment. If we do wait until we have achieved a high(er) level of certainty about outcome, and the patient happens to still be dependent on life support, the same questions about the intention of the doctor/parents would potentially arise.

One way out of the problem would be to argue that the doctrine of double effect does not apply to non-treatment decisions. As phrased above, and as sometimes interpreted, the doctrine is about *acts*, and decisions not to provide life-sustaining treatment are *omissions* (Williams 2009). But this does not necessarily solve the problem for two reasons. Firstly, it is not clear that treatment withdrawal decisions are really omissions. When the doctor switches off the ventilator, or removes the endotracheal tube, they are intervening in a clear way that changes the outcome for the child. It may well be that they are justified in doing so, but we should not pretend that they are not taking positive steps when they do this (Frey 2005b). Secondly, even if it is an omission to withdraw or withhold life-sustaining treatment, that does not necessarily mean that we are right to do so. We would judge harshly a doctor who omitted to provide life-sustaining treatment because he did not like the colour of a patient's skin, or because he stood to inherit money if the patient dies. We need some rule to cover which omissions are allowed and which are not. A number of descriptions of the doctrine of double effect suggest that it applies to both omissions and to acts (Gillon 1986; Kamm 1991).

A more radical response would be to suggest that we should not apply the doctrine of double effect for treatment withdrawal decisions on the basis of quality of life. The doctrine of double effect has been the subject of various criticisms over the years, and there are a number of problems with it (Gillon 1986; McIntyre 2004; Goldworth 2008). But here are several of the biggest problems. They relate to the second and third conditions of the doctrine.

The first problem is that the doctrine appears to encourage or at least permit doctors to reframe or redirect their intentions in a particular way. Imagine that a doctor is caring for a patient with a terminal illness who is suffering severe pain. If the doctor gives the patient palliative sedation with the intention of hastening the patient's death, her actions conflict with the DDE and are prohibited. But imagine now that the same doctor, faced with the same patient, and the same plan of palliative sedation realizes that she is not allowed to intend the patient's death. She repeats to herself— 'my intention is to relieve suffering, death is merely a side effect'. Then her treatment plan becomes permissible. The above discussion of different possible justifications of early withdrawal of treatment might seem to be an example of the same kind of sophistry. But it seems like a kind of ethical sleight of hand to be encouraging individuals to monitor their thoughts and change their intentions if they are ones that are not allowed. Does this really make a difference to the morality of withdrawing treatment, or providing palliative sedation? There is a related problem in policing the doctrine. The importance placed on the doctor's intentions makes it hard for a third party to know whether a particular course of action is allowed. How are we to know what the doctor's intentions are or were (Goldworth 2008)?

The second problem is whether the distinction between intention and foresight that the doctrine makes is psychologically plausible. Philosopher R.G. Frey has questioned whether the doctor can avoid intending the patient's death when she takes a course of action that is certain (or almost certain) to lead to death, and where she is willing for that death to occur (Frey 2005a). In a different example, imagine that a surgeon performs surgery to amputate a patient's leg with the goal of saving their life (they have gangrene in the foot, and risk overwhelming sepsis if the operation does not take place) (Gillon 1986). In that case, there is a good effect (saving life), and a bad effect (amputation), but it is hard to see how the surgeon would not intend to remove the patient's leg, even if she regrets that it is necessary to do so. The difficulty of removing this other intention may be one explanation for the relatively high proportion of doctors who (when asked anonymously) admit to intending the patient's death when making end-of-life decisions. A large survey asked UK doctors about the most recent patient who had died under their care (Seale 2009). One third of deaths involved decisions to give drugs or to withdraw or withhold treatment that the doctor expected would hasten the patient's death. In a quarter of those 800 or so cases doctors admitted to having, at least in part, an explicit intention to hasten death. (Some of the evidence cited above about morphine might cast doubt on this evidence of the intentions of doctors.

A number of those who expected that their actions may hasten death may have been mistaken.)

The third reason for casting doubt upon the DDE in some cases of treatment withdrawal is that it is not clear that the patient's death *is* a bad effect of withdrawing or withholding treatment. We would certainly judge death to be bad where there is a possibility of a patient living a longer life and of gaining benefit from that life. However, there appear to be cases where death is not, in itself, bad for the patient. Where a patient is suffering, and will soon die even if further treatment is provided, or where the patient's quality of life is sufficiently poor that it is preferable that they die rather than continue to live, death ceases to be something that must be avoided. In the same way, although it would be bad to cut off a patient's leg if they were able to survive without amputation and have full use of their limb, in the case described above it is not bad for the patient to lose a leg. It is, in a sense, the lesser of two evils.

If we reject the doctrine of double effect because of these problems, what are we left with for treatment limitation decisions? Are there any other rules that should govern whether or when such decisions are allowed, or is anything allowed? The problems listed above arose particularly from the second and third conditions of the DDE. However, the other conditions would still stand. A revised and simpler set of principles for treatment limitation decisions might be that

a. The act (or omission) must itself be one that is allowed, and
b. The good effects of the act (or omission) for the patient are enough to justify any bad effects that are anticipated.

This, much simpler, set of conditions would give us boundaries for end-of-life decisions without having to delve into the doctor's intentions. So, for example, on the basis of these principles it would be permissible to give a terminally ill patient in pain an analgesic dose of morphine, but it would not be permissible for a doctor to give a tenfold overdose of morphine or a dose of potassium. The latter actions are not generally accepted actions in end-of-life care. (There is an important separate question about what actions should be permitted, but the doctrine of double effect doesn't help us with that.) Similarly, a doctor would not be allowed to give a patient a standard dose of morphine because the doctor stood to gain an inheritance, or because he had judged (unilaterally and without justification) that their life was not worth living. What matters is whether, from the patient's point of view, the good of the morphine outweighs the bad, and we would have reason to doubt that in either of those circumstances. As another example, it would be reasonable for doctors to withdraw mechanical ventilation from a child or infant who is predicted to survive in a profoundly impaired state, whether early or later in the course of their illness. This is because this action (withdrawal of treatment) falls within the class of actions that we allow doctors to take, and because in this particular circumstance there is enough evidence to justify a judgement that the good of withdrawing treatment outweighs the bad. However, we would not need to know the intentions of the doctors or parents in taking this step.

The question that we started with was whether doctors and parents should be allowed to take into account the window of opportunity in their treatment limitation decisions? If delay will increase the risk of a child surviving with severe impairment, is it appropriate or ethical for decisions to be made earlier (at the cost of greater uncertainty)? We have looked at a range of different arguments against doing so—based on uncertainty, the prognosis of survivors, the burdensomeness (or not) of treatment, and on the doctrine of double effect. The latter concern may be the most significant argument against this way of dealing with uncertainty, but it is not decisive. There are ways of justifying the intent of treatment withdrawal that may avoid conflict with the doctrine (focusing on parents' wishes, and on the suffering of the child). More importantly, though, there are also good reasons to doubt whether we should be bound by the doctrine of double effect in treatment withdrawal decisions. If treatment is being withdrawn on the basis of predicted quality of life, the death of the infant must necessarily be judged to be better than continued life and treatment. It seems hypocritical to suggest that this cannot permissibly be one of the goals of action.

Withdrawal of Artificial Feeding from Children or Infants

An alternative solution to the window of opportunity problem, and a quite different way of dealing with the problem of uncertainty, is to wait until there is certainty (or at least a higher degree of certainty), and then to withdraw other, less intensive, treatments from infants or children who are no longer dependent on the ventilator. Along this line, Thomas Cochrane has argued that there is no urgency to make decisions about treatment, for example in adult patients following a stroke, because there is always the option of withdrawal of nutritional support. This would potentially remove one of the major disadvantages of the 'wait until certainty' strategy, the possibility of long-term survival in a highly compromised state. (It wouldn't reduce the other problem—of prolonged suffering, and in fact might worsen it.) Is this solution an option for children or infants? If it is ethical to withdraw feeding, in what circumstances should it be allowed?

Nutritional support can be provided to children and infants in a variety of ways. Food and fluids that are taken by mouth can be supplemented with calories or nutrients. Alternatively, those who are unable to take enough nutrition by mouth may have nutrition provided by a nasogastric tube (a tube inserted through the nose to the stomach), or gastrostomy (a surgically placed tube between the skin and the stomach). Finally, children who are unable to tolerate nutrition via the intestine may receive parenteral (intravenous) nutrition, usually via a central venous catheter. Almost all critically ill children receive artificial nutrition of one form or another while they are seriously ill. Few are in a position to eat and drink normally, and optimizing nutrition improves intensive care outcome. The reason that artificial nutrition becomes an issue in children who are recovering from critical illness and who are no longer sedated and mechanically ventilated, is that some of these children, particularly those who are left with long-term impairments, have ongoing difficulty taking nutrition by mouth. Brain injury and muscular weakness may make it difficult to control and coordinate the normal process of swallowing. This problem can be overcome or ameliorated by using artificial feeding as a supplement, or an alternative to food and fluids by mouth. However, when this occurs, artificial nutrition becomes a life-sustaining intervention. It prevents death from dehydration or malnutrition. It also reduces the risk of death from a chest infection, since neurologically impaired children who take food or fluid by mouth sometimes aspirate and choke because of difficulty protecting their airway while eating. For many of these children, if artificial nutrition were not available (as is the case still in other parts of the world), they would die.

Is it appropriate to withhold or withdraw artificial feeding from a child or infant? The question has provoked considerable debate and controversy

(Paris and Fletcher 1987; Miraie 1988; Paris and O'Connell 1991; Nelson, Rushton, et al. 1995; Stanley 2000; Carter and Leuthner 2003; Keown 2003; Levi 2003; Porta and Frader 2007). It is a particularly emotive question because the provision of nutrition is one of the most fundamental things that parents (or medical professionals) do for children. The idea of a child starving to death is disturbing and distressing to many. However, in recent years there has been explicit acceptance in professional guidelines that this *is* appropriate, at least in some circumstances. In the UK, the Royal College of Paediatrics and Child Health document on withdrawing and withholding treatment (discussed in Chapter 2), includes artificial nutrition in a list of treatments that may be withdrawn or withheld, depending on the circumstances, though does not set out what those circumstances might be (Royal College of Paediatrics and Child Health 2004). The more recent report by the Nuffield Council of Bioethics is more circumspect; it includes artificial nutrition and intravenous hydration as part of basic nursing care rather than a medical treatment, and concludes that it should only be withdrawn when it would cause discomfort and pain (for example, if there is little or no functioning bowel), or when death is imminent (Nuffield Council on Bioethics 2006). The recent General Medical Council (GMC) guidelines on treatment at the end of life concludes that what it calls 'clinically assisted nutrition' (whether by tube or via an intravenous 'drip') can be withheld or withdrawn if the burdens of treatment outweigh the benefits, and consensus is reached with parents and the rest of the healthcare team (General Medical Council 2010). In the USA, the American Academy of Pediatrics (AAP) released a report in 2009 that endorses withdrawal of artificial nutrition from children in certain circumstances (Diekema and Botkin 2009). Similar to the GMC guidance, it notes that nutrition may be withheld or withdrawn where the burdens of the intervention to the patient outweigh the potential benefits. The report provides three examples of situations where this might occur: firstly in children who permanently lack conscious awareness (for example newborn infants following severe HIE, or older children in a persistent vegetative state); secondly, infants or children who are in the final stages of dying; and thirdly, children with severe or total intestinal failure.

These guidelines, and the case law that they draw on in support of their recommendations, reject one argument against withdrawing nutrition, namely that nutrition is in a special category of treatment that may never be withheld or withdrawn. One of the distinctions that is sometimes made in the ethics of end-of-life decisions is between *ordinary* medical treatments and *extraordinary* medical treatments. The idea is that certain treatments represent a basic level of care that should be provided to all patients regardless of circumstances. For example, it would be unethical to fail to provide pain relief or comfort care to a dying patient, though it would be acceptable to decide not to provide a blood transfusion or antibiotics or breathing support. The former are ordinary treatments, while the latter are extraordinary, and thus optional. Some have argued that nutritional support represents an 'ordinary' treatment and thus may not be withdrawn (Clark 2006). This distinction between different categories of treatment has been discussed elsewhere (Lynn and Childress 1983; Glover 1990: 195–7) and the debate will not be revisited in detail here. Briefly though, the big problem with this way of thinking about treatments and withdrawal is that it seems to concentrate on the wrong thing. Many treatments seem to be either ordinary or extraordinary, depending on the situation. It would be perfectly acceptable to withdraw or withhold mechanical ventilation from a patient with disseminated malignancy and only a short time to live. But it would be completely inappropriate to withhold the same treatment from a patient with a chest infection and a very high likelihood of full recovery. What makes the difference is not the type of treatment; it is whether the positives of the treatment outweigh the negatives. For some treatments, it is hard to imagine situations where this is not the case; providing pain relief might be in this category. However, artificial nutrition is not like that. There are situations where providing enteral nutrition via tubes appears to offer no benefit to the patient (the dying or permanently unconscious patient), and others where it may harm them (for example the child with no functioning intestine).

The other argument that is sometimes made against allowing withdrawal of nutritional support is that this would violate the doctrine of double effect. We discussed above some of the problems related to the DDE for withdrawal of life-sustaining treatments, and some of the responses to them. Similar responses would apply to withdrawal of nutrition. Firstly, the intentions of the doctor (or parent) who withdraws or withholds artificial nutrition may not be that the infant dies, but may rather be to alleviate suffering, respect the wishes of the parent, or promote the interests of the infant. But secondly, as argued above, the doctrine of double effect may not provide the right boundary for ethical decisions at the end of life. The important questions are whether withdrawing artificial nutrition is in a category that is potentially permitted (the above arguments suggest that it is), and whether the good effects of withdrawing nutrition outweigh the bad.

It is sometimes appropriate to withdraw or withhold artificial nutrition from a child. But the next question is, *when* is it appropriate? In particular, how does this decision compare to decisions about other life-sustaining treatments like mechanical ventilation? The relevance for uncertainty and the window of opportunity problem is this. If there is complete symmetry between these two types of treatment withdrawal decision (call this the 'symmetry view'), there would indeed (as Cochrane suggested) be no need for urgency in decision-making. There would be no cases where it would be possible now to withdraw mechanical ventilation, but impermissible later to withdraw nutrition. The window of opportunity would not arise. On the other hand, if, as some of the guidelines above suggest, withdrawal of nutrition is a special sort of decision, with more stringent or limited conditions where it would apply, then we would still be left with this dilemma about whether mechanical ventilation should be withdrawn now (despite uncertainty) to avoid the risk of survival in a state of severe impairment. This would represent an 'asymmetrical' view about withdrawal of feeding.

The symmetry view: Withdrawal of mechanical ventilation and withdrawal of artificial feeding should be treated similarly. If it is permissible to withdraw or withhold ventilation, it would be permissible to withdraw or withhold artificial feeding.

The asymmetry view: Withdrawal of artificial feeding is a different type of decision from withdrawal of ventilation. There are cases where it would be permissible to withdraw or withhold ventilation, though it would not be permissible to withdraw or withhold feeding.

The AAP and GMC guidelines seem to support the symmetry view. Thus the GMC guidelines state: 'Nutrition and hydration provided by tube or drip are regarded in law as medical treatment, and should be treated in the same way as other medical interventions' (General Medical Council 2010). The AAP report contends that decisions about artificial nutrition should be made on the basis of the 'same principles' or 'same 2 conditions' as decisions about other medical interventions (Diekema and Botkin 2009). (The two conditions mentioned by the AAP report are either that a competent patient has refused treatment, or that the burdens outweigh benefits.) But in practice it doesn't appear that decisions about artificial nutrition and other treatments *are* treated symmetrically. Whereas decisions to withhold or withdraw mechanical ventilation are very common in newborn or paediatric intensive care, it is rare for artificial nutrition to be withheld or stopped. There are a large number of studies that have described the former decisions, but only rare reports of the latter. Sociologist Hazel McHaffie interviewed staff in six Scottish neonatal units in the 1980s (McHaffie and Fowlie 2001). Withdrawing or withholding decisions preceded the majority of deaths; however, in only one of the six units was withholding artificial nutrition an accepted practice. In a case series from a Canadian neonatal unit, artificial nutrition was withdrawn in only 5 per cent of deaths (Hellmann, Williams, et al. 2008). In one survey in the 1990s of American paediatricians-in-training, although all would withhold cardiopulmonary resuscitation from a child in a vegetative state, and 97 per cent would withdraw mechanical ventilation, only 35 per cent would withdraw nutrition (Rubenstein, Unti, et al. 1994).

Babies Pearson, Doe, and M

In the 1970s and 1980s in newborn intensive care units in the US, the UK, and Australia (and likely elsewhere too), it was privately thought acceptable to withhold artificial feeding from newborn infants whose parents had chosen not to pursue life-sustaining treatment. This practice received public attention in a series of highly controversial legal cases in the early 1980s. In the first of these in 1981 in the UK, a consultant paediatrician Dr Leonard Arthur was charged with murder for his role a year earlier in the death of a newborn infant with Down syndrome. The infant, John Pearson, did not appear to have any complications other than his chromosomal abnormality, but the parents had decided (after being informed of the diagnosis of Down syndrome) that they did not want to care for the child. Dr Arthur had ordered that nursing care be provided, and the infant was given only water and sedatives (dihydrocodeine), dying at sixty-nine hours of age. Dr Arthur was charged, but subsequently acquitted (Raphael 1988). (In contrast, in the same year, another infant with Down syndrome, 'B', was made a ward of the court after his parents refused to consent for surgery for a congenital blockage of his intestine (duodenal atresia). The court ordered that surgery and other life-sustaining treatment be provided because his life was not 'demonstrably intolerable' (Re B 1981).)

In the US, the following year, a similar case reached the courts and the media. In 1982, in Bloomington Indiana, doctors and parents discussed treatment options for Baby Doe, an infant with Down syndrome and oesophageal atresia with tracheooesophageal fistula (a serious but correctable connection between the airway and upper bowel combined with a blockage of the oesophagus) (Paris, Schreiber, et al. 2007). On advice from their obstetrician, Baby Doe's parents withheld consent for life-saving surgery; however, Baby Doe's paediatricians believed that surgery should be performed and went to the courts to overrule the parents. A series of courts upheld the parents' decision; an appeal was due to be heard in the Supreme Court, but Baby Doe died from aspiration pneumonia before the case could be heard. That case prompted the Republican President Ronald Reagan to commission a set of rules—known subsequently as the Baby Doe rules—that would prohibit American doctors from withholding treatment on the basis of disability. (A case the following year provided an interesting contrast, and a test of the Baby Doe rules. Baby Jane Doe had spina bifida, hydrocephalus, and microcephaly, and was predicted to have severe physical and cognitive impairment. Her parents and doctors decided not to attempt surgical closure of her spina bifida, but to treat her with antibiotics and bandages (Annas 1984). However, the court became involved when a third party (a right-to-life lawyer) sought an injunction to authorize surgery. The main issue at stake in the Baby Jane Doe case was not withdrawal of nutrition, but withholding of potentially life-prolonging surgery. A series of courts found in favour of the parents, and supported the decision to withhold surgery as this was in the best interests of the infant.)

The third prominent case involving a newborn infant and withdrawal of artificial nutrition took place in 1989 in Melbourne, Australia. Baby M was born with spina bifida, hydrocephalus, and vocal cord paresis. Like Baby Jane Doe, M's parents and doctors, after discussion, elected to treat her without surgery or antibiotics. She was given sedatives and analgesics, provided with oral feeds when she appeared to be hungry (but not supplemented with tube feeding), and intravenous fluids. She died at twelve days of age (Kuhse 1992). In another parallel with the Jane Doe case, this case reached public attention when third parties associated with a right-to-life movement attempted to intervene to prevent M's death. The police were called, interviewed doctors, and sought specialist second opinions—all of whom supported the treatment plan that was being provided. After the infant's death, a coronial inquest exonerated the doctors and parents of any wrong-doing.

At least some existing authoritative guidelines support the symmetry view on the basis that the principles for withdrawal of different types of treatment (including nutritional support) should be the same. But using the same ethical principles doesn't mean that *decisions* will be identical. If there are relevant differences in the benefits and burdens equation that apply for nutrition decisions compared to mechanical ventilation, then the same principles may yield different answers. What might those differences be?

One difference lies in the nature of the death, and possible harms from withdrawal of treatment. Death following withdrawal of mechanical ventilation usually ensues within a period of hours. In one study in a paediatric intensive care unit 85 per cent of children died within four hours of withdrawal of the ventilator (Burns, Mitchell, et al. 2000). In another study, 60 per cent of children in intensive care who had ventilation withdrawn (and who were potentially eligible to donate organs) died within one hour of withdrawal. In contrast, death following withdrawal or withholding of artificial nutrition may be delayed. In children, withdrawal of artificial feeding has been reported to result in death after ten to fourteen days (Cranford 1995). A similar duration has been reported in case reports and series in newborn infants, with an average survival of thirteen to sixteen days, though ranging from one to thirty-seven days (Carter and Leuthner 2003; Hellmann, Williams, et al. 2008; Siden 2010).

The significance of the longer period of survival after a decision has been made to withdraw treatment is twofold. Firstly, there is the possibility of infants or children suffering during the period between withdrawal of treatment and death. This has been argued to make decisions to withdraw artificial nutrition inconsistent with the infant's (or child's) best interests (Kuhse 1986). Secondly, there is a concern that this will lead to distress in parents or other staff. As for the first concern, there is little data on the nature or extent of distress or suffering in children or infants who have artificial feeding withheld. In adults, a number of papers and case reports have suggested that patients who refuse feeding, or who have artificial feeding and hydration withheld do not suffer from hunger or distress (Printz 1992; Brody, Campbell, et al. 1997). A survey of nurses working in hospices for dying adult patients found that one-third of nurses had cared for patients who had elected not to receive oral nutrition and hydration. The nurses reported these patients to have been peaceful, with low levels of pain and suffering (Ganzini, Goy, et al. 2003). In particular, these adults do not appear to have suffered from the sort of subjective distress and discomfort that we would associate with starvation in an otherwise healthy individual. It is not clear if the experience of children or infants who have artificial nutrition and hydration withheld is the same as that of adults who decline oral food and fluids. But there is some support for the idea that the experience would be similar. In a recent case series, five infants who had artificial feeding withheld were described as 'quiet', with 'no overt signs of hunger behaviour' (Siden 2010). So, although the dying process may be longer, it is not necessarily the case that children or infants would suffer unduly following withdrawal of artificial forms of nutritional support, compared to withdrawal of other treatments. It has been suggested that ketone release, which is a side effect of fasting, contributes to their level of comfort (Brody, Campbell, et al. 1997). There may also be a lack of a sensation of hunger or thirst in some of the severely brain-injured children (and adults) who have this type of treatment withdrawn. If a child or infant did start to become visibly distressed or uncomfortable, it would be possible to alleviate or ameliorate that with sedation or analgesia, in the same way that dyspnoea, distress, or discomfort is treated symptomatically after withdrawal of ventilation. It would, though, be impossible to guarantee that a child did not suffer any distress following withdrawal of artificial feeding, and this would potentially occur over a longer period.

On the other hand, there is evidence that parents find prolonged death following withdrawal of life-sustaining treatment distressing. In Hazel McHaffie's study of parents of newborn infants who had mechanical ventilation withdrawn, one-fifth of parents described distress at the length of time it took their child to die (McHaffie, Lyon, et al. 2001). (In that study, the longest duration of survival after treatment withdrawal was thirty-six hours.) Following withdrawal of feeding, parent distress has been reported to increase significantly, the longer the period of survival (Siden 2010). This may only be partly alleviated by counselling parents in advance that death will not necessarily be swift. Where death is delayed, parents often experience ongoing ambivalence or guilt about the decision that they have made, and this is exacerbated by concerns about whether or not the child herself might be suffering. While it is possible to support families through this period, it seems almost inevitable that this sort of death is more unpleasant for families than one that occurs following withdrawal of mechanical ventilation.

Another factor that may mark a difference between decisions about feeding and decisions about other types of treatment withdrawal is the particular meaning and emotional salience of feeding. The act of feeding a child, of putting them to the breast, is (in normal circumstances) often the first concrete act of caring and love that a mother provides for her newborn after birth. The infant is utterly dependent on others to provide nourishment in the newborn period, and following that, for the first years of life. There are good evolutionary reasons why adult humans have strong urges to provide that nourishment for dependent children. Conversely, the idea of starving a child is disturbing, even abhorrent to many. It is not surprising, then, that parents and medical staff sometimes find that withholding nutrition from a child *feels different* from withholding other types of treatment. One question is whether these gut responses can be overcome. If we have good reason to think that providing artificial nutrition to a child or infant would offer them no benefit, or would risk harm, then it may be a sincere act of compassion and caring *not* to provide it. Furthermore, if (as the limited evidence appears to suggest), infants or children do not suffer following withdrawal of artificial nutrition, then perhaps medical staff or parents should disregard their intuitive sense that this is a more worrying step to take. But on the other hand, if our gut feelings about withholding nutrition from children can't be overcome, then we may continue to treat these decisions differently, even if we are not, strictly speaking, justified in doing so.

A more important reason that would mark a difference between withdrawal of mechanical ventilation and withdrawal of artificial feeding relates to the burdensomeness of these two treatments. Long periods of support with a breathing machine may be unpleasant or painful for the patient, with the need for a tracheostomy and regular insertion of suction tubes into the airway to remove secretions, as well as occasional episodes of acute airway obstruction from secretions or tube dislodgement. The need for continuous respiratory support and nursing care may significantly limit mobility and independence. On the other hand, although gastrostomy or nasogastric feeding may cause discomfort (again, for example, when tubes are dislodged and need to be replaced), they are probably less commonly a source of pain or distress to the patient. If the burdens of treatment are greater for ventilation than for artificial feeding, then it would be easier for them to outweigh benefits. Simplistically, drawing on the earlier distinction between two types of quality of life justifications for withdrawing treatment (burdensome treatment or burdensome illness), withdrawal of mechanical ventilation could occur for either of these two justifications, but withdrawal of nutrition may be mostly, or entirely, based on a 'burdensome illness' judgement.

Finally, one concern that is sometimes expressed about withdrawal of artificial nutrition is that it may be abused. Allowing nutrition to be withdrawn from some infants or children with very severe illnesses or impairments may lead, via a 'slippery slope' to withdrawal of nutrition from other infants or children who are not so severely affected, where the burdens of treatment do not outweigh the benefits (Diekema and Botkin 2009). Because of the greater danger of this type of decision, we might either never allow it to occur, or allow it in more restricted circumstances than other types of treatment withdrawal (for example mechanical ventilation). But it isn't clear why such decisions *are* more prone to abuse. Doctors and parents might just as easily decide to withdraw ventilation for inappropriate reasons. Indeed, there would be one argument for regarding withdrawal of mechanical ventilation as a *more* dangerous decision. Since death usually follows within a relatively short period after extubation and removal of respiratory support, there would potentially be less time for others to scrutinize the decision, and less possibility of a third party intervening to prevent death. When it comes to withdrawal of other (more intensive) treatments, the possibility of abuse doesn't lead us to rejecting this type of decision—rather, the appropriate response is to make sure that treatment withdrawal occurs for the right reasons. Decisions are carefully documented, and a second opinion is often sought before withdrawing treatment. If those measures are enough to prevent abuse of ventilation withdrawal, why would they not be able to prevent abuse of withdrawal of nutrition?

Another reason for thinking that nutrition withdrawal would be more dangerous is that there are just more children who are dependent for a long period of time on artificial nutrition than there are children dependent on mechanical ventilation. So, even if abuse occurred only rarely, inappropriate withdrawal of artificial nutrition might affect more children. If that were the case, then perhaps we should be more restrictive about nutrition withdrawal decisions. But, on the basis of the same argument, withdrawal or withholding of antibiotics would appear to be an even more dangerous withdrawal decision. There are far, far more children who receive antibiotics than there are children who receive artificial nutrition. We should be even more restrictive about decisions to withhold antibiotics than decisions to withhold nutrition. But in fact there is usually much less attention or scrutiny paid to decisions about antibiotics, and the above-mentioned guidelines rarely mention them. In a survey of adult physicians, doctors preferred to withdraw blood transfusions and antibiotics over mechanical ventilation or tube feeding (Christakis and Asch 1993).

The final reason why decisions about withdrawal of nutrition are perceived as more prone to abuse is perhaps because of past cases, perhaps like the infants with Down syndrome Baby Pearson or Baby Doe mentioned above, where nutrition was withheld and infants allowed to die for reasons other than their best interests. It is now generally believed that such infants have lives that are worth living, and consequently that treatment cannot be withheld on the basis of their best interests. However, although there are no cases that have reached widespread attention like those, it is highly likely that in the 1970s or 1980s there were decisions to withhold or withdraw mechanical ventilation from infants with Down syndrome. In fact, the Down syndrome example provides evidence *against* the slippery slope. Although in the 1970s it was judged by a majority of paediatricians and paediatric surgeons to be acceptable to withhold surgery for intestinal blockage in such infants (Shaw, Randolph, et al. 1977), by the late 1980s few would support such decisions (Todres, Guillemin, et al. 1988). In one tertiary neonatal unit, from the 1980s to the late 1990s withdrawal of artificial nutrition became a far less common mode of death, and was undertaken in a far more restricted set of cases (Campbell 1999; Wilkinson and Fitzsimmons 2006).

So where does this leave us? There are relatively weak reasons to support the asymmetry view, and a different approach to withdrawal of artificial feeding compared with mechanical ventilation. Distress or discomfort following withdrawal of artificial nutrition might occur over a longer period, but (on current evidence) does not appear substantial, and would be treatable with medicines commonly used in palliative care. It would be possible for decisions to be made for the wrong reason, but this could equally occur with withdrawal of more intensive treatments, and does not mean that withdrawal should be prevented in cases where the burdens *do* outweigh the benefits. The biggest genuine difference is that the burdens of mechanical ventilation are potentially greater than the burdens of artificial feeding. Consequently there may be some cases where withdrawal of ventilation would be justifiable, but not withdrawal of artificial nutrition. Withdrawal of artificial nutrition would potentially only apply in the 'burdens of life' or 'lack of benefit' subgroups of quality of life treatment decisions.

Importantly, as discussed at the start of this chapter, the burdens of a short period of respiratory support are not great. It does not appear that the burdens of ventilation for a few days are necessarily greater than the burdens of artificial feeding. This would support withdrawal of artificial feeding as a solution to the 'window of opportunity' problem. On the basis of the above, if it is permissible to withdraw artificial ventilation from infants or children who are likely to only require short periods of respiratory support (and these are exactly the children where the 'window' appears to be a problem), it would be justified to withdraw artificial feeding.

The main reason in favour of treating such decisions differently is that parents may find a prolonged death more distressing, and that both parents and medical staff may intuitively find withdrawal of artificial nutrition harder. These concerns, relating to medical staff and parents, are not as strong as concerns that we might have about the child. But they cannot be easily or immediately dismissed. It is entirely understandable and appropriate that parents would find the idea of their child fading away from lack of nutrition over a period of days or weeks distressing. It is appropriate and desirable that medical staff should have strong intuitive desires to provide adequate nutrition for the infants and children in their care. It may be that with counselling and support parents' experience of this type of palliative care can be made less unpleasant, but it may still not be easy. If these responses to withdrawal of nutrition cannot be overcome, it would explain the different thresholds that doctors adopt for decisions about nutrition compared to decisions about more intensive treatments. Where medical staff or parents are reluctant or unwilling to withdraw artificial nutrition, or where there is explicit legal prohibition of withdrawing this type of treatment, the problems of uncertainty, and the 'window of opportunity' would remain.

Two Final Objections to Withdrawal of Feeding for Managing Uncertainty

There are two other arguments that might be made against withdrawal of artificial nutrition as a way of managing uncertainty in treatment decisions for children or infants.

The first relates to oral feeding—nutrition and fluids taken by mouth, without requiring nasogastric tubes, gastrostomies, or central venous catheters. We have discussed artificial feeding so far in this chapter, and the possibility of withdrawing nutritional support from patients who are not dependent on more intensive treatments like mechanical ventilation. But there may be a further group of patients who recover from their acute illness who are sufficiently impaired that it is questionable whether or not further life is a benefit to them, but who are not dependent on either ventilatory or nutritional support. If that is the case, then the option of withdrawal of artificial feeding wouldn't completely eliminate the window of opportunity problem.

Thomas Cochrane has suggested that for adult patients in this situation the option of not providing further food or fluids by mouth would prevent the perceived need for urgency in decision-making (Cochrane 2009). Cochrane argues that nutrition by mouth or by tube are equivalent, that a competent patient may decline either, and so too may their surrogate decision-makers if they are incompetent. Is this an option for children?

But it is not clear that this problem, or its proposed solution, apply to children. Cochrane provides the example of adults who suffer a stroke, and are left impaired, in a condition that previously they would have judged not worth living, but able to swallow. They would not have wanted to have had intensive care provided or continued if they had known that they would be left in this state. The justification for withholding oral nutrition now is based on the patient's previous wishes and judgement about what would make life worth living. But this doesn't apply to infants or children who have never been in a position to competently assess and express their view about future treatment and the type of life they would or would not be willing to live. In children we are guided instead by their best interests, and by whether or not their lives are (subjectively or objectively) worth living. Are there children who are able to take oral food and fluids, but for whom it would be appropriate not to provide mechanical ventilation and intensive care? It is theoretically possible, but if it occurs it must be very rare. The majority of children with severe chronic illness or impairment do receive nutritional support of one form or another. If they were sufficiently mildly affected not to require artificial nutrition, it is reasonably likely that they would gain significant benefit from life, and that treatment withdrawal would not be appropriate.

The second objection to withdrawal of nutrition as a way of managing uncertainty in treatment decisions is that it would be better, rather than withdrawing artificial nutrition, to euthanize children or infants whose quality of life is sufficiently poor that it is acceptable to allow them to die. Thus, Julian Savulescu has argued that treatment should be continued for adult patients in intensive care until there is prognostic certainty, and then euthanasia offered if the patient is likely to survive in a state that they would have judged worse than dying (Savulescu 1994). Helga Kuhse has similarly argued that euthanasia would be a better way to respect the interests of infants than to withdraw nutritional support, since they would be spared any suffering from the prolonged dying process (Kuhse 1986). This argument may be valid. However, as noted in Chapter 1, the focus of this book is on treatment withdrawal decisions, since analysis of these decisions is far more relevant for practice. In almost all jurisdictions around the world euthanasia of children or infants is not currently permitted, and consequently is not an available option for doctors or parents. In contrast, withdrawal of artificial nutrition is a sanctioned alternative. If it can take place without causing undue suffering for the infant (and with appropriate safeguards to prevent abuse), it may provide a legal and appropriate way of managing uncertainty in treatment decisions in intensive care.

In this chapter we have looked at two opposing ways of managing uncertainty in decisions in intensive care. But one further question is about how uncertainty interacts with some of the other interests at stake in treatment decisions. How does uncertainty affect the interests of the infant or of parents?

References

Airedale NHS Trust v Bland. [1993] AC 789.
Annas, G.J. (1984). 'The case of Baby Jane Doe: child abuse or unlawful Federal intervention? [21] ', *Am J Public Health* 74(7): 727–9.
Brody, H., M.L. Campbell, et al. (1997). 'Withdrawing intensive life-sustaining treatment—recommendations for compassionate clinical management', *N Engl J Med* 336(9): 652–7.
Burns, J.P., C. Mitchell, et al. (2000). 'End-of-life care in the pediatric intensive care unit after the forgoing of life-sustaining treatment', *Crit Care Med* 28(8): 3060–6.
Campbell, N. (1999). 'When care cannot cure: medical problems in seriously ill babies', in H. Kuhse and P. Singer (eds), *Bioethics: An Anthology*. Oxford: Blackwell, 243–54.
Carter, B.S. and S.R. Leuthner (2003). 'The ethics of withholding/withdrawing nutrition in the newborn', *Semin Perinatol* 27(6): 480–7.
Christakis, N.A. and D.A. Asch (1993). 'Biases in how physicians choose to withdraw life support', *Lancet* 342(8872): 642–6.
Clark, P. (2006). 'Tube feedings and persistent vegetative state patients: ordinary or extraordinary means?', *Christ Bioeth* 12(1): 43–64.
Cochrane, T.I. (2009). 'Unnecessary time pressure in refusal of life-sustaining therapies: fear of missing the opportunity to die', *Am J Bioeth* 9(4): 47–54.
Conlon, N.P., C. Breatnach, et al. (2009). 'Health-related quality of life after prolonged pediatric intensive care unit stay', *Pediatric Critical Care Medicine* 10(1): 41–4.
Cranford, R.E. (1995). 'Withdrawing artificial feeding from children with brain damage', *BMJ* 311(7003): 464–5.
Diekema, D.S. and J.R. Botkin (2009). 'Clinical report—Forgoing medically provided nutrition and hydration in children', *Pediatrics* 124(2): 813–22.
Edwards, M.J. (2006). 'Opioids and benzodiazepines appear paradoxically to delay inevitable death after ventilator withdrawal', *J Palliat Care* 21(4): 299–302.
Filan, P., T. Inder, et al. (2007). 'Monitoring the neonatal brain: a survey of current practice among Australian and New Zealand neonatologists', *J Paediatr Child Health* 43(7–8): 557–9.

Frey, R. (2005a). 'The doctrine of double effect', in R. Frey and C. Wellman (eds), *A Companion to Applied Ethics*. Malden, MA, Blackwell Publishing, 464–74.
—— (2005b). 'Intending and Causing', *The Journal of Ethics* 9(3): 465–74.
Ganzini, L., E.R. Goy, et al. (2003). 'Nurses' experiences with hospice patients who refuse food and fluids to hasten death', *N Engl J Med* 349(4): 359–65.
General Medical Council (2010). *Treatment and Care Towards the End of Life: Good Practice in Decision Making*. London: GMC.
George, R. and C. Regnard (2007). 'Lethal opioids or dangerous prescribers?', *Palliat Med* 21(2): 77–80.
Gillon, R. (1986). 'The principle of double effect and medical ethics', *Br Med J (Clin Res Ed)* 292(6514): 193–4.
Glover, J. (1990). *Causing Death and Saving Lives*. Harmondsworth: Penguin.
Goldworth, A. (2008). 'Deception and the principle of double effect', *Camb Q Healthc Ethics* 17(4): 471–2).
Hellmann, J., C. Williams, et al. (2008). 'Withdrawal of artificial hydration and nutrition in the NICU: a humane practice in tragic situations? (Abstract)', *Early Human Development* 84(Supplement): S130–1.
Kamm, F.M. (1991). 'The doctrine of double effect: reflections on theoretical and practical issues', *J Med Philos* 16(5): 571–85.
Keown, J. (2003). 'Medical murder by omission? The law and ethics of withholding and withdrawing treatment and tube feeding', *Clin Med* 3(5): 460–3.
Kipnis, K. (2007). 'Harm and uncertainty in newborn intensive care', *Theor Med Bioeth* 28(5): 393–412.
Kon, A.A. (2009). 'The "window of opportunity": helping parents make the most difficult decision they will ever face using an informed non-dissent model', *Am J Bioeth* 9(4): 55–6.
Kuhse, H. (1986). 'Death by non-feeding: not in the baby's best interests', *J Med Humanit Bioeth* 7(2): 79–90.
—— (1992). 'Quality of life and the death of "Baby M": a report from Australia', *Bioethics* 6(3): 233–50.
Lantos, J.D. and W. Meadow (2006). *Neonatal Bioethics: The Moral Challenges of Medical Innovation*. Baltimore: Johns Hopkins University Press.
Levi, B.H. (2003). 'Withdrawing nutrition and hydration from children: legal, ethical, and professional issues', *Clin Pediatr (Phila)* 42(2): 139–45.
Lynn, J. and J.F. Childress (1983). 'Must patients always be given food and water?', *Hastings Cent Rep* 13(5): 17–21.
Mason, J.K., G.T. Laurie, et al. (2011). *Mason and McCall Smith's Law and Medical Ethics*. Oxford: Oxford University Press.

Mazer, M.A., C.M. Alligood, et al. (2011). 'The infusion of opioids during terminal withdrawal of mechanical ventilation in the medical intensive care unit', *J Pain Symptom Manage* 42(1): 44–51.

McHaffie, H. and P.W. Fowlie (2001). *Crucial Decisions at the Beginning of Life: Parents' Experiences of Treatment Withdrawal from Infants*. Abingdon: Radcliffe Medical Press.

McHaffie, H.E., A.J. Lyon, et al. (2001). 'Lingering death after treatment withdrawal in the neonatal intensive care unit', *Arch Dis Child Fetal Neonatal Ed* 85(1): F8–F12.

McIntyre, A. (2004). 'The double life of double effect', *Theor Med Bioeth* 25(1): 61–74.

Mercuri, E., A. Guzzetta, et al. (1999). 'Neonatal neurological examination in infants with hypoxic ischaemic encephalopathy: correlation with MRI findings', *Neuropediatrics* 30(2): 83–9.

Miraie, E.D. (1988). 'Withholding nutrition from seriously ill newborn infants: a parent's perspective', *J Pediatr* 113(2): 262–5.

Morita, T., J. Tsunoda, et al. (2001). 'Effects of high dose opioids and sedatives on survival in terminally ill cancer patients', *J Pain Symptom Manage* 21(4): 282–9.

Nelson, L.J., C.H. Rushton, et al. (1995). 'Forgoing medically provided nutrition and hydration in pediatric patients', *J Law Med Ethics* 23(1): 33–46.

Nuffield Council on Bioethics (2006). *Critical Care Decisions in Fetal and Neonatal Medicine: Ethical Issues*. London: Nuffield Council on Bioethics.

Ouellette, A. (2006). 'Disability and the end of life', *Oregon Law Review* 85: 123–82.

Paris, J.J. and A.B. Fletcher (1987). 'Withholding of nutrition and fluids in the hopelessly ill patient', *Clin Perinatol* 14(2): 367–77.

—— and K.J. O'Connell (1991). 'Withdrawal of nutrition and fluids from a neurologically devastated infant: the case of baby T', *J Perinatol* 11(4): 372–3.

—— M.D. Schreiber, et al. (2007). 'Parental refusal of medical treatment for a newborn', *Theor Med Bioeth* 28(5): 427–41.

Porta, N. and J. Frader (2007). 'Withholding hydration and nutrition in newborns', *Theor Med Bioeth* 28(5): 443–51.

Portenoy, R.K., U. Sibirceva, et al. (2006). 'Opioid use and survival at the end of life: a survey of a hospice population', *J Pain Symptom Manage* 32(6): 532–40.

Printz, L.A. (1992). 'Terminal dehydration, a compassionate treatment', *Arch Intern Med* 152(4): 697–700.

Racine, E. and M.I. Shevell (2009). 'Ethics in neonatal neurology: when is enough, enough?', *Pediatr Neurol* 40(3): 147–55.

Raphael, D.D. (1988). 'Handicapped infants: medical ethics and the law', *J Med Ethics* 14(1): 5–10.

Re B (a minor) (wardship: medical treatment). [1981] 1 WLR 1421.
Royal College of Paediatrics and Child Health (2004). *Withholding and Withdrawing Life-Saving Treatment in Children: A Framework for Practice*. London: Royal College of Paediatrics and Child Health.
Rubenstein, J.S., S.M. Unti, et al. (1994). 'Pediatric resident attitudes about technologic support of vegetative patients and the effects of parental input—a longitudinal study', *Pediatrics* 94(1): 8–12.
Savulescu, J. (1994). 'Treatment limitation decisions under uncertainty: the value of subsequent euthanasia', *Bioethics* 8(1): 49–73.
Seale, C. (2009). 'Hastening death in end-of-life care: a survey of doctors', *Soc Sci Med* 69(11): 1659–66.
Shaw, A., J.G. Randolph, et al. (1977). 'Ethical issues in pediatric surgery: a national survey of pediatricians and pediatric surgeons', *Pediatrics* 60(4 Pt 2): 588–99.
Siden, H. (2010). 'Prolonged survival frequent after withdrawal of neonatal nutrition and hydration (Abstract)', 18th International Congress on Palliative Care.
Stanley, A.L. (2000). 'Withholding artificially provided nutrition and hydration from disabled children—assessing their quality of life', *Clin Pediatr (Phila)* 39(10): 575–9.
Swamy, R., S. Mohapatra, et al. (2010). 'Survival in infants live born at less than 24 weeks' gestation: the hidden morbidity of non-survivors', *Arch Dis Child Fetal Neonatal Ed* 95(4): F293–4.
The Multi-Society Task Force on PVS (1994). 'Medical aspects of the persistent vegetative state (2)', *N Engl J Med* 330(22): 1572–9.
Thorns, A. and N. Sykes (2000). 'Opioid use in last week of life and implications for end-of-life decision-making', *Lancet* 356(9227): 398–9.
Todres, I.D., J. Guillemin, et al. (1988). 'Life-saving therapy for newborns: a questionnaire survey in the state of Massachusetts', *Pediatrics* 81(5): 643–9.
Tyson, J.E., N.A. Parikh, et al. (2008). 'Intensive care for extreme prematurity—moving beyond gestational age', *N Engl J Med* 358(16): 1672–81.
Wilkinson, D. (2011). 'The window of opportunity for treatment withdrawal', *Archives of Pediatrics & Adolescent Medicine* 165(3): 211–15.
Wilkinson, D.J., J.J. Fitzsimons, et al. (2006). 'Death in the neonatal intensive care unit: changing patterns of end of life care over two decades', *Archives of Disease in Childhood Fetal and Neonatal Edition* 91(4): F268–71.
Williams, G. (2009). 'Medically assisted death', *Med Law Rev* 17(3): 491–7.
Wyatt, J. (2005). 'Quality of Life', <http://www.cmf.org.uk/literature/content.asp?context=article&id=1702>.

7

Interests and Uncertainty

In Part I of this book, we looked at certain predictions of impairment from the hypothetical Carmentis machine and the interests of children and parents. We are working towards a framework for decision-making about life-sustaining treatment in a world where prognosis is not an exact science. This highlights another question for us to address. How does uncertainty about the future impact upon the interests of children and their parents? We will spend some time thinking about these in turn, before finally looking at a different type of uncertainty that lies at the heart of disputes about treatment— moral uncertainty.

Interests of Parents and Uncertainty

We looked, in Chapter 4, at the nature of parents' and other family members' interests, and how these may be affected by the survival or death of the child. I assessed the relative weight of these interests against those of the child when they come into conflict. But this separation of the interests of parents and child may appear artificial or unrealistic. In the real world the interests of parents and of the child often overlap. They intertwine in ways that make it hard to separate them. This is potentially one reason why parents' views are taken into account in decisions about children in intensive care even when the interests of the child are ostensibly the only focus of decisions. But why is there an overlap, why do these interests intersect? The answer relates to uncertainty.

Influencing the Outcome

One possibility is that the interests of parents, in some cases, influence or determine whether or not the infant has an interest in continuing life. Part of our uncertainty in prognosis relates to how much support parents are actually going to be able to provide for the child. When parents express their wishes about treatment this potentially reflects both their desire to provide care for the child and their capacity to provide what the child will probably need. Some parents, for example, devote enormous amounts of time, energy, and financial resources into the care of their severely impaired children. They are able to enrich the lives of such children and help them experience benefits despite enormous challenges. Though it might usually be the case for a child with such severe impairment that life-sustaining treatment is not in their best interests, the strength of these particular parents' interest in the child surviving makes the difference for the child between a life that is worth living and one that is not. (Blaine Yorgason's adopted daughter Charity in Chapter 4 perhaps fits into this category.)

Conversely, other parents who have limited financial and personal resources, perhaps who have other existing children, are unable to devote as much attention to a child with very severe impairment. They do not neglect the child, but nor are they able to care for them to the degree of the parents described above. The benefits of life for that child may be outweighed by burdens, though in other environments they could have had a life worth living. For those families, the negative impact on their own interests makes it less likely that the child's life is of overall benefit to them.

Mutual Interests

The second way that the interests of parents and child overlap is through interdependence. Parents have an interest in promoting the welfare of their children (it is usually good for parents when their child is happy, and bad when they are not), but children also usually have an interest in promoting those of their parents (it is good for a child when their parents are happy, etc).

There are two ways that we could justify this mutual interest. We might point to the future desires of the child. Most children will have a desire that their parents are happy. Alternatively, (recalling the different theories of interests summarized in Chapter 4) we could point to a 'rational desire' (a desire the child would have if they were fully rational and fully informed) or include this in our list of objective interests for the child.

What is the relevance of mutual interests? Imagine, for example, a child in whom the burdens of life just outweigh the benefits. Perhaps Angelos from

Chapter 2 is in this category (the child with severe muscle weakness and intellectual disability, dependent on a ventilator)? If we considered only Angelos it seems that we should not continue life support. But imagine in this case that Angelos' parents have a very strong desire that treatment continues. Then it seems possible that his interest in his parents' wellbeing could tip the balance in favour of continued life. Because his parents want treatment to be provided, it now becomes in Angelos' interest to provide treatment.

It is difficult to know how strong the interdependent interests of a child are. Could they outweigh the harm of ongoing treatment for a child like Angelos? In another context, we could imagine a patient with a sufficiently severe and debilitating illness that they are led to contemplate ending their life (they judge their life to be not worth living). Yet they decide not to do so for the sake of a partner or other family member who would be devastated if they died. There may be a limit to this effect. It is difficult to imagine that a child's interest in his parents' happiness would be enough to make it in his interests to suffer severe or protracted pain.

Could these mutual interests work the other way? Imagine now that the balance of benefits and burdens is slightly positive for Angelos (life is overall a benefit for him, but only just), but his parents do not want treatment to continue. Could this tip the balance against treatment? Here it may make a difference why we think that there are mutual interests. If they are based on future desires, there is a problem, since if Angelos dies these future desires will not come to fruition. We are justifying not providing treatment (at least in part) on desires that we are ensuring will never actually exist. On the other hand, if the mutual interests are based on rational preferences or on the idea that objectively it is good for Angelos if his parents are happy then this may still count in favour of withdrawing treatment. (For children with severe cognitive impairment, mutual interests must be based on rational preferences or on the objective value of parental happiness, since they will never be in a position to have explicit desires about the happiness of their parents.)

Shared Values

The third possible cause of overlapping interests is that the *values* of parents are at least partly shared with the child, and thus influence what would be in their best interests. In previous chapters we have discussed controversial questions without clear correct answers including which theory of well-being we should use, the moral status of infants, the best way of assessing quality of life. Given such disagreement it is difficult to know how to make decisions. For adults, we would use the patient's own values to guide treatment. Would the patient have wanted to be kept alive in this particular state? Which values would they apply to decisions if they could? For older children or adolescents we may have some evidence about their own values, distinct from their parents, and can use this to inform our choice. But for infants and young children this is not an option. In many cases of children who are critically ill in intensive care we are not going to have good evidence about the values that they would apply to this sort of question, nor is there a value-neutral perspective that we can fall back on.

One option is to adopt the parents' values, or at least to give them extra weight in deliberation. There are perhaps two reasons to do this. The first is that this respects the point of view of parents, and reflects their interests (it also avoids privileging the perspective of the doctor, who may have a very different cultural background and world view.) But we might also do so because the values that the child will or would adopt (if they survive) are likely to be influenced by those of their parents (Glass, Bengtson, et al. 1986). They will not necessarily share the values of their parents, but this is at least somewhat more likely than not. Consider, for example, a child with very severe physical impairment but no cognitive impairment, such as Baby Amelia from Chapter 2. If Amelia's parents had a strong attitude of optimism and a determination to overcome physical adversity, we might anticipate that this will influence their care for her, and the balance of benefits and burdens in her life (see above). But it also seems plausible that this will make it more likely that she will share a similar positive outlook on life. It would potentially influence her future judgement about whether life is tolerable.

Would this factor work in the opposite direction? That is a little less clear. If parents had very negative views about severe disability, it is possible that this might be shared with the child, and lead to the child having a more negative perception of her own life. Imagine that Amelia's parents had very high standards of achievement, and as a consequence she is led to feel more frustrated by her physical condition and inability to do things like other children. That might affect the balance of benefits and burdens in her own life. But it would seem troubling if parents' views made a child feel that her life were not worth living. We might reasonably think that parents should instead revise their expectations if they were caring for a child with impairment. (Indeed it seems likely that many would in fact do this if the child survives (Hartshorne 2002; Heiman 2002; Boström, Broberg, et al. 2010).) If they cannot revise their expectations perhaps the child's care should be transferred to someone else? On the other hand, it may not be that parents have a particularly pessimistic view of impairment and disability. It may simply be that they lack the optimism and determination of other families, and weigh up as impartially as they can the positives and negatives in life. In that case it would be more reasonable to ascribe a similar perspective to evaluating the child's life.

One related question is whether parents' religious views and values should be ascribed to the child. It is possible that parents' religion is a major reason for them to want life-sustaining treatment to continue. Some religions have a vitalist perspective, and regard it as 'playing God' to withdraw life-sustaining treatment where there is the possibility of keeping a child alive, or reject the idea that the burdens could outweigh benefits in the setting of severe impairment (or both). Alternatively, they may feel strongly that prayer and divine intervention will change the outcome for the child. If parents have strong religious views it is fairly likely that the child will grow up to have similar views (McAllister 1988; D'Onofrio, Eaves, et al. 1999). So perhaps, from the infant or child's point of view, we should give extra weight to a vitalist perspective, if parents have this belief? However, there are problems with extending religious values to the child. One problem is that, again, a significant proportion of the children from whom we may be contemplating withdrawing life support will never be in a position to consciously share the religious (or non-religious) values of their parents. They cannot come to share their parents' values if they do not survive. (This would count against decisions to stop treatment, but not against decisions to continue treatment.) In addition, children with moderate or greater cognitive impairment will never be able to understand, choose, and express those values. A second problem is that in many societies a significant proportion of children do not come to share the religion of their parents. For example, data from a large recent British survey indicated that where both parents shared a religious belief, there was only a 50/50 chance of their young adult children sharing that belief (Voas and Crockett 2005). On the other hand, in the same survey, a lack of religious belief among parents was transmitted more frequently to children. More than 90 per cent of young adults whose parents both had no religious affiliation themselves reported no religious belief. Perhaps parents' non-religious values are more likely to be shared with a child than their religious values? However, the survey information only provides average data across a population. There may be subgroups (for example within particular ethnic communities), where there is a much higher chance of religious views being shared between parents and child.

Shared values give us some reason to pay attention to parents' judgements about life and about treatment—from the child's perspective. But for children who will never be in a position to choose and express their own values it is hard to justify giving the parents' values extra weight when we assess what would be in the child's interests.

Greater Knowledge

Finally, there is a sense in which parents are sometimes in a particularly good position to assess the interests of the child (Diekema 2004). This may be particularly relevant for older children, where parents are usually going to be in the best position to know the child's preferences, desires, dislikes, and ability to tolerate physical suffering. If parents are the primary caregivers they will potentially have a good sense of how much pleasure the child is able to gain from life, and how much pain, discomfort, and distress they experience on a day-to-day basis. But this factor could also have some relevance to infants. In the case of MB discussed in Chapter 2, the judge placed significant weight on the evidence of parents about the experience of the paralysed infant, and the degree that MB was aware of, and able to appreciate, his environment (An NHS Trust v MB 2006). The parents had spent large periods of time at his bedside and had done so since birth. As a result they were perhaps in a better position than medical or nursing staff who cared for multiple different patients over the same period. Parents may also be better able to anticipate the future environment for the child and their own ability to care for him or her than a third party.

The above four factors make it hard to separate the interests and desires of parents and the interests of the child. In practice, when there is conflict, even if it appears that the interests of parents and the interests of the child are opposed, it is almost always claimed by parents that they are representing the child's interests. Thus, for example, parents who wish to continue treatment against the advice of doctors usually claim that it is in their child's interest to continue to live. Parents who wish to discontinue treatment despite the belief of doctors that it should be provided usually claim that such treatment is not in their child's interest (see for example (Kopelman 2007)). The third and fourth factors listed above (shared values and greater knowledge) provide some reason to give extra credence to the assessment or value judgement that parents have made. The first and second factors (influencing outcome and mutual interests) may serve to bring the child's interests closer to the parents' and resolve the apparent conflict.

The overlap in interests between the child and his or her parents partly arises from uncertainty about the experience and outcome for the child. But it also arises from a different type of uncertainty, *moral uncertainty*, about the values that we should apply to such decisions. (We will look at moral uncertainty in more detail shortly.) Is this overlap any different for children of different ages? There are some reasons why it may be greater for infants than for older children. The link between parents' interests and the child's outcome may be greater for infants because of a longer period of dependency. Shared values are potentially more significant for infants and younger children because their own values are yet to develop. On the other hand, the mutual interests of the infant and his parents do not appear any stronger than those of an older child's and his parents. They might be weaker, if those interests are based on a conscious desire of the child for his parents' happiness, since very young children are not likely to have that desire. And parents of an older child may be in a better position to assess the child's interests than those of a young infant, since they will have had time to know the child, to be aware of her likes and dislikes, capacities and limitations.

Some writers have argued against taking parents' views into account when we are assessing the interests of children and newborns. They point out that parents may not be in the best position to assess the child's future interests (Fost 1981; Dare 2009). Parents may be mistaken about the effect of impairment on the child's life and on their own ability to care for the child. For example their view about the child's experience may be overly positive because of a range of factors including guilt, a need to maintain hope, belief about the value or sanctity of life, or a psychological need to justify the sacrifices that they have made and continue to make to care for the child. Their view might be unduly negative because of stress or depression

(White-Koning, Arnaud, et al. 2007), or because of unrealistic impressions about quality of life in individuals with disability. Alternatively they may be swayed by consideration of their own well-being and interests. The conflict between their interests and those of the child means that parents are not always impartial judges of the child's best interest (Fost 1981; Fost 1986). These reservations are valuable, and should be taken into account. Sometimes parental interests will not overlap with the child's in the ways that I have described. But that does not mean that parental views can never or should never influence our assessment of the interests of the child. If we paid no attention to parents' views about the child's interests we would potentially lose valuable information about the child's experience and future, and would risk imposing values on the child that they may not share, or come to share. Instead, it is important for doctors and parents to be aware about potential errors and biases in their assessments and value judgements, and to work hard to limit these. Once we have set this aside, at least in cases where there is genuine uncertainty about whether the child's life is worth living, parents' interests and views are relevant to whether it is in the interests of the child to provide life-sustaining treatment.

The Interests of the Child and Uncertainty

How could uncertainty affect the interests of the child? One obvious answer to this is that uncertainty may affect the options that it is ethical to pursue. If we were certain that a very bad outcome for a child were inevitable, we may feel that it would be unreasonable to continue treatment even if parents request it. But if we are *uncertain* about the outcome, if there is some chance that things wouldn't be so dire, we may be less sure whether the right thing to do is to overrule parents' wishes. Similarly, if we could be absolutely certain that a child would have a life worth living, again we may not feel justified in limiting treatment. But what if there is a risk that keeping the child alive would harm them overall? Should we then go against the parents' decision? Is it always in a child's interests to continue treatment if there is a chance that they would survive to have a life worth living? And is this any different for a newborn infant compared to an older child?

In Chapter 2 we looked at the interests of the child and when it is in the best interests of the child to withdraw treatment. There were two different (but overlapping) ways of answering this question that emerged from legal cases and ethical guidelines. The first was the idea that it would not be in the best interests of the child to provide treatment if this would be intolerable for the child. The second approach was to weigh up the benefits and burdens in a child's future. If the burdens outweigh the benefits it is not in the child's best interests to provide treatment.

These two approaches have much in common, but the first appears to emphasise the subjective judgement of the child or infant (or perhaps the adult that they would become), while the second attempts to impartially trade off the positives and negatives for the child. Both of these approaches want to draw a line or a threshold that marks the difference between cases where it is appropriate to withdraw treatment and those where it is not. If we imagined a graph depicting the future quality of life or well-being of the child, there is a point below which quality of life becomes sufficiently poor that treatment may be withdrawn (Figure 7.1). On the balance sheet account this would be a point where burdens are equal to benefits—there is neither net positive nor net negative well-being. I will refer to this as the 'zero point' on the quality of life or well-being spectrum. Using the concept of intolerability, this point would be where tolerable becomes intolerable and vice versa.

But where there is uncertainty about a child's prognosis and future interests, it is inevitable that decisions will sometimes be in error. There are two ways that we could go wrong. We could withdraw life-sustaining treatment and the child dies, though in fact they would have had a life of

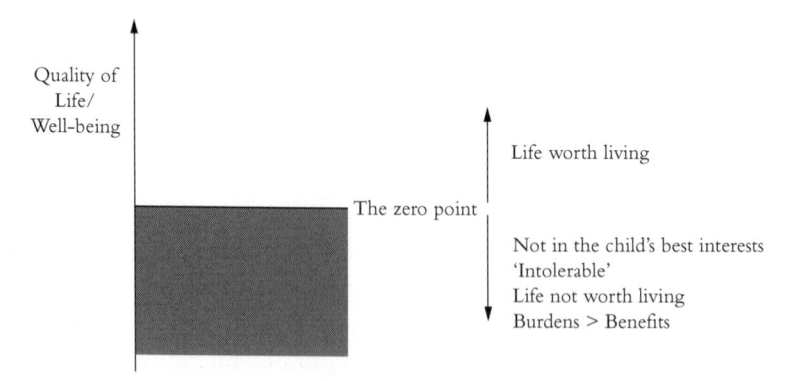

Figure 7.1 Decisions about life-sustaining treatment and the zero-point of well-being.

overall benefit, a life worth living (we could call this a *let die mistake*). Alternatively, there is a risk that we continue treatment and the child survives, though in fact the burdens outweigh the benefits, a life not worth living from her perspective (call this a *keep alive mistake*). How likely is each of these mistakes? That will depend on where we draw the line. But in theory at least, at the zero point, 50 per cent of the time we would make a let die mistake, and 50 per cent of the time a keep alive mistake. Is this the right cut-off point?

Imagine, as an analogy, that we are testing a new body scanner to determine if an airline passenger has a fever. At the height of the concern about swine flu in 2009, airports deployed thermal image scanners to detect skin temperature. If the level of infrared radiation measured from the skin was more than a certain level, passengers were judged to be likely to have a fever, pulled aside to have their temperature measured formally, and were interviewed to assess whether they could have the flu. They might be prevented from flying. What cut-off point should we use to decide which passengers to interview? It would be important to know the relationship between the level of infra-red radiation and actual core body temperature. We could look at the infra-red level that corresponds to a core body temperature of 38 degrees, for example. Given the imprecision involved in external thermal scanning, there will be a spread of actual body temperatures. But we might choose as a cut off the infra-red level that corresponds to a median body temperature of 38. Of those who have this infra-red reading, half will actually have a body temperature of more than 38 degrees, and half will have a temperature of less than 38 degrees. Furthermore it is inevitable that some passengers with slightly lower levels of infra-red would actually have a fever. And there would be some passengers with a higher infra-red level who, on formal testing, turn out not to really be febrile.

To know where we should set the cut-off point for screening body temperature we need to know how to weigh up different types of mistakes. Which type of error is worse? For airport screening we want a test that is particularly sensitive so that very few passengers who do actually have a fever are missed. If we are interested in preventing the spread of pandemic influenza it is probably worse to miss incoming passengers who have the flu, than it is to conduct unnecessary screening on passengers who aren't sick. On that basis we might choose as a cut-off an infra-red level corresponding to a temperature below 38 degrees. The second piece of information that is relevant for this type of screening test is the proportion of passengers who do have a fever—since this will affect the predictive value of the test. If it is very rare for passengers to have a fever, most of those who are flagged by infra-red screening will actually not be febrile, and will have been falsely identified.

The airport situation is different from making decisions about critically ill children. Chapter 5 pointed to the lack of data on the frequency of children who have lives that are of very poor quality among those with significant predicted disability. This means that we can't assess the predictive value of different cut-offs. But we may be able to assess the other important question. Which is a worse mistake—a let die mistake, or a keep alive mistake? How we weigh up these mistakes affects where we should draw the line for decisions (Figure 7.2). For example, if we think that they are equally bad mistakes to make, this would support drawing a line at the zero point (7.2a). But we might think that a let die mistake is worse. If that is the case, we should draw a line for decisions below zero—this will make it less likely that we allow children to die who could have had lives worth living (7.2b). Alternatively, if a keep alive mistake is the worse one to make, we might draw the line above the zero line (7.2c).

One possibility is that the way that we should weigh up these mistakes depends in part on the child's age. This relates to the argument in Chapter 4 that death is less of a harm for a newborn infant than an older child.

For a child or an adult, death is bad because it deprives them of a valuable future. They fail to experience all the good things in life that they would have enjoyed if they had lived. But death is also bad because it cuts short desires, plans, and hopes of the individual, and severs the links that the child or adult has established with others and with the world around them. A let-die mistake is, therefore, very serious, and something that we should try hard to avoid. How serious it is will vary depending on how good the child's future life would have been. It would be very bad to deny someone a long, full, and enriching life. On the other hand, if their life would have been very short, or so full of pain and discomfort that it is close to the point of being intolerable or not worth living, a let-die mistake would be lessened. But a keep-alive mistake is also serious. To save the life of someone for whom the burdens of medical treatment and of life outweigh the benefits is to harm them. They experience ongoing and unrelieved pain or distress, uncompensated for by the good things in their lives. Indeed, if we reflect on those cases where overwhelming illness or suffering leads adults to feel that

INTERESTS AND UNCERTAINTY   247

(a)

Quality of Life/Well-being

The zero point

Let die mistake   Keep alive mistake

(b)

Quality of Life/Well-being

The zero point

Cut-off point for withdrawing treatment

Let die mistake   Keep alive mistake

(c)

Quality of Life/Well-being

Cut-off point for withdrawing treatment

The zero point

Let die mistake

Keep alive mistake

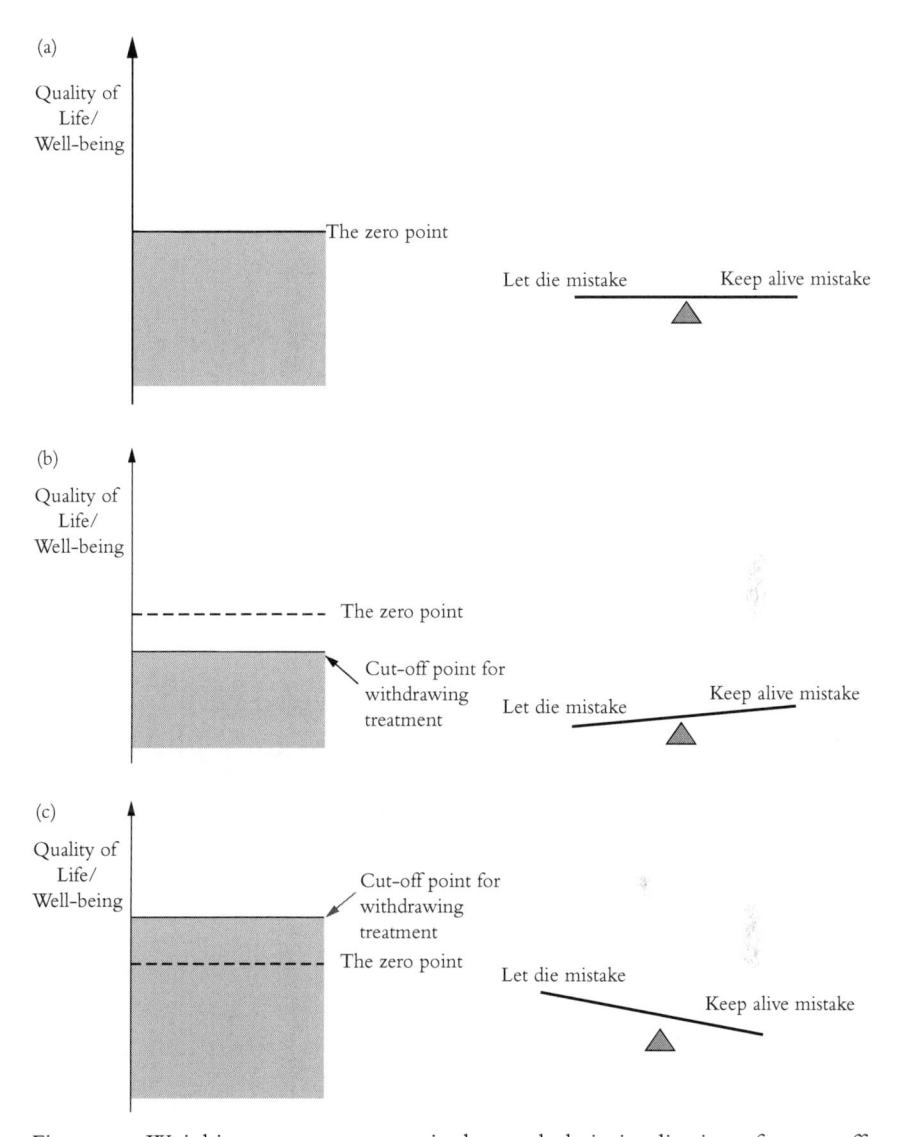

Figure 7.2 Weighing up treatment mistakes and their implications for cut-off points for withdrawing treatment in the face of uncertainty.

their life is not worth continuing, we might be tempted to think that keeping alive someone in such a state is one of the worst mistakes that we could make. Again, just how bad this mistake is will vary. If a child had a life where the burdens only just outweigh the benefits, or where they were going to survive for only a short time (after having their life saved with treatment), it would be a lesser mistake than if a child were destined to survive for a long period with burdens that overwhelmed all potential benefits.

It is not straightforward how we should weigh up these two mistakes for a child or an adult. Both are serious. They may be equally weighty, or perhaps (especially if there is a possibility of a long and fulfilling life) a let-die mistake is worse. We should perhaps draw a threshold for decisions at the zero point or even below.

But what about infants? In Chapter 4 we discussed the harm of death for a newborn infant. I argued there that death is not as bad for a newborn as for an older child because they have not yet established relationships, nor developed preferences, plans, and hopes. It deprives them of their future life. However, because they will never be aware of that loss, nor regret it, there is a sense in which this loss is tempered. From the infant's perspective, death is bad, but it is bad in a similar way that death is bad for a fetus. It is the absence of experience rather than the experience of a negative. This reduces the significance of a let-die mistake. In contrast, a keep-alive mistake would be at least as bad as for an older person. The harm of life for an infant who is kept alive, though in fact they have a life not worth living, a life of net burden, *is* conscious, is experienced, and may come to be regretted, both by the infant, and by the infant's family. A keep-alive mistake is potentially worse for a newborn infant than for an older child or adult if the newborn would survive in a negative state for a very long period of time. (The length of survival may depend on whether there are options such as those discussed in Chapter 6 to withdraw artificial nutrition.)

In the airport screening case, the harm of missing a passenger with true influenza is greater than the harm of incorrectly delaying a passenger (who does not in fact have a fever). This imbalance or *asymmetry* in the relative harms means that we should err on the side of caution, and set a lower threshold for screening passengers. In the case of infants with significant predicted impairment, there is a different asymmetry. The harm of a keep-alive mistake is greater than the harm of a let-die mistake. We should therefore choose a *higher* threshold in the face of uncertainty for decisions about treatment. The cut-off point will be above the zero point.

Where exactly we should draw the line is a question that we will return to in Chapter 8, but asymmetrical harms would support a threshold that is somewhere above the zero point. However, the threshold would probably not usually be a long way above the zero point. There are two reasons for this. Firstly, the greater a child's or infant's future well-being, the more they have to lose from a let-die mistake. If an infant is predicted to have a life that is comfortably above the zero point, there would be a significant harm in allowing them to die. Secondly, the risk of the worst outcome, surviving with a life that is intolerable, becomes much smaller the better a child's future life is predicted to be. Close to the zero point it would take relatively little for the balance to be tipped to the negative; life is finely balanced, but the development of extra complications or a worsening of the child's condition by a small degree might lead them to experience a life not worth living. Conversely, as we consider situations that are more positive, and further from the zero point, the risk of burdens outweighing benefits in life is much less. As an example, children with Down syndrome have moderate cognitive impairment; it is generally thought that they have lives worth living. Occasional children with Down syndrome have very substantial health problems, including complex congenital heart disease, pulmonary hypertension, and gastrointestinal abnormalities. Rarely, the combination of these illnesses, and the treatment needed for them, might tip the balance for a child with Down syndrome against further treatment. But at the start, the probability of this being the case would be small, and the loss to the child significant. On this basis we might reasonably judge conditions like Down syndrome to be above our threshold for treatment decisions.

Another way of thinking about these decisions would be to draw on a thought experiment suggested by political philosopher John Rawls (Rawls 1999). Rawls' idea was that in formulating the rules that would govern a just society we should try to imagine a set of law makers who did not know where they would be in society. The law makers would have to consider the possibility that they would be amongst the most disadvantaged. Behind what Rawls called a 'veil of ignorance' it would be rational for legislators to set up rules that would be fair for all. In particular, if you did not know whether you were going to be rich or poor, healthy or sick, black or white, it would make sense to ensure that the worst-off in society were in as good a position as possible. Rawls referred to this principle as 'maximin'. Rawls' principle was designed to apply to politics and societal structure, but a similar principle is sometimes used in other areas of ethics.

If we apply maximin to treatment decisions we would again need to weigh up the gravity of different types of mistakes (Kipnis 2007). For older children or adults, the loss of future life would weigh heavily. We might well choose to have the sort of rule that is often applied to decisions in intensive care, with a presumption in favour of providing life-sustaining treatment unless it is clear that continued life would be not worth living. However, we would potentially get a different answer for newborn decisions. Behind the veil of ignorance, it would be rational to choose to reduce the chance of the worst outcome. If it is indeed worse to survive with a life not worth living than to die prematurely in the newborn period, we should choose to set our decision threshold above the zero point.

The Puzzling Asymmetry of Conception

Asymmetrical harms have been discussed widely in relation to decisions about conception or bringing children into existence (McMahan 2009). There is a fairly commonly held belief that it isn't wrong to decide not to conceive a child (who would have had a life worth living). But it *is* generally thought to be wrong to bring a child into existence who will have a life not worth living. This difference in judgements is usually explained by the existence of an individual to whom harms could be attached. If potential parents make a decision not to have a child, there is no child who suffers from that loss, no person who fails to come into existence. It is true that if the child had been born he would probably have been glad that his parents conceived him. But if he is never conceived, there is no one who is harmed by that loss. Conversely though, if a child comes to exist but is so severely impaired that they have a life not worth living, there *is* a child who is harmed.

One of the puzzles about these decisions is that if we turn around the question to look at who *benefits* from these decisions, we would reach the opposite conclusion. So, if we make a decision not to bring a child into existence who would have had a terrible life, there is no child who thereby benefits, no one who is spared future suffering. But if we conceive a child who has a good life, there is an identifiable individual who is benefited. But it isn't clear that this alternative way of looking at decisions has as much force. Many people intuitively worry more about causing harms than about causing benefits.

The asymmetry in bringing people into the world continues to puzzle philosophers. One apparent implication of the asymmetry, if we take it seriously, is that it appears to provide a moral imperative for us not to have children. After all, we harm no one by not bringing them into existence, but we do risk harming them if they are brought into the world. If we are faced with uncertainty about whether or not a child that we conceive might have an intolerable life, then perhaps we should always err on the side of not bringing them into existence? Philosopher David Benatar has provocatively argued along these lines, in his book *Better Never to Have Been* (Benatar 2006). Benatar takes the argument to its logical extreme, arguing that it would be better if the human race were to become extinct! (A similar conclusion is implied by so-called 'negative utilitarianism'—the view that we should choose whichever course of action will reduce or avoid suffering to the greatest possible degree.) Other philosophers have challenged this pessimistic conclusion, suggesting that it either means that we should reject the asymmetry view of conception, or revise it in some way (Doyal 2007; Baum 2008; McMahan 2009).

If we only take into account future harms, and ignore future benefits, then we might well be led to Benatar's view that it would be better if we had no children. But there is one possible way of avoiding such a nihilistic conclusion. Although we often worry more about causing or alleviating harms than about bringing about benefits, there can often be moral reasons to bring about benefits too, even if perhaps we choose to alleviate harms first where there is a choice. Imagine that a government agency is contemplating how to spend a sum of money left over in its budget for improving reading skills in six-year-olds in a community. In this hypothetical example they have a choice between a health intervention to reduce ear infections in early childhood (there is a high incidence of early ear infections in this community) (intervention A), or a school intervention to increase reading skills (intervention B). We should imagine for this example that both interventions would be equally effective in the short and medium term. Intervention A would prevent a harm, and lead to 10 per cent of children not having a 20 per cent reduction in their reading skills at age six. Intervention B would cause a benefit—and lead to 10 per cent of children at age six having a 20 per cent improvement in their reading skills. If asked simply to choose between the interventions, we might choose A, on the basis that it is better to prevent a harm than to create a benefit. But imagine now that the agency does not have option A available, and it has to choose whether to implement intervention B or nothing (the money if unused would disappear into general government coffers, or be used to service debt). Surely there is a good reason to improve six-year-olds' reading skills if we can? If that is the case, we could imagine different versions of the dilemma where intervention B is more effective than intervention A (it affects more children). If the difference between A and B is great enough, we may choose to fund intervention B even though it generates a benefit rather than prevent a harm.

The asymmetry of conception decisions is different from a general harm/benefit asymmetry. In the reading intervention example, if the agency failed to fund intervention B (and allowed the money to go to a different educational priority) there are existing children who would be worse off, who would fail to improve their reading. There are individual-affecting reasons to fund intervention B. In contrast, there are no individual-affecting reasons (for the sake of the children at least) to conceive children who will have good lives. Yet it may still be bad *impersonally* if individuals (who would have had good lives) are not brought into existence. Impersonal reasons help to make sense of cases like the Teratogen case discussed in Chapter 3. Benatar's view is based on an absolute asymmetry between benefits and harms: it is never bad to fail to realize a benefit, whereas it is always good to prevent a harm. But another possibility is that there is a *relative asymmetry* between benefits and harms as in the reading example above. On this view, harms count for more than benefits, but failure to realize benefits would still count for something. Imagine, for example, that the harms of future life counted twice as much as benefits. If that were the case we would err on the side of not bringing a child into existence if the chance of a child having a life below the zero point were equal to or even somewhat greater than the chance of them having a life worth living. But if the chance of the child having a life worth living were high enough (odds of more than 2:1 in this example), we would then have a moral reason to bring them into the world.

Moral Uncertainty

We have looked at the different ways in which uncertainty could affect the interests of parents and children. But before we move on it will be worthwhile distinguishing between different types of uncertainty. (See Table 7.1)

Table 7.1 Different types of uncertainty.

Type of Uncertainty	Definition	Example
Prognostic uncertainty	Uncertainty about outcome	Possible outcomes include A or B or C
First-order prognostic uncertainty	Uncertainty about which of two or more outcomes will occur	There is a 90% chance of outcome A, but a 10% chance of outcome B
Second-order uncertainty	Uncertainty about the probability of different outcomes	There is a 75–95% chance of A, and a 5–25% chance of B
Experiential uncertainty	Uncertainty about the nature of the experience of the patient if they have a particular outcome	If the patient does have outcome A, how difficult will they find this, how much pain will they experience, how happy or unhappy will they be?
Moral uncertainty	Uncertainty about what we ought to do	It is unclear whether we should continue life-sustaining treatment or allow a child to die
Value uncertainty	Uncertainty about our evaluation of different outcomes	How bad would it be for the patient to die, how bad is survival with severe impairment?
Ethical uncertainty	Uncertainty about which ethical theory or rules should apply to decisions	Should we be guided by utilitarianism or by virtue ethics, by the 'four principles' of medical ethics, or by reference to the rights of the child?
Second-order moral uncertainty	Uncertainty about how to respond to moral and prognostic uncertainty	Should we aim to maximize overall value or should we aim to ensure that the worst outcome (if it occurs) is as good as possible (maximin)?

Prognostic uncertainty makes decision-making complicated. One of the reasons for this is that it makes it challenging to know which course of action to take. We need to know which outcomes are good, and which bad. (That is not exactly straightforward when we are talking about states of severe impairment.) We also need to know what the probabilities are of those different outcomes. That raises further problems because we may have uncertainty about uncertainty—it may be very difficult to put a figure on the likelihood of different degrees of impairment. In Chapter 5 we looked at the difficulty in knowing what states of severe impairment are like for children (we could call this 'experiential uncertainty' (Table 7.1)). But there is yet another type of uncertainty that affects decisions. We need to know how to respond to states of prognostic uncertainty. As highlighted in the section above on parental interests, there are a range of different values and views that people apply to decisions. It is often not clear which value is the right one. Whose values or views should count? This is a manifestation of *moral uncertainty*.

One example of the range of values was discussed in Chapter 5. Saroj Saigal and colleagues surveyed ex-premature adolescents and their parents and doctors about their judgement of the quality of life of several hypothetical children (Saigal, Stoskopf, et al. 1999). One of these, 'Pat', had sensory impairment, some motor impairment (needed equipment to walk), and cognitive impairment. She was described as learning very slowly and needed special assistance at school, and with personal care (bathing/toiletting). The description is somewhat imprecise, but it seems that Pat has moderate motor and moderate or severe cognitive impairment. One of the interesting findings from Saigal's survey was that there was variation between doctors and parents and ex-premature children in their judgements about Pat's quality of life. Doctors were the most pessimistic, giving Pat on average a score just below zero using a standard gamble. (Scores below zero represent a judgement that the condition is worse than death.) Parents were the most positive, giving Pat a score of 0.2 on average. The teenagers gave similar, though slightly more negative answers to their parents (average score of 0.16). But the other interesting finding was that the range of answers varied enormously in all three groups. Some answered extremely negatively, judging Pat's state to be as low as − 0.95, while others rated it akin to almost perfect health (+ 0.95).

How should we interpret such variation in assessments of quality of life? If there were a clear correct answer to the question of which chronic states are worse than death, the variation in judgements would not matter so much. We should be guided by that correct answer, and take the variation in responses as indicating a need to educate people about how to judge quality of life. But, as I argued in Part I of this book, even if prognostic uncertainty is eliminated using the Carmentis machine, it is unclear for more severe conditions, which are above and which below a zero point of well-being. There is significant moral uncertainty ('value uncertainty', Table 7.1) about just how good or how bad these states are.

A second type of moral uncertainty relates to the ethical theory or approach that we should take ('ethical uncertainty'). Should we follow a set of rules about decisions, or should we focus on the outcome? How much do the intentions or attitude or virtues of the individual agent matter? If we are to be guided by rules, which rules should we follow, and which are the most important? I have largely avoided focusing in this book on a particular ethical framework. But some parents and doctors may be influenced by a rights-based framework in their thinking, others may be more consequentialist or utilitarian, others still may apply rules or principles derived from religious teaching. There is no consensus about which of these is the correct approach, nor does it seem likely that one will emerge in the immediate future.

Yet another example of moral uncertainty relates to the response to risk and prognostic uncertainty. People vary in their attitude to risk. This can be seen in everyday decisions, about purchasing insurance, buying lottery tickets, or taking part in dangerous sports. Some people are risk-takers, happy to take a gamble, even if the chances of a positive outcome are very small. Others are risk averse, preferring to pay a price or forego some chance of benefit if there is a chance of major losses. Which of these is the better strategy? This variation affects major health decisions that people make for themselves and for their loved ones (Nightingale and Grant 1988). We looked above at the way that uncertainty might affect the interests of a newborn infant. I argued that it is potentially worse for a newborn infant to be kept alive with an intolerable life than to be allowed to die (though they would have had a life above the zero point). On this basis some would choose to err on the side of not providing life-sustaining treatment where there is a risk of an outcome worse than death. Others, though, would not agree. They might want to err on the side of providing treatment to avoid a let-die mistake. Again, although there are arguments in favour or against these different strategies, it is not clear which of them is correct.

Prognostic uncertainty makes decisions difficult. The appropriate response to that sort of uncertainty is to attempt to reduce it (for example by improving prognostication, by working on the development of a Carmentis machine). But there is also a need to decide how to respond to uncertainty until we achieve this. Similarly, with moral uncertainty we should strive for greater certainty about which is the correct approach, which are the correct values to apply. (This book represents one attempt to do this.) But we may be even less confident of reaching such a solution, and hence we need to decide what to do in the meantime.

Broadly, there are a couple of different options. One option, which we could perhaps call a 'democratic' option, would be to determine the values, principles, and way of responding to uncertainty of the majority in society, and use that to derive our policy. A survey like Saigal's study mentioned above could be used to inform such a policy, since it provides a set of average quality of life judgements for a range of conditions. If the majority supported withdrawal of life support or continuing life support for Pat, then this would determine what doctors should do.

There is a lot to be said for a democratic way of responding to variation in opinion and values. But democracy also has its flaws when it comes to ethically complex and fraught decisions. It isn't always clear that we should settle such questions by opinion poll. We might find that the population is capricious, sometimes supporting and sometimes opposing proposals. Should policy change with each shift in opinion? Another problem is that polling can be distorted or manipulated fairly easily. It can be hard to provide enough balanced information for individuals to make informed decisions. The answer that is obtained depends on the exact question that is asked of respondents, as well as how it is asked. A further problem is that if there is significant disagreement within the community about what is the right answer, then a large sub-section of the community may find their views unrepresented in policy. Why should the values of others be applied to the decisions that people make for themselves or their family members? For example, a majority of the population might feel that life-sustaining treatment should not be provided to patients who are in a persistent vegetative state (PVS). We could decide, on this basis, that it is not appropriate to provide treatment for adults or children in PVS. But there could well be a substantial minority of the population who, for religious or non-religious reasons, would want at least some life-sustaining treatments provided if they or their loved ones were in PVS. Should the views of the majority affect the treatments available to those who do not share those views? When it comes to personal matters about how our own lives are lived, and particularly about how they end, it seems inappropriate to enforce on all the values of the majority. If we have a largely secular society should those values be applied to those with religious views? Conversely, in a society with a majority of the population who are religious, should the religion of the majority dictate the rules that apply to those of different religions, or of no religion? None of these options would be consistent with religious tolerance, a value that is central to most western democracies.

A second option in the face of uncertainty would be to adopt a 'liberal' strategy. Given a range of values and viewpoints, we could allow individuals to apply their values to their own lives. As long as their decisions did not harm others, we should respect the right of individuals to make decisions for themselves (Mill 1956). This strategy would lead to different end-of-life decisions for different individuals. Life-sustaining treatment might be continued for patients in a PVS who had previously evinced a strong vitalist perspective, and believed that life was still valuable even in the absence of consciousness. On the other hand, life-sustaining treatment might be withdrawn from patients who would not see value in prolonging life if they had little or no chance of even experiencing consciousness. The advantage of the liberal strategy is that it respects the choices and values of different individuals. This liberty is not boundless; if there are issues of limited resources, individual choices may be restricted by the availability of treatment. However, in the absence of limited resources, we might generally respond to moral uncertainty by emphasising individual freedom to decide.

But the problem with the liberal solution to moral uncertainty when it comes to paediatric decision-making is that the key question *is* about harm to another individual, the child, and whether or not further treatment would be harmful. Is it a harm for a severely impaired child or newborn infant to survive? Is it more of a harm for them to die? We can't usually ask the child for their views. As noted in the first section of this chapter, there may be some overlap in the values of parents and those of the child, but these will not necessarily coincide, and it arguably does not make sense for parents' values to be ascribed to a severely cognitively impaired child. What should we do then?

The answer, in my view, is to apply a modified form of liberalism to parental decisions. This third strategy would set limits to the freedom of parents to decide. Where there is genuine and legitimate disagreement about whether or not treatment is in the interests of the child we should reasonably defer to the views of parents or caregivers. We should respect parents' assessment because of the ways in which their own interests are affected by decisions, because of the overlap between their interests and those of the child, and perhaps also because there is considerable value in giving parents the freedom to bring up their children in the way that they believe is appropriate. This does not mean that parents are given free rein to make any decision for their child. Where parents' views fall outside the bounds of reasonable disagreement, where their decision appears likely to cause substantial harm, we should override their choices (Diekema 2004).

Conclusions

In this chapter we have seen just why uncertainty complicates decisions about life-sustaining treatment for children. Uncertainty about how much support families will be able to provide for a child, about how much the child will or would care about the interests of his parents, about the values that he would apply to his own life, all make it hard to predict whether treatment is in a child's best interests. These uncertainties also lead to an inevitable blurring between the interests of the parents and the child. Furthermore, uncertainty about future harms makes it challenging to know whether treatment is in the interests of the child. I have argued that for very young infants the harms of different mistakes are not equally weighty. This would justify a different threshold for treatment withdrawal decisions in newborn infants compared to older children. However, I also acknowledged that there are likely to remain different views about this. There is moral uncertainty about the nature of different harms, about how we should weigh them against each other, and fundamentally, about how we should respond to uncertainty in treatment decisions.

In the last section of this chapter we have looked at the different types of moral uncertainty that affect decisions. The presence of disagreement does not mean that we should give up on trying to determine what the right answer is for treatment decisions. As with the prognostic variety, we should work to try to reduce moral uncertainty, where it exists. We can imagine that at some point we will have substantially less moral uncertainty (though a moral version of the Carmentis machine that tells us exactly what we should do seems extremely far-fetched). But we also need to decide how to act given moral uncertainty, about how to manage the different competing views of those in society. I have argued that we should respect reasonable differences in values, ethical theories, and in responses to uncertainty. We will look in the next chapter at ways to set out the limits to parental discretion, but one answer would be to look for democratic ways of determining what counts as a reasonable or legitimate decision for parents to be allowed to make. We might then try to decide collectively not which values the majority shares, but which values the majority is able to respect.

References

An NHS Trust v MB. [2006] 2 F.L.R. 319.

Baum, S.D. (2008). 'Better to exist: a reply to Benatar', *Journal of Medical Ethics* 34(12): 875–6.

Benatar, D. (2006). *Better Never to Have Been: The Harm of Coming into Existence*. Oxford: Clarendon.

Boström, P., M. Broberg, et al. (2010). 'Parents' descriptions and experiences of young children recently diagnosed with intellectual disability', *Child: Care, Health and Development* 36(1): 93–100.

D'Onofrio, B.M., L.J. Eaves, et al. (1999). 'Understanding biological and social influences on religious affiliation, attitudes, and behaviors: a behavior genetic perspective', *J Pers* 67(6): 953–84.

Dare, T. (2009). 'Parental rights and medical decisions', *Paediatr Anaesth* 19(10): 947–52.

Diekema, D.S. (2004). 'Parental refusals of medical treatment: the harm principle as threshold for state intervention', *Theor Med Bioeth* 25(4): 243–64.

Doyal, L. (2007). 'Is human existence worth its consequent harm?', *Journal of Medical Ethics* 33(10): 573–6.

Fost, N. (1981). 'Counseling families who have a child with a severe congenital anomaly', *Pediatrics* 67(3): 321–4.

—— (1986). 'Treatment of seriously ill and handicapped newborns', *Crit Care Clin* 2(1): 145–59.

Glass, J., V. Bengtson, et al. (1986). 'Attitude similarity in three-generation families: socialization, status inheritance or reciprocal influence?', *American Sociological Review* 51(5): 685–98.

Hartshorne, T.S. (2002). 'Mistaking courage for denial: Family resilience after the birth of a child with severe disabilities', *Journal of Individual Psychology* 58(3): 263–78.

Heiman, T. (2002). 'Parents of children with disabilities: Resilience, coping, and future expectations', *Journal of Developmental and Physical Disabilities* 14(2): 159–71.

Kipnis, K. (2007). 'Harm and uncertainty in newborn intensive care', *Theor Med Bioeth* 28(5): 393–412.

Kopelman, L.M. (2007). 'The best interests standard for incompetent or incapacitated persons of all ages', *J Law Med Ethics* 35(1): 187–96.

McAllister, I. (1988). 'Religious change and secularization: The transmission of religious values in Australia', *Sociology of Religion* 49(3): 249–63.

McMahan, J. (2009). 'Asymmetries in the morality of causing people to exist', in M. Roberts and D. Wasserman (eds), *Harming Future Persons: Ethics, Genetics and the Nonidentity Problem*. New York, Springer, 49–70.

Mill, J.S. (1956). *On Liberty*. New York: Bobbs-Merrill.

Nightingale, S.D. and M. Grant (1988). 'Risk preference and decision making in critical care situations', *Chest* 93(4): 684–7.

Rawls, J. (1999). *A Theory of Justice*. Oxford: Oxford University Press.

Saigal, S., B.L. Stoskopf, et al. (1999). 'Differences in preferences for neonatal outcomes among health care professionals, parents, and adolescents', *JAMA* 281(21): 1991–7.

Voas, D. and A. Crockett (2005). 'Religion in Britain: Neither believing nor belonging', *Sociology* 39(1): 11–28.

White-Koning, M., C. Arnaud, et al. (2007). 'Determinants of child-parent agreement in quality-of-life reports: a European study of children with cerebral palsy', *Pediatrics* 120(4): e804–14.

8

The Threshold Framework

In Chapter 2 I looked at existing guidelines for decision-making in infants and children. Those guidelines were vague, and difficult to apply in practice, even where the prognosis for a child was known with certainty. Guidelines were also ambiguous about the role of parents in decisions. They seemed to imply that parents should make decisions; however, they also appeared to undermine parents' role by emphasising that decisions had to be made in accordance with the child's best interests. Over the last few chapters we have built up a picture of some of the additional challenges for decision-making arising from uncertainty. Those challenges make it hard in individual cases to know what course to take. They also make it difficult to develop recommendations for decision-making.

In this last chapter I will grasp the nettle and seek to develop a substantive framework for decision-making about life-sustaining treatment in children and infants. This framework is a first step towards developing more detailed and specific guidelines. It will defend the important role of parents in decisions, but also seek greater clarity about the limits to that role. I will outline different alternatives for fleshing out this framework and the process that might be used. Somewhat more tentatively, I will provide an example of guidelines for infants and children. Since these represent the view of one individual, these suggestions should be seen as a starting point. For reasons that I will discuss in the final section, they may not be appropriate in other societies or cultures.

I start by outlining what I call the *threshold framework*, and illustrate why it is attractive. We will look at different versions, but I will defend the idea that there are at least two thresholds, an upper and lower threshold setting out the boundaries of parental discretion in decisions. I will explore four different methods for determining the boundaries of decisions in the threshold framework. Those methods will help defend the framework against a number of potential objections. Finally, I will look at applying the framework in newborn intensive care, and point to the work that still lies ahead in defining the different thresholds for different types of decisions, in different countries, and in different groups of children.

The Framework

To briefly recap, these are the principle conclusions from earlier chapters that are relevant to a framework for decisions:

1. It is extremely difficult to define the point where life becomes 'intolerable' for the child, or where benefits are outweighed by burdens. (Chapter 2)
2. Parental views about decision-making should carry some weight because their interests overlap with those of the child. (Chapter 7)
3. Parental interests should also carry independent weight in decisions because of the substantial potential impact on the interests of parents and other family members if a child survives with very severe impairment. (Chapter 4)
4. Where there is prognostic uncertainty, we should give some weight to the chance that an infant or child will survive in a state that is negative or harmful. (Chapter 7)
5. There is moral uncertainty about some of the key elements of decisions, for example about how to weigh interests, about when life is worth living, and about the best course of action in the face of uncertainty about a child's outcome. (Chapter 7)
6. Where there is moral uncertainty about harms to a child, we should allow parents to make decisions, within limits. (Chapter 7)

There are a number of challenges for decision-making that we have discussed in the previous chapters of the book. Here is another challenge: how do we reconcile decisions to limit treatment for some children or newborns with decisions to continue treatment in other children or newborns with very similar conditions. The following pair of examples highlights this challenge.

Henry was born at forty-two weeks gestation. When his mother arrived at the hospital in labour, the fetal heartbeat was found to be worryingly slow, and an emergency caesarean section was performed. Henry was born in poor condition and required extensive resuscitation. He was put on a mechanical ventilator and transferred to intensive care. He was floppy, comatose, and had abnormal electrical patterns on electroencephalogram. At 72 hours of age Henry remained dependent on the breathing machine, but his condition had stabilized. It appeared likely that he would survive if intensive care were continued. Magnetic resonance imaging of his brain at that time revealed abnormal signal in the basal ganglia, and absence of the normal signal in the internal capsule. His parents were told that based on his clinical condition and brain scan appearances Henry had a very high likelihood of developing severe spastic quadriplegic cerebral palsy with at least moderate cognitive impairment.

Michael is aged seven. He has severe spastic quadriplegic cerebral palsy, microcephaly, and epilepsy. He is cortically blind, and has severe intellectual disability. Michael appears to recognize the voices of his parents and teachers and responds with a smile. He also smiles and sometimes laughs in response to familiar music. Most of the time he does not appear to be in pain or discomfort. But he is not able to communicate verbally, nor with the aid of communication tools. He has a specially fitted wheelchair, but has no control over it. He is fed via a gastrostomy. Michael was in the newborn intensive care unit for a month after birth with severe birth asphyxia, and has had several hospital admissions since that time with prolonged seizures or chest infections. Michael's capacity for interaction is unlikely to change over time but his life expectancy is hard to predict. It is possible that he will survive into adult life, perhaps for several decades.

These cases are fictional, though they are fairly typical and represent situations encountered frequently in neonatal and paediatric care. The problem that they pose is that in cases like Henry's doctors will often allow treatment to be withdrawn if parents agree to this. This is most commonly justified in terms of the best interest of the child, and implies that doctors and parents believe that it would be better for Henry if he were to die rather than continue to live. But this judgement clashes with evidence from children like Michael and from some of the quality of life literature referred to in Chapter 5. Although Michael has very significant impairment, it does not appear that his life is so bad that it would be better if he were to die. Talking with those who care for children like Michael with severe impairments, most caregivers do not believe this to be the case. If Michael becomes critically ill and requires a brief period of life-sustaining treatment, it would often be provided.

The second challenge is that although some parents in the first situation will choose comfort care and withdrawal of life-sustaining treatment, others want to have treatment continued. But if it is not in Henry's best interests to have treatment continued (and hence it is appropriate to withdraw life-sustaining treatment), how can parents be allowed to choose continued treatment?

There are a couple of different ways of reconciling the conflicting judgements in these two cases. One option is to question whether life support *should* be withdrawn from infants with severe impairment like Henry. Although difficult, his life would likely be worth living; we would be wrong to let him die. Parents should therefore not be given the option of limiting life-sustaining treatment. The opposite response would be to revise our judgement about the quality of life of surviving children like Michael. We might feel that caregivers are biased in their assessment of his quality of life, and systematically overemphasise the positives while underestimating the negatives for him. Michael would actually have been better to die in infancy. If we take that view we would be wrong to continue life support in the newborn period at parents' request, and wrong to provide life-prolonging treatments to Michael now if he becomes seriously ill. But there is a third possible response. That response says that it would be appropriate to either withdraw or to continue life-sustaining treatments for critically ill infants or children like Henry. Henry's future is not so bad that he would be harmed if life continues, he may indeed have a life of some benefit, and his parents should be supported if they want to continue active treatment. But the probability of survival, or the benefit to Henry if he survives, is sufficiently small that parents and doctors are also justified if they decide to withdraw life-sustaining treatment and allow Henry to die. The framework for decision-making that I will describe takes this third path.

There are two key elements to the revised framework for treatment limitation decisions in children. The first of these is derived from the above and from the role that parents play in decision. Although we should aspire to make the right decision for every child, decisions are necessarily going to vary between families. There is a spectrum of cases where it would be appropriate either to provide life-sustaining treatment, or to decide not to provide that treatment, and where families' wishes are relevant. This spectrum encompasses conditions with a range of severity, but it has limits.

How does the spectrum relate to the best interests of the child, and a life worth living? This is the second element to the framework that we are developing. There are a number of different possibilities. The first is that within the spectrum life-sustaining treatment is neither in the best interests of the child, nor contrary to their interests. How could this be? It has some similarities with a very old philosophical problem called the Sorites paradox (also known as the paradox of the heap).

The Sorites Paradox and Solutions

A man with one hair on his head is called 'bald'.

If a man with one hair is bald, a man with two hairs must also be bald. (The difference between being bald and being hirsute can't come down to a single hair.)

But then, if a man with two hairs is bald, a man with three hairs on his head must also be bald.

If a man with three hairs is bald, a man with four hairs is bald...

We continue this series until we reach the conclusion that a man with 10,000 hairs on his head is bald! But surely that cannot be right?

The earliest description of this paradox is ascribed to the ancient Greek Philosopher Eubulides (Hyde 2008). The Sorites problem is related to the philosophical problem of 'vagueness'. Certain concepts are hard to pin down or define. Is this merely a problem of language, or are certain concepts genuinely vague in themselves? Examples that are often cited of genuine vagueness are the boundaries of a cloud or the edge of a mountain. Where does the cloud or mountain begin and end? There is no answer.

There are several ways that philosophers have attempted to resolve the Sorites paradox:

1. Linguistic: One option would be to *create* a clear boundary by defining terms in a specific way. For example we could say that having less than 100 hairs on your head is the definition of 'baldness'. The problem is that such distinctions are fairly readily seen to be artificial, even absurd. They may also seem arbitrary. Why is 100 hairs the criterion for not being bald, and not 99 or 101, or 200, or 1000? There may be considerable practical value in having a precise definition (for example in legislation). But we are likely to still worry about the truth of the matter, and where to place the boundary.

2. Many-valued or fuzzy logic: An alternative approach is to suggest that the alternatives are not binary (true or false, bald or non-bald). Instead we could include a third category: bald, non-bald, or indeterminate. This would take into account the problem of a single hair making the difference between being bald and not-bald. But this might in turn create further uncertainty about the boundary between bald and indeterminate, indeterminate and non-bald. Fuzzy logic takes this solution further by positing that there are degrees of truth to statements. Someone with no hairs is bald with a truth value of 1. Someone with 10,000 hairs is bald with a truth value of 0 (i.e. they are not bald). But in between there is a spectrum. Adding a single hair will change the truth value of baldness by a small amount until eventually we reach certainty that the individual isn't bald.

3. Supervaluationism: There is a related alternative, which is to suggest that the answer to the question 'Is John bald' is not 'Yes' or 'No', but 'it depends'. The idea is that for vague terms, whether or not John is called bald depends on our definition of baldness. Is John bald if he has 101 hairs? Yes if the definition that we use for baldness includes having 101 hairs, no if we use a more stringent definition of baldness. But we will also sometimes answer 'yes' or 'no' without the qualification. If John has zero hairs on his head, then he is bald no matter what our definition of baldness is.

4. Epistemicism: The last way of responding to the Sorites paradox is to suggest that there *is* an answer to the question of whether or not a man is bald—it is just that we don't know what it is. On this view, the problem is not that the words that we use are vague or vary in meaning depending on the circumstances, nor that there is some in-between or partially true state in between baldness and non-baldness. The problem is simply that we cannot get to the truth.

The Sorites paradox arises from the vagueness of language. Many of the terms that we use (think of tall vs small, thin/fat, old/young), do not have precise boundaries. The concept of the best interests of the child appears to have a similar degree of imprecision.

One way of trying to resolve the problem is to suggest an intermediate state between opposing terms (Figure 8.1a). Perhaps there are a group of infants and children with 'closely balanced interests'? Those cases where parents may make decisions about life-sustaining treatment could correspond to such an intermediate state. This might appeal to some because some of the different values at stake in a best interests judgement appear incommensurable, i.e. they cannot be readily traded off against each other. Can we really weigh up the value of life against the harm of suffering? Can we balance the child's interests in their own future against the child's interests in parents' well-being? A second argument in favour of this interpretation of the 'grey zone' is based on relativism. Relativism is the belief that different ethical viewpoints are equally valid or acceptable; they are relative to the societal, cultural, religious, or philosophical perspective of the individual. There is no single correct answer to ethical questions. Extreme forms of relativism are untenable, since they appear to suggest that there is nothing ultimately to be said about the wrongness of genocide, slavery, rape, or murder. This is implausible. However, there are also more moderate forms of relativism. Although some questions are clear-cut, others appear indeterminate. We might be confident that life-saving treatment is in the best interests of a patient who is certain to recover to full health if treatment is provided. (There can't be anything 'relative' about this judgement.) However, other cases, such as the ones discussed in Chapter 2 are contestable and unclear.

Intermediate categories help a little, since they allow us to sit on the fence, and avoid being forced to classify someone as definitely bald or hairy, or treatment as being definitely in or contrary to the patient's interests. They don't, however, completely solve the problem, since the boundary between 'bald' and 'balding' is also fairly readily seen to be vague, and so we might find it difficult to define our new intermediate category.

A different solution to the problem argues that there is a sharp distinction to be drawn around these apparently vague concepts; it is just our limited understanding of the world, and the right way to classify things that leads to our difficulty in determining the boundaries. This second alternative is attractive for a judgement about best interests. Although it seems slightly

(a)

Quality of Life/ Well-being

Treatment must continue

} Parental discretion about life-sustaining treatment

Treatment must be withdrawn

(b)

Quality of Life/ Well-being

Treatment must continue

Cut-off point for withdrawing treatment

Treatment may be withdrawn or may continue

(c)

Quality of Life/ Well-being

Treatment may be withdrawn or may continue

Cut-off point for withdrawing treatment

Treatment must be withdrawn

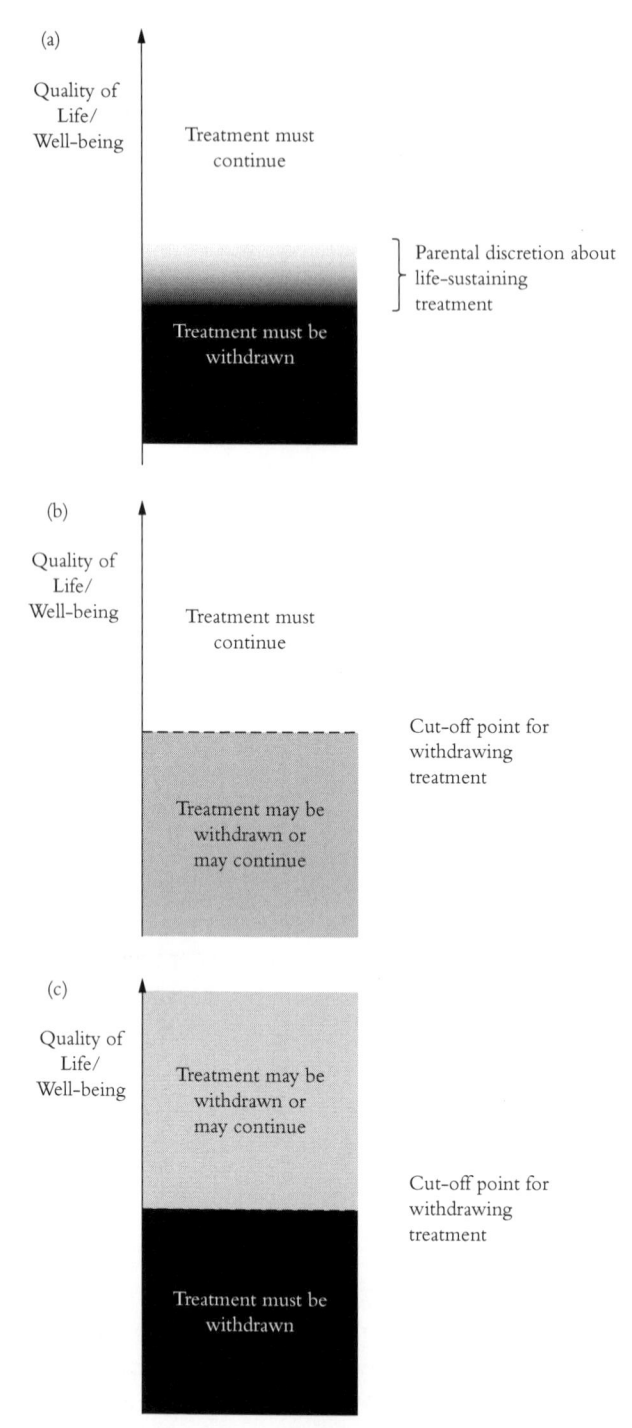

Figure 8.1 Different views about parental discretion for life-sustaining treatment.

implausible that there might be a true but unknowable boundary between 'tall' and 'small', perhaps there is something to the idea that if we knew all of the relevant facts and were extremely wise, we would know whether or not treatment were in a patient's best interests. If there were no true answer to the best interests question, we would be wasting our time in trying to determine which course would be best for the child. But if there is an answer to be found, perhaps we can continue to seek it, even if we cannot always be confident that we have succeeded.

If there is a fact of the matter about best interests, how does the idea of a range of cases where parents might decide about treatment relate to this? One possibility that might have some appeal is shown in 8.1b. It illustrates the view that parental discretion might involve a veto over treatment limitation, but not over treatment continuation. There is an upper boundary, but no lower boundary. On this view, parents might be permitted to insist that treatment continue or be provided even if doctors believe that this would be harmful to the child. However, they would not be permitted to request treatment limitation where treatment is thought to be in the interests of the child.

There are some features of practice that encourage an asymmetrical view of this sort. For example, there is often a legal requirement to obtain parental consent prior to withdrawal of treatment, but no requirement to obtain parental consent when treatment is being continued. There is also a general presumption in favour of providing life-sustaining treatment. This is because death is usually regarded as a great harm, but also because it is always possible to reconsider decisions to continue treatment at a later stage. (If treatment has been stopped (or withheld), and the child has died, there is obviously no way of going back and revisiting the decision.) Furthermore, there is often more sensitivity about stopping treatment against parent's wishes than about continuing treatment. Newspaper headlines tend to be particularly unkind to doctors who limit treatment against parents' wishes, but much less so when treatment continues over parents' objections.

Yet, on further questioning this view seems problematic. Surely we would not want to allow parents to insist on treatment continuing no matter how harmful to the child, and no matter what the cost? Would we really want to allow doctors to provide or continue to provide a treatment that caused a child severe pain, but yielded no significant benefit? Although there are not infrequent disputes about artificial ventilation, and whether doctors may withdraw treatment that is believed inappropriate, there is another, more invasive, life-sustaining procedure that does not generally lead to the same disputes. Extra-corporeal membrane oxygenation (ECMO) provides a form of heart-lung bypass for children or adults with lung or heart failure, using large, surgically placed vascular catheters, and an external machine to circulate the blood. There are occasional disputes about whether or not ECMO should be offered or provided if a family requests it, but these are rare (Paris, Schreiber, et al. 1993). Another example is that of cardio-pulmonary resuscitation (CPR). CPR is commenced after a child has a cardiac arrest. Cardiac compressions and artificial ventilation are able to maintain some degree of oxygenation and circulation. However, at some point, for example after ten or twenty minutes of resuscitation, sometimes longer (depending on the cause of the arrest), if there is no return of the spontaneous circulation, CPR is ceased. If there were no lower boundary to decision-making, if parents always had the option of vetoing decisions to discontinue treatment, that would seem to imply that ECMO or CPR might need to continue indefinitely at parental request. But that would surely be absurd. Although we may want to allow parents some freedom to decide when further treatment would be harmful and should not be provided there must be some limit to this right. There must be a lower boundary—the question is where that boundary should be.

A second possible framework is shown in Figure 8.1c. This view takes the concerns about harming a child for the sake of parents to its logical extreme by not permitting any harm of the child for the sake of parents. If treatment would not be overall in the interests of the child it should never be provided or continued, no matter what parents' views were. On the other hand, parents might have a right to refuse potentially beneficial treatment for their child. One reason for supporting this view is that this appears to be an extension of laws relating to consent for treatment. If an adult is judged to be legally competent most legal jurisdictions and ethical frameworks would not permit enforced treatment against the patient's will. Treating the patient, against his or her express wishes, would be judged to be a form of assault. This is the case even if the treatment would be unequivocally in the patient's best interests (for example, a blood transfusion in the setting of major blood loss). However, patients are not given the same freedom to *request* treatment. In the UK, the courts and other professional bodies have endorsed the view that there is no obligation for a doctor to provide treatment that they do not believe would be appropriate (i.e. that it would not be in the patient's interests) (General Medical Council 2010). Discretion about treatment for adult patients, then, appears to resemble 8.1c, with a lower boundary but no upper boundary for treatment. If the situation were similar for children, parents might have absolute discretion to refuse treatment, but limited or no discretion to request non-beneficial treatment.

But again, this does not seem the right framework for children. Patients are allowed to refuse treatment for themselves because of the high value placed on individual autonomy. The freedom to make choices about our own lives is extremely important to most people. As long as our choices do not harm other people, we should be allowed to pursue our own goals, and to make decisions about our own lives. But the qualification 'as long as our choices do not harm other people' means that there is something different about parents' choices on behalf of a child. Parents' choices can and sometimes do result in harm for their children. We don't (or shouldn't) allow parents to abuse their children, to neglect them, or to make decisions on their behalf that are likely to result in substantial harm to the children. There must be an upper limit to parental discretion about treatment.

It appears from the above arguments that there must be upper and lower limits to parental discretion about treatment. At one extreme, the prognosis for the child is sufficiently good that treatment must be provided, even if parents do not wish this. At the other extreme, prognosis is so poor that life-sustaining treatment should not be provided, even if parents request it. These extremes mark the boundaries of permissible treatment limitation decision, and represent two treatment thresholds: a threshold of mandatory treatment (call this the *upper threshold*), and a threshold of inappropriate treatment (call this the *lower threshold*). We could set either of these at the zero point of best interests. For example, we could give parents discretion only over treatment below the zero point—they have some freedom to decide, but may not refuse or decline beneficial treatment. Alternatively we could give parents discretion only over treatment *above* the zero point— they may decline some beneficial treatment, but may not insist that harmful treatment is provided. These possibilities appear more plausible than the two frameworks discussed above. However, arguably neither of these frameworks is correct either. Setting either the upper or lower threshold at the zero point raises serious problems for practice because of the difficulty in defining when the benefits of treatment are equivalent to the burdens. But moreover, the above arguments about the overlapping interests of parents and child, the independent weight of parents' interests, and about moral uncertainty that affects the evaluation of benefits and harms, all suggest that there should be some degree of parental discretion about treatment on either side of the zero point. This framework for treatment decisions is illustrated in Figure 8.2.

Figure 8.2 shows a comparison between a pure best interests framework, as outlined in Chapter 2, and the threshold framework. The spectrum of cases where parents may have discretion about treatment straddles the zero point. Within this spectrum there will be some cases where the infant or child will (if they survive) probably have a life of overall benefit and treatment would overall be in their interests. There will also be some cases where the burdens of life probably outweigh the benefits.

I have spent some time working towards a model that is likely to be familiar to a number of those who work in intensive care. The language of the threshold framework is very similar to a model of decision-making that is often applied to decision-making about extremely premature infants. Infants who are born sixteen or seventeen weeks prematurely (at around twenty-three or twenty-four weeks of gestation) have a high mortality rate, even in centres with considerable specialized expertise in the care of very premature infants. Approximately one quarter of surviving infants born at this gestation have severe impairment (Tyson, Parikh, et al. 2008). Consequently parents and doctors sometimes elect not to actively resuscitate infants born this prematurely. There have been numerous guidelines written about treatment decisions for extremely premature infants (MacDonald and Newborn 2002; Lui, Bajuk et al. 2006; Verloove-Vanhorick

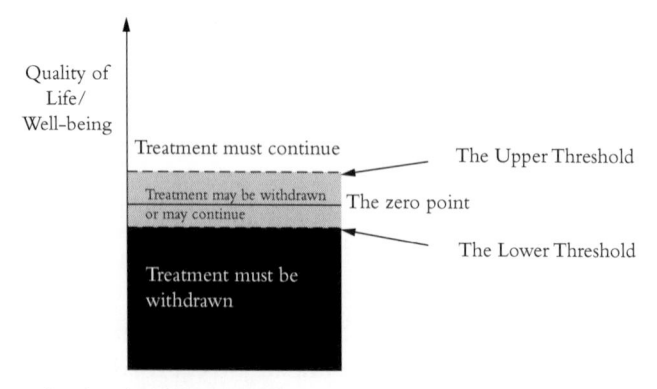

Figure 8.2 The threshold framework.

2006; Wilkinson, Ahluwalia, et al. 2009; Kattwinkel, Perlman, et al. 2010; Moriette, Rameix, et al. 2010) and there is striking common ground between guidelines in different countries (Meadow 2007). Almost all of these guidelines suggest that there is a point (usually below twenty-two or twenty-three weeks gestation) where the chance of survival without severe impairment is so small that resuscitation should not be offered. There is another point (usually above twenty-four or twenty-five weeks gestation) where the probability of survival without severe impairment is sufficiently high that resuscitation should always be provided. In between these points (from twenty-three to twenty-four weeks gestation) parents' views and interests have the most impact on decisions about whether or not to resuscitate. This area of sanctioned parental discretion in decisions is sometimes referred to as the 'grey zone', implying that decisions are not black or white for infants with such a high chance of death or impairment. Jon Tyson and John Paris, referring to the same types of decisions, have distinguished between groups of infants in whom treatment is 'mandatory', 'optional', or 'unreasonable' (Tyson 1995; Paris, Schreiber, et al. 2007).

However, the distinctive feature of the framework as described here is that it makes it clear how the grey zone relates to a pure best interests model, and why there should be parental discretion in end-of-life decisions. There is surprisingly little explicit justification in the medical literature for why parents should be allowed discretion over decisions for extremely premature infants. Guidelines usually refer vaguely to the relevance of uncertainty. The issues discussed earlier in this book, and summarized above help to answer this question. It is the combination of prognostic and moral uncertainty that justify this approach, along with the importance of family interests for (particularly) neonatal decision-making. But these ethical arguments do not just apply to extremely premature infants. The framework applies also to critically ill infants and children with other medical conditions. There will be a range of cases in which parents' views are highly relevant to decisions about treatment.

Defining the Thresholds

I have argued that there must be a degree of parental discretion about treatment decisions, but there must also be limits to this discretion. Is it possible to define these limits? In the next section we will explore several different alternatives.

Analysis

The first possibility is that we might use ethical analysis to help determine where the thresholds should be. Here is one attempt to do so. The reasons that I have argued underpin the relevance of parental views about treatment could be used to set out ethical criteria for the boundaries of parental discretion. These principles for the upper boundary are outlined below.

Criteria for the upper threshold

Treatment withdrawal is permissible for infants or children with conditions that
C1. Reduce benefits or involve substantial burdens for the child (or both) AND
C2. Are anticipated to be close to the zero point (i.e. to the point where life becomes not worth living), AND EITHER
C3. Involve a significant risk of a life not worth living OR
C4. Impose a substantial burden of care on others.

According to these criteria treatment withdrawal does not require that the burdens of treatment outweigh the benefits, or that life is intolerable (objective or subjective ways of assessing whether life is worth living—from Chapter 2). Instead it requires that the future for the child or infant is low and close to this point. The child's illness or impairment reduces the benefits of life for the child to such an extent or imposes such substantial burdens that the overall benefit of life is small. The proximity to the balance or 'zero point' is important, since conditions that are close to the zero point involve a significant risk of life overall being harmful. It is also in cases close to the zero point where the benefits to the child are relatively small, and it is most likely that the benefits to others outweigh the benefits to the infant or child. Finally, as noted in the previous chapter, in genuine borderline cases (i.e. where the child's future life is close to the zero point), the overlapping nature of interests would justify giving some weight to parental interests and views. On the other hand, treatment withdrawal would not be permitted for children with significant impairment who nevertheless have a clear benefit from treatment. The greater benefit for the child would outweigh the potential burdens of care for parents, and would make it unlikely that the child would be harmed overall by treatment.

The listed criteria suggest that withdrawal of treatment may be allowed *either* if there is a risk of overall harm *or* if treatment imposes a large burden on caregivers. But would it really be justified to withhold treatment where there was no risk of the child's life falling below the zero point, and where the only reason is because of the impact on the family? Such a conclusion would be highly worrying to some people. They might worry about these criteria being used to justify treatment limitation for reasons of social convenience in children with relatively minor impairments, for example Down syndrome. However, the criteria as set out would not permit this to take place. This is firstly because the second condition requires that the child's condition is close to the level of a life not worth living. This isn't the case for children with minor or moderate impairments such as Down syndrome. Most children with Down syndrome are able to communicate, flourish, and experience a wide range of the valuable features of human life (Gillon 1986; Berube 1996). Their lives are not even close to being intolerable. Secondly, the type of family impact discussed in Chapter 4 is not mere social convenience. (In that chapter I suggested that the negative impact on the family should be discounted where it is within the control of the family, or likely to be alleviated by social change. However, it is legitimate to consider the likely impact on the family even if society is imperfect. Third, in practice infants or children who have such severe illness or impairment that their lives are close to the point of not being worth living have a risk that they will be harmed by treatment, *and* their care substantially affects the interests of others.

It is possible, however, to imagine cases where these reasons do not go in the same direction. One example might be that of a child in a persistent vegetative state (PVS). If this condition has been present for a sufficient period of time it is highly unlikely that the child will ever recover. It appears reasonably clear that patients in PVS do not experience pain (Laureys 2005). It does not appear that there is a significant risk that the child will be harmed by continuing treatment, so if we allow parents to elect for withdrawal of treatment this must be based on other factors—such as the burden of care.

There may be some uncertainty about whether survival in PVS is a harm or benefit to the child. Some within the community might judge that simply being alive confers a net benefit to the child, while others might regard the indignity of surviving without the capacity for consciousness as a net harm. Or perhaps we are wrong about the lack of painful experience? Recent studies using functional neuroimaging raise the possibility that a small proportion of those in a persistent vegetative state retain at least intermittent conscious awareness of their surroundings (Monti, Vanhaudenhuyse, et al. 2010). That may be a good thing if it enables those patients to communicate, or to access treatments to improve their profoundly impaired state. On the other hand, it may be that being in PVS is much worse for the patient than we have thought, because there is a chance of retaining awareness of pain, discomfort, anxiety, but of having no means of communicating that distress (Wilkinson, Kahane, et al. 2009).

Let's imagine instead a different example, where the Carmentis machine predicts profound cognitive impairment (the child will have the cognitive capacities of a three-month-old infant), but good physical health. This might be the infant Chloe described in Chapter 2 with polymicrogyria. The machine indicates that Chloe is not going to suffer from illness or require painful medical interventions. It seems that her life will be potentially worth living, from her point of view. She will have a small (perhaps very small) amount of benefit from life, but little on the burden side of the equation. If Chloe's life would not be intolerable, or the benefits would outweigh the burdens, the best interests views described in Chapter 2 would appear to mean that life-sustaining treatment must be provided. Should the interests of Chloe's family be taken into account? In Chapter 4 we looked at some of the potential costs for families in terms of psychological and physical illness as well as marital discord and break-up. Continuing treatment for a child with profound impairment of this degree could have a substantial negative impact on the interests of parents, while providing a relatively small benefit to the child. Although parents are expected to be willing to make some sacrifices for their children, the sacrifice involved in such cases is much more than most parents ever have to make. Perhaps it is more than should be required of them? One fairly commonly held view is that some actions, while good and praiseworthy, go above and beyond the call of duty. Where aiding another individual would require substantial personal sacrifice and effort, that action is sometimes referred to as *supererogatory* rather than obligatory (Wolf 1982; Kamm 1985). For example, it may be good for individuals who are well off to donate a proportion of their income to support those in poorer countries who are suffering from famine, illness, or natural disaster. There may even be a moral obligation for people to do so. However, while it would be even better for someone to donate *all* of their income to charity, or to give up their comfortable life and go and work as an aid worker in developing countries, we would not expect everyone to do so. There are various accounts of the level of personal sacrifice that would make an act supererogatory (Flescher 2003: 54, 72; Heyd 2008). On most accounts, though, an action would fall into this category if it involves substantial imbalance in its effects, where the costs to the individual are great while the benefits achieved are small. Some levels of sacrifice by parents appear to be supererogatory rather than obligatory; the situation for Chloe appears to be like this. According to the framework that we are developing, it would be appropriate to support Chloe's parents if they did not want life-sustaining treatment to be continued.

What about the lower boundary of parental decision-making? When should doctors refuse to continue treatment even if parents wish it to be provided? A set of corresponding criteria for the lower threshold are given below.

Normative criteria for the lower threshold

Treatment continuation is not permissible for infants or children with conditions that
C1. Reduce future benefits or impose substantial burdens on the child (or both) AND
C5. Mean that the child's will not be close to the level of a life worth living AND
C6. Render it highly likely that the infant or child will have a life not worth living and be significantly harmed by continuing treatment.

Again, the proximity to the zero point (or lack of proximity) is important. It means that above this point the harms and benefits for the child are relatively closely matched. In borderline cases parental interests may overlap with those of the child, and their views are highly relevant because of moral uncertainty about the evaluation of benefits and harms. As we discussed in Chapter 4 (in the section on Death/Life conflicts and the interests of the child), above this point the benefit to the parents of continuing treatment for their child may outweigh the harms to the child—where those harms are relatively small. Beyond the lower threshold, though, the harm is so great that parents' interests are insufficient to outweigh the costs to the child. Overlapping interests cannot plausibly make it in the child's interests to keep them alive. We should not allow parents to choose continued treatment in this situation.

Although these ethical criteria may be helpful in justifying parental discretion in decision-making, one very real concern may be about whether they are of any practical assistance. It can be difficult to know how to determine whether or not treatment is in the best interests of a child, whether life would be intolerable, or whether the burdens of treatments outweigh the benefits. But the criteria that I have listed above are not necessarily any easier to apply. What is a 'significant' risk, or a 'substantial' burden of care? What does it mean to say that future life is 'close' to the zero point? How close must it be, and how would we know? One thought is that it is potentially easier to identify borderline cases, where a child's future is close to the level of a life worth living (LWL) than to be sure exactly which fall above and which below the best interests line. In a sense, then, it may be easier to identify cases that sit in between the thresholds than to use best interests to decide difficult cases. But this solution potentially just moves the goal posts, since we still have to decide which conditions are between the two treatment thresholds, and which are outside. Which conditions are *close enough* to the level of an LWL to allow parents a say in treatment? Is it possible to develop more practically applicable criteria for the thresholds?

Convergence

One approach to developing more specific guidelines for the boundaries of parental discretion would be to seek a consensus view. It would, perhaps, be challenging to try to reach agreement on how far above a hypothetical zero point we should draw the upper threshold, or how far below it the lower threshold. But we can approach the thresholds in a more practical way. The upper threshold is the point at which resuscitation or life-sustaining treatment becomes mandatory. This means that parents who wish treatment not to be provided above this point would be overruled. What level of prognosis is sufficiently positive that it would be appropriate to take over the care of a child and to organize for adoption or foster care? Our answer to this depends on our judgement about which decisions are unreasonable, but also on how confident we are that courts will side against parents, and on the availability of adoption or foster care. At the other end of the spectrum the relevant question is this: how bad does prognosis need to be to overrule parents who wish treatment to continue and to unilaterally withdraw or withhold treatment? Again, this judgement includes a number of related factors, for example, the availability of intensive care beds, and the likelihood that if treatment is continued for this child, that another child will be harmed. If we are able to reach agreement about when to overrule parents' wishes, what remains becomes, by definition, the area for parental discretion.

There is a precedent for such a process of consensus. As noted previously, although decisions about resuscitation of extremely premature newborn infants are often thought to be controversial, there is considerable agreement between different guidelines about where active treatment is optional, mandatory, or unreasonable. Some of these guidelines have specifically sought a range of views in determining treatment thresholds. One relevant example was a conference held in New South Wales in Australia in 2006 (Lui, Bajuk, et al. 2006). That conference brought together over 100 neonatologists, neonatal nurses, obstetricians, ethicists, allied health professionals, and parents. Information was presented to participants on local survival figures for extremely premature infants, and there was time devoted to ethical, parental, and legal views about resuscitation decisions. In a large group format a number of clinical scenarios were discussed, with questions or issues brought out for discussion in smaller groups. Those smaller groups then worked to develop guideline statements for inclusion in a consensus statement. Their statements were brought back to the whole group, where a voting process established the proportion of participants who agreed or disagreed with them. Statements that more than 75 per cent of participants agreed or strongly agreed with were regarded as reaching consensus. On the basis of the results the conference was able to provide a set of guidelines for resuscitation decisions, including the boundaries of decisions by parents that should be respected.

We shouldn't underestimate the challenge, however. The lower threshold corresponds to a concept that is often referred to by doctors, but which has proved strikingly difficult to pin down, that of 'futility' (Wilkinson and Savulescu 2011). The term 'futile' is used to describe treatment that doctors believe has such a low chance or magnitude of benefit for the patient that it should not be provided even if the patient or family requests it. There has been a large amount written about futility over several decades (mostly in relation to adult patients), but it remains contentious. One example definition that has been proposed is that treatment is *quantitatively futile* when it has not been of benefit in the last 100 consecutive cases (Schneiderman, Jecker, et al. 1990). Although a guideline of this nature appears intuitively plausible, this definition of a lower threshold is not uniformly accepted. One concern is that it is very difficult to know when the quantitative criteria have been met. How similar does a case have to be to previous ones for it to be reasonable to group them together? The problem of self-fulfilling prophecies (Chapter 5) means that there is a difference between treatment that *has not been* successful, and treatment that *could not have been* successful (if continued). A second reason for dissent about this futility definition is that although a doctor may judge treatment to be futile if there is less than 1 per cent chance of success, patients may consider this chance worth grasping (where the alternative is certain death).

Another problem for any attempt to reach consensus on the thresholds for treatment is who to involve in the process. The New South Wales conference involved mostly medical professionals but also a small number of others, including parents. Doctors do not reach the same conclusions about when treatment should be provided as members of the wider community. In one survey, when asked whether they would choose cardiopulmonary resuscitation (CPR) for themselves, healthcare professionals were 10–20 per cent less likely than patients to want CPR across a range of hypothetical conditions (Kerridge, Pearson, et al. 1999). This might be partly as a result of better knowledge about the relevant medical facts, including the chance of CPR being successful. But it is also likely to reflect different values placed by doctors on survival and impairment in different states. As noted in previous chapters, doctors' assessment of the quality of life of individuals in severely impaired states is more negative than that of parents or children. So there is good reason for thinking that the perspectives of others are needed. The practical challenge is that the smaller or more similar the group that is involved in the process of developing consensus guidelines, the easier it is to reach agreement. The broader the group, the harder it will be, and the more likely it is that agreement will prove impossible.

Divergence

Agreement about where to place the upper and lower thresholds for treatment is likely to be difficult to achieve. But it may be possible to define boundaries for decisions despite disagreement. In fact we could draw on the fact of disagreement to help generate guidelines. Figure 8.3a shows in schematic form the different position of the upper and lower thresholds by a group of individuals. Each is asked to indicate where they would not permit parents to make decisions about withdrawing treatment (solid lines

THE THRESHOLD FRAMEWORK 281

(a) Quality of Life/Wellbeing

(b) Quality of Life/Wellbeing

Treatment must continue

Treatment may be withdrawn or may continue

Treatment must be withdrawn

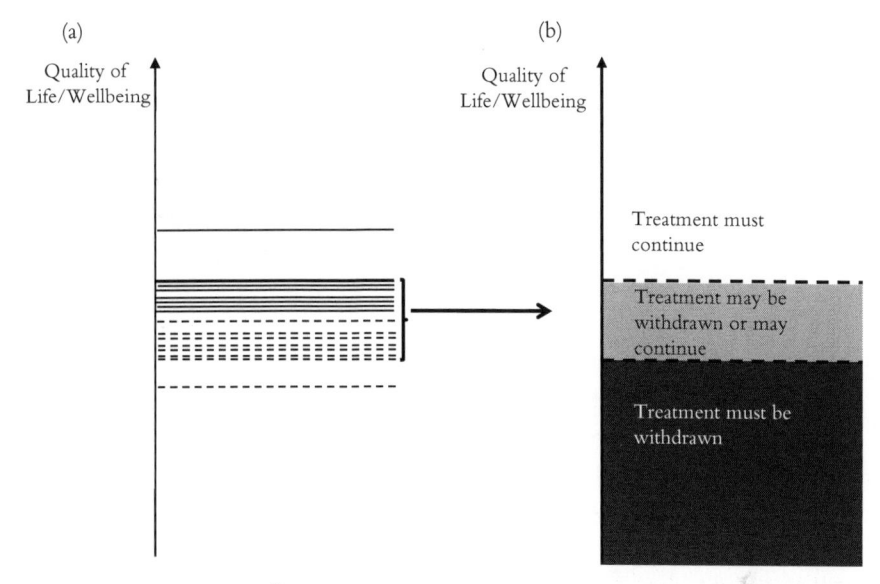

Figure 8.3 Agreeing to disagree.

indicate the upper boundaries for these decisions, while the dotted ones are the lower boundaries). In the figure, the lines vary from person to person, reflecting the views of different people. Some draw the upper threshold higher, giving parents more scope to make decisions; others would draw it lower down. Moral uncertainty is one of the reasons for this spread of views about when treatment limitation should be allowed or disallowed. Moral uncertainty is also one of the main reasons why it is legitimate to involve parents in decision-making. But then, the distribution of different views about treatment helps to map out where there is moral uncertainty about treatment. If we ignore outliers, 8.3b indicates the position of the upper and lower thresholds derived from this spectrum of views. Parents would be provided with a choice about treatment where at least some of the community shared their view that this is a reasonable course of action.

Another analogy for this way of developing guidelines is the concept of clinical (or sometimes called 'community') equipoise (Weijer, Shapiro, et al. 2000).

Equipoise
   Normally there is an ethical requirement for doctors to recommend or provide treatment that they believe would be best for the individual

patient. But when a patient is in a randomized controlled trial something different takes place. A coin is tossed, or some other means of random selection is employed in order to determine which treatment the patient receives. This may mean that the patient receives a treatment that the doctor doesn't believe is the most suitable for them. Is it ethical to perform a randomized controlled trial, and if so when is it appropriate?

One answer to this question refers to the concept of equipoise. If a doctor is ambivalent between two treatments, such that they do not know which of them is superior, it appears acceptable for the decision to be made on the basis of random chance. This is consistent with the doctor's ethical obligations to the patient, since in this theoretical state of equipoise there is no conclusive reason for the doctor to choose one or the other treatment.

Yet in practice there are several challenges to equipoise. The first is that it is very rare for doctors to be in a state of complete ambivalence about treatment options. When choosing between new treatment X, and standard treatment Y, there is often a range of factors favouring one or the other treatment. There may be encouraging pre-clinical or clinical results for the effectiveness of X, or there may be considerable experience and confidence with the safety of Y. Doctors are often in a position of preferring one treatment over another. In this situation, the justification for randomization is a combination of equipoise and uncertainty. Uncertainty about the potential benefits or harms of the different treatments leads the clinician to discount their preference for one treatment, and to adopt a position of relative equipoise. The second challenge, though, occurs when a clinician individually lacks both equipoise and uncertainty. They are confident that treatment X is superior to treatment Y, and would be uncomfortable providing Y to their patients. Yet, other members of the medical community hold the opposite position, and would always provide treatment Y. In this setting, individual equipoise is absent, but the presence of divergent views across the community means that patients could receive either treatment, depending on which doctor they happen to attend. There is a balance of views about the different treatments across the medical community (it may not be equally balanced), and this is sometimes referred to as community (or clinical) equipoise.

Community equipoise does not usually apply outside the specialized context of research. But it might be relevant, for example, if a patient were to request treatment Y from a doctor whose normal practice is to prescribe X. Although this doctor's preference may be otherwise, there is a case for allowing the patient to have treatment Y, or at the least referring the patient to another physician who is willing to provide Y. Similarly, the presence of divergent practice across the medical community potentially creates an obligation for doctors to inform patients of the different treatment options available. The range of different reasonable views within the medical community is relevant to informed consent.

There is a sense in which there is community equipoise about the thresholds for providing or limiting life-sustaining treatment. Although the medical community is not likely to embark on a randomized controlled trial, it may be appropriate to recognize and incorporate the range of existing views about treatment into guidelines that set out the boundaries of acceptable practice.

This approach to developing guidelines for decision-making would potentially allow progress to be made despite disagreement. The threshold framework itself would help since it does not seek a single answer about when treatment is indicated or not indicated. Rather it seeks to set out the range of treatment decisions that it is reasonable to support.

It is important to note though, that not all disagreement arises from moral uncertainty. Some divergence in views may arise from misunderstanding or incorrect facts. It would be important, before using the range of views as supporting a range of decisions, to know that those involved had been given all available accurate and relevant information. Those who prescribe treatment Y might do so because they haven't read the latest research papers or the systematic reviews that support treatment X. But it is also possible that some have a full understanding of the relevant facts, and yet hold views that should not be respected. It is possible, for example, that some within the community would never want to overrule parents and withhold or withdraw treatment against their wishes, even if the child were predicted to suffer substantially as a result of treatment or had no chance whatsoever of benefit. They might do so because of a fear of negative publicity, or because of a belief that parents have an absolute right to decide. It is also possible that some would allow parents to elect for withdrawal or withholding of treatment in the face of predicted mild disability. (As noted in Chapter 6, it was once thought acceptable by many in the medical community to withhold surgery from infants with Down syndrome if parents did not wish it to take place.) Yet the arguments and the ethical criteria provided in this book suggest that neither of these views fall within the range of moral uncertainty and legitimate difference of opinion. One approach to determining which views should be included might use a simple statistical approach, like the rejection of outliers in the figure, or perhaps using an inter-quartile range, covering the views of 75 per cent of surveyed individuals. Alternatively, or additionally, the ethical criteria developed earlier in this chapter could be applied to the results of deliberation to ensure that guidelines are appropriate.

Procedural Solution

One final alternative to setting out the boundaries of decisions works around the difficulty in getting people to agree in advance about contentious and controversial questions. There have been numerous attempts to define the concept of 'medical futility' in order to provide a justification for overruling parents or surrogates who are requesting a treatment that doctors believe is not beneficial (Youngner 1988; Schneiderman, Jecker, et al. 1990; Brody and Halevy 1995). In some parts of the world futility statutes have been developed that attempt to do this. But it has proved extremely difficult to arrive at a clear definition of futility that applies to these cases of conflict and that would be robust enough to be incorporated into law. The vagueness of existing definitions means that decisions not to provide treatment are sometimes appealed, resulting in lengthy and costly court deliberations (Pope 2007).

Because of this difficulty, a different approach has recently developed that focuses on the *process* rather than the substance of futility disputes. This model has been adopted in Texas as part of a broader act looking at end-of-life decision-making (Fine 2009; Stewart 2011). The Texas Advance Directives Act sets out a number of steps that must be followed in resolving futility disputes. Clinicians may request ethics consultation by the institutional ethics review committee if they judge treatment to be inappropriate. Family members are then given at least forty-eight hours notice of the planned committee meeting. If the committee agrees with the clinicians that further treatment should not be provided, families are given ten days to try to find an alternative healthcare provider who is willing and able to provide treatment. The family may appeal for a longer period, or may appeal the decision if the arbitration process as set out by the act has not been followed. However, in the absence of an alternative doctor and hospital willing to provide treatment, after ten days treatment may be withdrawn, and clinicians are protected from civil or criminal prosecution.

The concept of futile or medically inappropriate treatment corresponds to the lower threshold in the threshold framework. A procedural solution like that described might be particularly attractive for drafting law relating to treatment decisions, because it avoids the need to set out specific medical details in legislation, and allows the court to assess procedure rather than making medical judgements. But this sort of solution is also compatible with the development of more specific guidelines for decisions; it may be appropriate and desirable to have some guidance for clinicians about the sorts of situation that would fall above or below the lower threshold, *and* to have a clear process for dealing with cases that are uncertain.

Could a similar procedural solution be applied to the upper threshold? As with the approach described above, it would be possible to use existing structures to do this. Where families do not want treatment continued, but the responsible doctors disagree, either doctors or the family could seek review by the hospital ethics committee or by the court. The committee could review the relevant facts, and hear from both the family and the medical team why they have reached differing opinion. This process may be enough in itself to resolve misunderstandings about the facts, or about the issues at stake. (In Texas, the majority of disputes are resolved in this way) (Fine and Mayo 2003). The committee may end up siding with the family or with the doctors, but one additional safeguard is the possibility of the family finding another doctor who agrees with them. In futility disputes, families are able to have treatment continued if they are able to find another health care provider who is willing and able to provide it. In continuation disputes, treatment might be limited if families are able to find another health care provider who is willing to provide palliative care. The advantage of this safeguard is that it overcomes concerns with the procedural approach about committee composition and the fallibility of committee decision-making (Stewart 2011). Imagine, for example, that doctors and an ethics committee in a hospital funded by a religious group are unwilling to agree to treatment withdrawal. In this circumstance, both physicians and the ethics committee may draw on religious values that are not shared by the patient and/or his family. However, the presence of others within the medical community who have differing views would potentially allow the family's views to be respected.

I have listed above four alternative ways of defining or determining the thresholds for treatment limitation decisions. In fact, these should be seen as complementary rather than mutually exclusive. Attempts to develop more specific guidelines for decisions might seek consensus, but respect reasonable disagreement where this is not possible. Ethical analysis might be used to develop criteria that could provide a check or counterbalance for guidelines that are developed within a community. Finally, procedures for dealing with conflict could and should be used to resolve disagreements and uncertainties that remain despite guidelines.

Counter-Arguments to the Threshold Framework

What arguments might be raised against this framework for decision-making? I will discuss several, and suggest responses to each in turn.

Difficulties in Definition or Interpretation

One concern about the threshold framework has been alluded to above: it may be difficult to define or determine which conditions fall in between the thresholds. The ethical criteria outlined in the early part of this chapter may be just as difficult to apply as pure best-interests-based rules for decisions. If these ethical criteria were the only basis for decisions, then it may be hard for individual clinicians or parents to know how to interpret them. But we have explored above their potential use as a basis for the development of more specific consensus (or dissensus) guidelines. Such guidelines would not be binding, and would not preclude decisions being influenced by specific factors applying in individual cases. But they could provide a valuable point of reference for decisions.

Arbitrariness

A second potential concern with the threshold view is that the exact position of the upper and lower thresholds are arbitrary. How far above and below the zero line should these thresholds lie? Some might view the space between these thresholds as very wide, while others might see them as being close together.

There are, though, different senses of arbitrariness. A cut-off point may be arbitrary in the sense that it could be defensibly drawn at a different level. Or it could be arbitrary in the sense that there is *no reason* to make the distinction. There are numerous policies or laws that are arbitrary in the first sense; in South Australia teenagers are able to obtain a driving license when they are seventeen, while in the state of Victoria, the minimum age is eighteen, and in the Northern Territory it is sixteen and a half. There are similar variations between different states in North America, and there seems little clear reason to prefer one point to another. But there is good reason to draw a line somewhere, and a number of reasons why a point in the late teenage years is an appropriate place. Driving age rules are not arbitrary in the second sense. Similarly, there are multiple plausible places to draw a threshold for treatment withdrawal. If we draw on the example of extremely premature infants again, in some parts of the world the lower threshold is set at twenty-three weeks, but others would draw it at twenty-four or even twenty-five weeks' gestation (Pignotti and Donzelli 2008). A line drawn at one of these points, or at other possible ones such as twenty-three weeks and one day or twenty-two weeks and five days, etc., is arbitrary in the first sense. But such thresholds are not arbitrary in the second sense. There is good reason to think that the cut-off point for resuscitation (if there is a cut-off point) should be somewhere between twenty-one and twenty-five weeks of gestation. Likewise, there are a number of reasons why the upper threshold should be set above, but close to, the best interests zero point.

Furthermore, there is a sense that the alternative is also arbitrary. We discussed in Chapter 2 the difficulty in pinning down just how severe future impairment needed to be to allow treatment limitation. On the basis of the child's best interests some clinicians might allow treatment withdrawal for baby Amelia (the infant with predicted severe motor impairment but relatively preserved intellect), while others would not. Some clinicians would resuscitate a premature infant with a gestational age of twenty-two weeks and six days, while others would only resuscitate infants of more than twenty-four weeks gestation. Although the best interests rule itself is not arbitrary, decisions made on the basis of best interests may be arbitrary—in the first sense.

Even if the thresholds are arbitrary, there is a further question about whether this should lead us to reject the threshold framework. Given the important practical need to determine when treatment withdrawal is permissible, and the reasons that I have outlined in favour of setting out a range of cases in which parents' views may be taken into account, it is possible that the disadvantages of arbitrariness are outweighed by the other advantages of having a clear framework for practice.

Finally, the adjective that often accompanies a claim that a particular rule is 'arbitrary' is that it is 'capricious'. The preceding description of ways to develop guidelines based on the framework should make it clear that the thresholds are not being decided on mere whims, nor on the opinion of single individuals. They are based on considered, reasoned judgements of a community caring for sick children and infants.

Particularism and Rules

The threshold framework tries to map out the boundaries for decision-making, and to set out criteria for when treatment is obligatory, or when it is unreasonable. But one argument against a framework of this sort is that guidelines do not (and perhaps cannot) take into account the particular factors that are relevant in an individual case. It might be thought reasonable to consider the interests of the child including the risk of harm from treatment, and the interests of families. However, given the varying strength of these competing factors, a defined line, no matter where it is drawn, is unlikely to be able to adequately separate cases where it is permissible to withdraw treatment from those where it is not (Chen and Chen 2011).

This concern is similar to one that might be expressed about rules or guidelines for any morally complex decision. There is a tension between providing clear enough guidelines to ensure that practice is appropriate (and consistent), but also flexible enough to allow those involved in decisions to take into account factors that can't be predicted or specified. The more specific the rules that are applied, the less likely it is that decisions will be made outside those parameters. This will limit or prevent decisions that shouldn't be made, but may also prevent decisions that should be made but don't fit into the neat boxes that have been created. (The philosopher Jonathan Dancy has argued in favour of a broader ethical view that there aren't in fact common ethical rules or principles that adequately cover different cases. He endorses a view sometimes called 'moral particularism', which holds that moral judgement applies to and arises from individual cases, and that overarching principles can't be derived from them (Dancy 2004).)

But the problem with taking a particularist approach to end-of-life decisions is that it risks considerable differences in interpretation and inconsistency in decisions between different doctors. Considerable variation in willingness to make end-of-life decisions has been documented in intensive care (Ravenscroft and Bell 2000; Poulton, Ridley et al. 2005; Wunsch, Harrison, et al. 2005; Lee, Tieves, et al. 2010). In some adult intensive care units in the UK very few deaths followed decisions to withdraw active treatment, while in others almost all the patients who died had had treatment withdrawn (Wunsch, Harrison, et al. 2005). In a large European survey of doctors working in neonatal intensive care there was variability in self-reported experience of withdrawal of life-sustaining treatment between countries, but also within countries (Cuttini, Nadai, et al. 2000). In another study 270 paediatric intensive care physicians and oncologists were presented with a set of cases involving a six-year-old child with severe viral pneumonia and a previously diagnosed haematological malignancy (Randolph, Zollo, et al. 1999). Physicians were given a series of options for the aggressiveness of further treatment. In six of the eight cases less than half of the surveyed physicians agreed on which course of treatment was appropriate. In three of the cases more than 20 per cent of physicians chose treatment plans that were diametrically opposed. There is some evidence that these different views translate into actual decisions. Critical care nurses in several surveys have indicated that consultants vary significantly in their threshold for withdrawal of life-sustaining treatment (Gresiuk and Joffe 2011; Ravenscroft and Bell 2000). One potential contributor to doctors' variation in offering treatment limitation is the vagueness of existing guidelines.

Although the above discussion refers to rules or guidelines, it is perhaps important which of these we are talking about. Legal or professional rules for behaviour are necessarily prescriptive. To be enforceable they must be specific, and encompass all situations that are likely to arise; they are usually binding and authoritative. Guidelines, however, have a different relationship to practice; they may be more or less specific, they do not necessarily cover all situations, they are usually non-binding, and admit of exceptions. The concern about individual cases applies especially to rules. It is one reason why there are relatively few laws specifically relating to treatment withdrawal decisions. But guidelines, by their nature, do not aspire to prescribe behaviour in every situation. Their aim is to inform and guide decisions, but they acknowledge that it may be appropriate to reach different decisions in particular cases. Given that the threshold framework as I have described it relates to treatment guidelines rather than laws or rules, the 'particular case' concern may be less of a problem.

It also matters how we manage exceptions. When drafting rules or guidelines, policy-makers could attempt to cover all possible situations. This would be vulnerable to the particular-case concern, though it might also be that for some policies this is the right approach. If exceptions are rare enough, the value of having binding and clear rules could outweigh the fact that in some cases they yield the wrong answer. Our approach to some questions in end-of-life care is like this. For example, criteria for determination of brain death are explicit and detailed. There might be rare exceptions to these criteria, but part of their value is in being unambiguous. A second approach to exceptions would be to use guidelines which aim to cover the usual cases, but to leave exceptional cases to the clinician. The main disadvantage of this approach is that it potentially undermines the value of having guidelines. Part of the aim of having guidelines is to promote consistent decision-making. But if doctors are allowed to step outside of guidelines whenever they believe that the individual circumstances merit this, it may encourage or permit considerable variation in practice. There is a third possibility. Clinical guidelines or rules could set out how decisions should be reached in standard cases. They could also set out a process for managing exceptional cases. This might involve seeking a second or third opinion from a colleague, ethics committee, or the courts. The procedural alternative I outlined above attempts to do this.

The Technical Criteria Fallacy

One final concern about the treshold framework is that it may end up looking like other attempts by doctors to define which children should be treated, and which should not. Neonatologists have in the past developed criteria for treatment, for example on the basis of gestational age (Wilkinson, Ahluwalia, et al. 2009), or on the basis of specific medical features in infants with spina bifida (Lorber 1972). Gestational age guidelines have been criticized on a number of grounds (Janvier, Barrington, et al. 2008; Meadow and Lantos 2009; Turillazzi and Fineschi 2009; Batton 2010). Back in the 1970s American bioethicist Robert Veatch criticized spina bifida guidelines on the basis of what he called the 'technical criteria fallacy'.

> In principle it is a mistake, so I would claim, to assume that any set of technical criteria will be able to make a definitive separation between babies to be treated and those not to be treated. (Veatch 1977: 15)

Veatch objected to the criteria advanced by John Lorber and others on the grounds that they appeared to medicalize questions that are fundamentally value judgements. Those who outlined such criteria provided no ethical argument for adopting their criteria rather than an alternative set. Moreover, such criteria appeared to leave no place for other values, such as those of parents.

Is the threshold framework guilty of this fallacy? The framework might risk being reduced to a set of medical opinions about treatment. Yet, the ethical criteria outlined above are openly based on normative (ethical) judgements. Furthermore, the threshold framework makes explicit the importance of taking into account parental views, albeit within limits. Finally, as discussed in the previous section, the framework is designed to help develop guides for decisions, not to apply rigid rules that doctors or parents must follow. There are likely to be other relevant factors in individual cases that should be taken into account.

Putting It All Together

Treatment Guidelines for Birth Asphyxia

What would the threshold framework look like in practice? What sort of guidelines might be developed using the framework? In this final section I will make some provisional suggestions for the condition that has been used as an example in several places in the book, and with which I am most familiar from my own practice, neonatal birth asphyxia. As noted already, this represents the view of only one individual. It may, nevertheless, provide a useful starting point for discussion. Figure 8.4 and Table 8.1 are an attempt to apply the framework to prognostication in this condition.

292   PART II

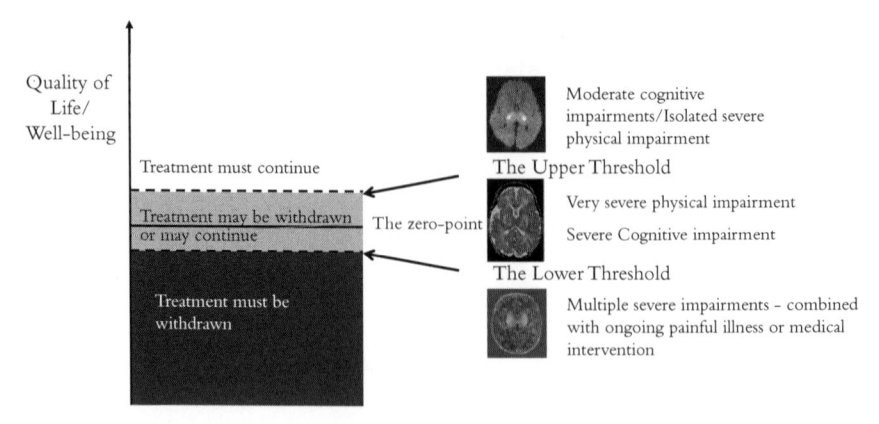

Figure 8.4 The threshold framework as the basis for treatment limitation guidelines in birth asphyxia.

Table 8.1 Patterns of imaging and treatment limitation decision in birth asphyxia.

Pattern on conventional MRI	Usual Outcome	Treatment limitation
Normal scans, mild basal ganglia or moderate white matter changes	Normal outcome (may include minor behavioural or learning problems)	Not permitted
Focal basal ganglia changes with bilateral signal abnormality in the PLIC	Moderate to severe motor problems (often dystonic/athetoid cerebral palsy), cognitive development may be normal	Usually would not be permitted (depending on likelihood of coexistent cognitive impairment and severity of predicted motor impairment)
Severe white matter changes	Moderate to severe motor impairment, as well as moderate to severe cognitive impairment	Permitted—if parents agree
Severe and diffuse basal ganglia changes	Severe motor impairment, severe cognitive impairment, microcephaly, often cortical blindness	Permitted if parents agree. (If severe global injury and infant is ventilator-dependent treatment continuation would not be permitted)

The figure and table indicate that children predicted to have moderate cognitive impairment (for example a predicted IQ more than 35 (see Chapter 5)) or isolated severe physical impairment (e.g. cerebral palsy with a Gross Motor Functional Classification System (GMFCS) level 4 or better, see Chapter 5) would be above the upper threshold. Why choose these levels of impairment? Children with isolated severe physical impairment (for example with cerebral palsy but normal intelligence) are usually able to have some degree of physical function. They may have serious ongoing challenges because of their impairment; however, they are likely to be able to communicate, to interact, to develop relationships, and achieve some measure of independence. They have access to a wide range of the goods of human life. Children and adults with moderate cognitive impairment (IQ 35–50) are usually socially interactive and able to communicate at least to the level of basic needs, and often can carry on simple conversations. Both types of impairment would be consistent with a broad range of goods on either subjective or objective theories of well-being. For both of these groups of children it is not usually thought that they have lives that are not worth living, nor that there is a significant risk of this befalling them. Treatment withdrawal or palliative care should not normally be an option where either of these alternatives (or less severe impairments) is likely for the child.

In contrast, for individuals with very severe physical impairment (GMFCS 5) or with severe cognitive impairment (IQ <35) (particularly where these are combined) it is more questionable whether their lives fall above the zero point, and more reasonable to worry that they may have a life not worth living. Children with the most severe forms of spastic quadriplegic cerebral palsy may be able to communicate or to control an electronic wheelchair. However, they often have a range of significant and painful comorbidities, including seizures, gastro-oesophageal reflux, contractures, recurrent aspiration, scoliosis, etc. For infants and children with severe cognitive impairment, it appears most clear that the benefits of life are diminished (Wilkinson 2006; McMahan 2009). It is for infants with this level of impairment that there is most debate about whether or not treatment is in their best interests. Although Henry (the baby at the start of this chapter with hypoxic brain injury) may be expected to have a life that is worth living, there is a risk that his impairments will be more severe than anticipated, or that other medical problems arise. Treatment for children in these groups may be continued or may be withdrawn.

Finally, I have suggested that treatment for children who have combinations of severe impairment and ongoing painful illness or interventions falls below the lower threshold. For example, this might include children with severe global brain injury following birth asphyxia who have ongoing refractory seizures, or who remain dependent on mechanical ventilation. In these children, the very dramatic reduction in benefits from life combined with evidence that they may be suffering makes it very likely that continuing life-sustaining treatment would harm them. Continuing treatment in this circumstance would be inappropriate.

What about when there is uncertainty about prognosis? I have not indicated a specific statistical threshold for withdrawing treatment, but the arguments about the risk of harms and the interests of the child would suggest that it is reasonable to give weight to at least modest chances of significant harms. Is it possible to be more specific? One way of capturing this idea without using specific numerical thresholds would be by borrowing the language of the law. Civil cases are often settled on the basis of the *balance of probabilities*, while criminal conviction is usually required to establish guilt *beyond reasonable doubt* (Murphy 2007: 111). The latter is unsatisfactory, since there is always some doubt about prognosis. Stipulating the former would permit treatment withdrawal in infants with a slightly less than 50 per cent chance of survival without severe impairment, which may give too great a weight to survival with impairment. In the absence of a better standard, I suggest that it would be permissible to withdraw treatment if there is *clear and convincing* evidence that an infant will have severe impairments as described above. The clear and convincing evidence standard is used in some American legal cases, and indicates a high degree of probability—more than 50 per cent, but less stringent than beyond reasonable doubt (Murphy 2007: 111). Similarly, if there is *clear and convincing evidence* that continuing treatment would harm an infant, it should not be provided, even if parents request it.

Setting out clearly those conditions where I believe that it is appropriate to limit life-sustaining treatment may betray my own view about well-being. In Chapter 4 I briefly referred to the ongoing philosophical controversy about what makes for the good life. It is beyond the scope of this book to engage seriously with that debate, or to advance a substantive position about well-being. Nevertheless, it is perhaps worth briefly outlining what I take to be the most plausible view. My own view has some common features with Aristotelian views about the constituents of human flourishing, and with Sen and Nussbaum's capabilities framework (Sen 1993; Nussbaum 2000). The subjective experience of the individual is a critical component of how well their life is going. That is the reason why the views of the individual are so important in quality of life research. However, subjective levels of happiness or satisfaction are not the only important features. Nussbaum lists capabilities including practical reason, cognitive capability, affiliation with other human beings, humour, and play (Nussbaum 1992). She suggests that the lack of basic capabilities calls into question whether an individual is truly human, and that this would justify different attitudes towards treatment (Nussbaum 1992: 228). Other writers have suggested that a lack of the ability to develop relationships or engage in social interaction are minimum features to ascribe an individual with interests, or that such a life lacks 'meaning' or 'purpose' (McCormick 1974; Engelhardt 1978; Arras 1984; Doyal 1998 Royal College of Paediatrics and Child Health 2004). These authors are all correct in suggesting that it is appropriate to limit life-sustaining treatment for children or infants with a severe cognitive impairment. However, I believe that their justification for doing so is not the right one. A child like Michael, or Charity (Chapter 4), or Chloe (Chapter 2) is clearly human in the ordinary biological sense. Furthermore, when we pay attention to their lived experience it is clear that they have interests—they can be benefited and harmed. Moreover, it is not correct that their lives lack meaning or purpose—this is not true from the point of view of their caregivers, and we have no way of knowing whether the children themselves derive meaning or purpose from their lives. But what is important is that severe cognitive impairment very seriously reduces for the child the benefits of life that they can access. This loss of the ability to take part in features of life that are almost universally felt to be valuable features of human life underpins the common intuition that these are bad states for an individual to be in.

The importance of cognitive function for decisions about life-sustaining treatment reflects the centrality of cognition to human flourishing. Many objective list theories of well-being include elements that are related to cognitive function, including communication, knowledge, aesthetic appreciation, the development of deep reciprocal relationships, the achievement of goals or ambitions (Parfit 1984: 493–502; DeGrazia 1995; Veatch 1995; McMahan 2009). (It is perhaps worth noting that although a minimum level of cognition is needed to be able to enjoy these goods, having higher (above minimum) levels of cognitive capacity does necessarily make for a better life. Geniuses may be better at some things, but they do not necessarily have greater access to many of the goods of life—they may do worse on some—such as the development of relationships with others.)

Not all would agree with the conclusions that I have reached above. Some who prefer subjective theories of well-being would reach a different answer. It is not necessarily the case that an individual with severe cognitive impairment would have less pleasure or more pain than an unimpaired individual, nor that fewer of their desires or preferences would be satisfied. Consequently, on those views, a severely cognitively impaired child would have no less good a life than a cognitively normal individual. Such a view, however, would also imply that there is *nothing* bad for the infant and nothing to regret for their sake about a medical condition in infancy that causes brain damage and leaves the child severely cognitively impaired. This seems highly implausible. Furthermore, even if some hold this view and are prepared to accept its counterintuitive implications, the more objective view outlined above represents a reasonable alternative accepted by many, and reflected in many existing guidelines. In the face of moral uncertainty about which view of well-being is the correct one we should permit those who hold the objective view to apply it to their own lives and those of their children.

The great advantage of the threshold framework is that making guidelines like the provisional ones outlined above does not commit us to saying that the lives of children with severe impairments are not worth living. Unlike a view drawing on best interests in isolation it does not commit us to the judgement that if parents refuse to allow withdrawal of life support from an infant like Henry, they, and by extension any doctors who go along with their request, are harming the infants. It is consistent with the approach adopted currently in many intensive care units. In cases like those listed above doctors do not force parents to agree to withdrawal of life support. In my experience they often do not even try to persuade parents that treatment should be withdrawn. On the contrary, withdrawal of life support is offered to parents as an alternative that they may choose to embrace (Wilkinson 2010). With rare exceptions, doctors usually comply with parental requests to continue life support.

A second advantage is that it makes it possible to separate judgements about what *ought* to be done—for the sake of the child alone—and what should be *permitted*. It provides scope for recommendations about decisions, but permission for alternative decisions to be made. It is consistent with the threshold framework for a doctor to believe that, for the sake of Henry, life-sustaining treatment *should* be continued, even to recommend that it be provided, and yet ultimately to respect his parents' decision to allow him to die.

Multiple Thresholds

In the above description of treatment limitation guidelines I did not specify which treatment was to be withdrawn. Does that matter? In Chapter 6 I argued that there is no significant ethical difference between decisions to withdraw mechanical ventilation (when this would be required for only a short period), and decisions to withhold artificial nutrition. The thresholds should be the same for both. However, I also pointed to two practical differences that may lead to some difference between these decisions. Parents and staff may find withdrawal or withholding of artificial nutrition more distressing or personally challenging than withdrawal of mechanical ventilation. There may also be a higher likelihood of legal sanction if nutritional support is withheld. If these factors cannot be overcome a different threshold for decisions about artificial nutrition would be inevitable. The American Academy of Pediatrics' (AAP) clinical report on foregoing artificial nutrition suggests that it would be appropriate to withhold nutritional support from children who are in a persistent vegetative state, or who 'will never possess conscious awareness' (Diekema and Botkin 2009). It is not clear whether the AAP would endorse a different threshold for other types of life-sustaining treatment. However, if these recommendations were endorsed the upper threshold for decisions about withholding feeding would be lower and closer to the zero point than I have suggested that it should be for decisions about mechanical ventilation.

What about other types of end-of-life decisions in newborn infants? I have referred in this book almost exclusively to decisions about withdrawing or withholding life-sustaining treatment, for reasons set out in Chapter 1. But it is perhaps worth briefly digressing to discuss the use of additional thresholds in countries that legally sanction euthanasia in newborn infants. In the Netherlands, euthanasia of newborn infants is theoretically permitted in very limited circumstances. Doctors in a medical centre in Groningen developed a set of legal and medical criteria for this practice. They do not guarantee that doctors will not be prosecuted, but if adhered to make this unlikely (Verhagen and Sauer 2005a and b). The first two criteria in the Groningen Protocol include that the infant has a certain diagnosis and prognosis, and that 'hopeless and unbearable' suffering is present (Verhagen and Sauer 2005b). These criteria are stringent, and clearly would not apply to most of the cases discussed throughout this book. Cases where newborn infants were euthanized included infants with severe epidermolysis bullosa (de Vries and Verhagen 2008) and osteogenesis imperfecta (Verhagen, Dorscheidt, et al. 2009). Indeed, the criteria appear much closer to the lower threshold as described earlier in this chapter than to the upper threshold. If euthanasia is ever permissible in newborn infants, cases where infants are experiencing a life not worth living, and are likely to continue to suffer despite provision of appropriate palliative care, are the ones where the justification for this decision would be strongest. However, for other types of treatment decisions in neonatal intensive care, Dutch neonatologists use different criteria. Studies in the Netherlands indicate that predicted poor quality of life is a common reason for withdrawing or withholding life-sustaining treatment, and physicians point to future suffering or to an inability to communicate as factors justifying such decisions (Verhagen, van der Hoeven, et al. 2007; Verhagen, Dorscheidt, et al. 2009). For these decisions clinicians in the Netherlands apply criteria that may be closer to the upper threshold. Neonatal euthanasia is, in fact, rare in the Netherlands, and the majority of deaths in newborn infants follow decisions to limit life-sustaining treatment (Verhagen, Dorscheidt, et al. 2009). If euthanasia is permitted, but is seen as a more serious decision, requiring stronger justification and tighter controls than decisions to withdraw life-sustaining treatment, it is appropriate that different thresholds are used for this decision than for other end-of-life decisions.

Should there be different thresholds for older children than for newborn infants? I have suggested as much in earlier chapters of the book when I defended the idea that a newborn's interests should be assessed differently from an older child's. If that is correct, the thresholds may move as a child ages. This would be more apparent for the upper threshold than for the lower threshold, since it is the newborn infant's interest in continuing life that may be weaker (but not their interest in avoiding suffering). It is appropriate for parents' interests to be given more weight in decisions in newborn intensive care than in paediatric intensive care. How would this difference work in practice? If infants' interests are different from an older child's, it is likely that they evolve continuously. Just as there is no point when a bald man suddenly becomes hairy, there is no point at which infants suddenly gain the interests of an older child or adult. This makes it challenging to develop practical guidelines, and is perhaps one reason why existing guidelines all support the idea that decisions in newborn infants and older children should be made on the same basis. (Though this does not appear to be reflected in practice.) One option would be to accept that there is a continuum between the infant and the older child. Thresholds might be developed for newborn infants and different thresholds for older children, with acknowledgement that in later infancy/early childhood something in between would be appropriate. A second option would be to draw an arbitrary line (for example at two months of age), and to apply different criteria before and after this point. This second option would clearly be vulnerable to the arbitrariness objections raised earlier; it would, however, be easier to implement.

Should there be different thresholds in different places? (Figure 8.5a–c.) The guidelines that I have proposed for birth asphyxia may be appropriate for a wealthy country like Australia or the UK. However, guidelines developed from consensus opinion (or from differing opinions) may well be different in different parts of the world. This is probably inevitable given the different values and backgrounds of parents and clinicians around the world. What counts as a reasonable view about well-being or about the interests of the child will vary. But there is another factor that is highly likely to influence where thresholds are drawn—the availability in society of resources to care for the child and the priorities that are set by society for the distribution of those resources. For the most part in this book I have focused on the child and his family. I have set aside issues of resources. (There are enough uncertainties to think about if we confine ourselves to the child and their family.) But the provision of treatment for one child may mean that another child is denied treatment. It is not possible to ignore the importance of resource constraints as a source of limitations on decisions in intensive care. Theologian and ethicist Charlie Camosy has recently argued

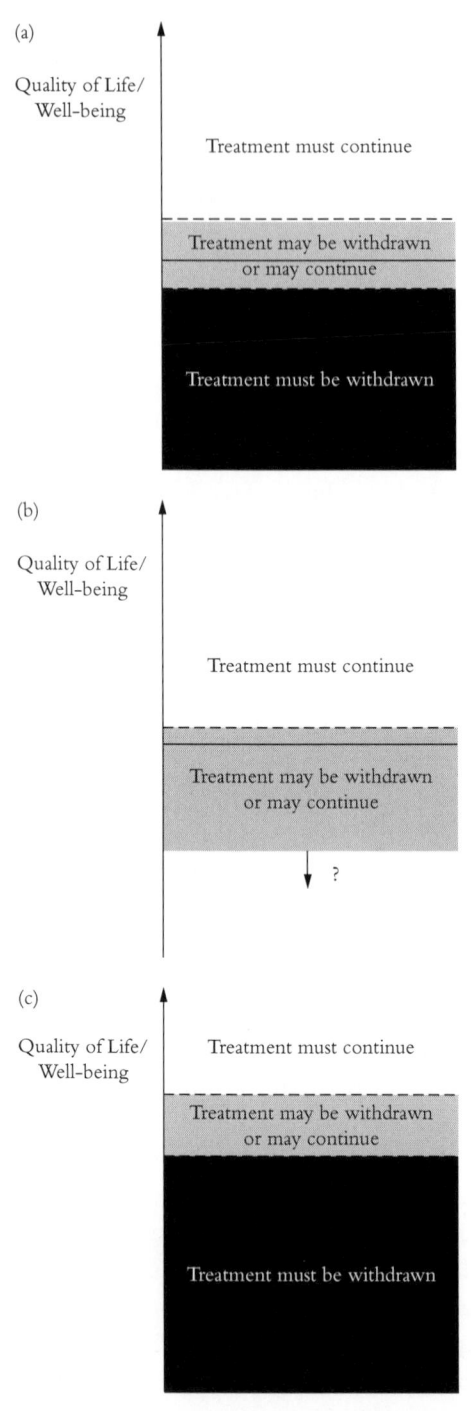

Figure 8.5 The threshold framework and resources. Figure a represents the framework as described earlier. Figure b represents a threshold framework in a theoretical country with unlimited healthcare and social care resources. Figure c represents a threshold framework in a country with very limited healthcare resources.

in his book *Too Expensive to Treat? Finitude, Tragedy and the Neonatal ICU* that costs should be a primary consideration in treatment decisions for newborn infants and older patients (Camosy 2010).

Resources are perhaps most important when we are discussing the lower threshold for treatment. They represent the strongest reason to resist providing 'futile' treatment for a patient (Wilkinson and Savulescu 2011). Treatment would not only fail to serve the interests of the patient, but it also risks harm to other patients since it may lead to them being denied access to intensive care. In a country with considerable intensive care resources and no pressure on beds there might be greater willingness to continue treatment at the behest of families—particularly if it could be ensured that the patient herself was not suffering unduly as a result (Figure 8.5b). The opposite might also be true—in a country with very few resources the lower threshold might be considerably higher, it may even be above the zero point. In parts of the world where even basic services are limited, and basic healthcare is absent for many patients, parents may not be permitted to request provision or continuation of life-sustaining treatment even though this would be clearly in the best interests of the child (Figure 8.5c).

Resources are also relevant to the upper threshold (Figure 8.5). I alluded to this in Chapter 4, and in the earlier section on 'convergence'. The availability of resources to provide medical care for the child and support for the family will influence how well or badly a child's life may be. It may determine whether or not she has a life worth living. It is likely to influence the degree to which a family's interests are affected by the survival of a child. Resources also determine whether there is likely to be foster care or adoption available to care for the child if the parents are unable or unwilling to do so. In countries with very limited social care, and very limited possibilities for adoption (perhaps where there are a large number of orphaned children without impairment) it may be appropriate to set the upper threshold higher than would be the case in wealthier countries (8.5c). Conversely, if there were no issue of resources, if there were unlimited foster families available and willing to care for very severely impaired children, the upper threshold may be much lower than I have indicated, closer to the zero point (8.5b). Parents' interests could still be given weight, but this would lead to adoption rather than to withdrawal of life-sustaining treatment.

Through a Scanner Darkly

> What does a scanner see? he asked himself. I mean, really see? Into the head? Down into the heart? ... Any given man sees only a tiny portion of the total truth. (Dick 1977: 146–7)

Let us return to the thought experiment that started this book—the fabled Carmentis Machine, able to provide perfect prognosis for critically ill infants and children. The Carmentis Machine is a myth, but like the version of the Roman priestess Carmentis who appears in history books, there may be a kernel of truth behind it. It is not clear whether there really was a priestess, or a temple, or how often parents took their newborn infants to have their futures foretold. It appears unlikely that there will even be a machine that is completely accurate in the way that I have imagined. But newborn intensive care units are now being built (and are in use in some parts of the world) with magnetic resonance imaging scanners at their heart, so that critically ill infants can have imaging performed early in their illness without the need for transfer to other parts of the hospital. In many paediatric intensive care units, neurologists, with their prognostic toolkits at hand, are regularly called upon to act as seers, gazing into the future for children who have suffered near-drowning, or who have progressive degenerative disorders. Current technology is imperfect, but studies are already being performed with higher intensity MRI, functional magnetic resonance imaging, diffusion tensor imaging, and optical imaging. Future developments are likely to substantially improve the ability of doctors to prognosticate for ill children and infants, even if some uncertainty remains.

This book has analysed some of the ethical issues arising from neuroimaging for prognosis in critical care. This analysis reveals the same broad themes that are apparent in other areas of neuroethics, and which were outlined in Chapter 1. Firstly, at present a certain degree of scepticism is warranted about the ability of technology to provide predictions of future impairment (and particularly of quality of life). This is partly as a result of limitations of scientific studies that have been carried out. It points to the need for more, and better research studies into prognosis. Secondly the development of prognostic technology raises a number of practical questions that are not addressed by existing guidelines. Thirdly, these developments bring to the fore old questions about treatment decisions in infants and children and the role of parents in such decisions.

Uncertainty plagues prognosis. That is one reason why there continues to be attempts to improve the ability of doctors to predict outcome for seriously ill patients. However, prognostic uncertainty will remain, and so there is a need for careful attention to decision-making in the face of uncertainty, and how we should make decisions when we are not sure what the outcomes of different courses of action would be. Part II of this book has attempted to do that, to think through the ways in which uncertainty influences decisions, and how we should respond to it. But, as has become obvious in the last couple of chapters, there is a further type of uncertainty, moral uncertainty, which also plagues decision-making for children and infants. Having recognized the problem of moral uncertainty we need to seek ways of reducing it; we also (since it is unlikely to go away) need ways of dealing with it in practice.

I have criticized guidelines for treatment decisions that focus on the best interests of the child, since it seems to me that such guidelines are unable to provide practical guidance to clinicians. In many cases it simply is not clear whether or not it would be in the best interests of the child to keep them alive. Nevertheless, the model that I have developed for decision-making retains an important role for best interests. Treatment decisions *should* be guided by what would be best for the patient. However, this is not the only consideration. It is the starting point, but not the finishing point for reflection about treatment withdrawal from infants and children in intensive care.

The framework for decision-making that I have developed in this last chapter would not necessarily lead to a major change in practice in intensive care. It would not (in countries like those that I have been fortunate to work in, with well-resourced public health care systems) lead to the withdrawal of life support from infants or children with a reasonable chance of a good life. But it potentially provides a more robust and more practical basis for the difficult decisions that are made daily in intensive care units. It provides a way of moving forward with developing guidelines, guidelines that reflect the fundamental ethical underpinnings of decisions, but also respect the range of different views within a community about how we should evaluate the risks and benefits of future life, and of death. There is considerable work still to be done in translating this analysis into practical recommendations, and into setting out the thresholds for different groups of children, different types of decision, and different parts of the world.

I cannot predict (my personal crystal ball is too hazy) whether this framework will be used in intensive care units. I hope, though, that it will provoke debate, and thought, and clearer reasoning about the most difficult and devastating decisions that we who work in intensive care have to face—a decision whether or not to allow a child to die.

References

Arras, J.D. (1984). 'Toward an ethic of ambiguity', *Hastings Cent Rep* 14(2): 25–33.

Batton, D. (2010). 'Resuscitation of extremely low gestational age infants: an advisory committee's dilemmas', *Acta Paediatr* 99(6): 810–11.

Berube, M. (1996). *Life As We Know It: A Father, A Family and An Exceptional Child*. New York: Pantheon Books Inc.

Brody, B.A. and A. Halevy (1995). 'Is futility a futile concept?', *J Med Philos* 20(2): 123–44.

Camosy, C. (2010). *Too Expensive to Treat? Finitude, Tragedy and the Neonatal ICU*. Grand Rapids: Michigan, Eerdmans.

Chen, Y.C. and Y.Y. Chen (2011). 'A Moderate Zero Line Approach: Opposing Thresholds Beyond the Zero Line', *The American Journal of Bioethics* 11(2): 41–2.

Cuttini, M., M. Nadai, et al. (2000). 'End-of-life decisions in neonatal intensive care: physicians' self-reported practices in seven European countries. EURO-NIC Study Group', *Lancet* 355(9221): 2112–18.

Dancy, J. (2004). *Ethics Without Principles*. Oxford: Clarendon Press.

de Vries, M.C. and A. Verhagen (2008). 'A case against something that is not the case: the Groningen Protocol and the moral principle of non-maleficence', *The American Journal of Bioethics: AJOB* 8(11): 29–31.

DeGrazia, D. (1995). 'Value theory and the best interests standard', *Bioethics* 9(1): 50–61.

Dick, P. (1977). *A Scanner Darkly*. New York: Vintage books.

Diekema, D.S. and J.R. Botkin (2009). 'Clinical report—Forgoing medically provided nutrition and hydration in children', *Pediatrics* 124(2): 813–22.

Doyal, L. and G. Durbin (1998). 'When life may become too precious: the severely damaged neonate', *Seminars in Neonatology* 3: 275–84.

Engelhardt, H. (1978). 'Medicine and the concept of a person', in T.L. Beauchamp and S. Perlin (eds), *Ethical Issues in Death and Dying*. New Jersey, Prentice-Hall: 271–84.

Fine, R.L. (2009). 'Point: The Texas advance directives act effectively and ethically resolves disputes about medical futility', *Chest* 136(4): 963–7.

—— and T.W. Mayo (2003). 'Resolution of futility by due process: early experience with the Texas Advance Directives Act', *Ann Intern Med* 138(9): 743–6.
Flescher, A. (2003). *Heroes, Saints and Ordinary Morality*. Washington, DC: Georgetown University Press.
General Medical Council (2010). *Treatment and Care Towards the End of Life: Good Practice in Decision Making*. London: GMC.
Gillon, R. (1986). 'Philosophical medical ethics. Conclusion: the Arthur case revisited', *Br Med J (Clin Res Ed)* 292(6519): 543–5.
Gresiuk, C.S. and A.R. Joffe (2011). 'Variability in the pediatric intensivists' threshold for withdrawal/limitation of life support as perceived by bedside nurses: a multicenter survey study', *Annals of Intensive Care* 1(1): 31.
Heyd, D. (2008). 'Supererogation', in E. Zalta (ed.), *The Stanford Encyclopedia of Philosophy*, < http://plato.stanford.edu/entries/supererogation/>.
Hyde, D. (2008). 'Sorites paradox', in E. Zalta (ed.), *The Stanford Encyclopedia of Philosophy*, <http://plato.stanford.edu/entries/sorites-paradox/>.
Janvier, A., K.J. Barrington, et al. (2008). 'Ethics ain't easy: do we need simple rules for complicated ethical decisions?', *Acta Paediatr* 97(4): 402–6.
Kamm, F.M. (1985). 'Supererogation and obligation', *Journal of Philosophy* 82(3): 118–38.
Kattwinkel, J., J.M. Perlman, et al. (2010). 'Neonatal resuscitation: 2010 American Heart Association Guidelines for Cardiopulmonary Resuscitation and Emergency Cardiovascular Care', *Pediatrics* 126(5): e1400–13.
Kerridge, I.H., S.A. Pearson, et al. (1999). 'Impact of written information on knowledge and preferences for cardiopulmonary resuscitation', *Med J Aust* 171(5): 239–42.
Laureys, S. (2005). 'The neural correlate of (un)awareness: lessons from the vegetative state', *Trends Cogn Sci (Regul Ed)* 9(12): 556–9.
Lee, K.J., K. Tieves, et al. (2010). 'Alterations in end-of-life support in the pediatric intensive care unit', *Pediatrics* 126(4): e859–64.
Lorber, J. (1972). 'Spina bifida cystica. Results of treatment of 270 consecutive cases with criteria for selection for the future', *Arch Dis Child* 47(256): 854–73.
Lui, K., B. Bajuk, et al. (2006). 'Perinatal care at the borderlines of viability: a consensus statement based on a NSW and ACT consensus workshop', *Med J Aust* 185(9): 495–500.
MacDonald, H. and A.A. o.P.C.o.F.a. Newborn (2002). 'Perinatal care at the threshold of viability', *Pediatrics* 110(5): 1024–7.
McCormick, R.A. (1974). 'To save or let die. The dilemma of modern medicine', *JAMA* 229(2): 172–6.

McMahan, J. (2009). 'Radical Cognitive Limitation', in K. Brownlee and A. Cureton (eds), *Disability and Disadvantage*. Oxford: Oxford University Press, 240–59.

Meadow, W. (2007). 'Babies between a rock and a hard place—neonatologists vs parents at the edge of infant viability', *Acta Paediatr* 96(2): 153.

—— and J. Lantos (2009). 'Moral reflections on neonatal intensive care', *Pediatrics* 123(2): 595–7.

Monti, M.M., A. Vanhaudenhuyse, et al. (2010). 'Willful modulation of brain activity in disorders of consciousness', *N Engl J Med* 362(7): 579–89.

Moriette, G., S. Rameix, et al. (2010). 'Very premature births: Dilemmas and management. Second part: Ethical aspects and recommendations', *Archives de pediatrie: organe officiel de la Societe francaise de pediatrie* 17: 527–39.

Murphy, P. (2007). *Murphy on Evidence*. Oxford: Oxford University Press.

Nussbaum, M. (1992). 'Human Functioning and Social Justice: In Defense of Aristotelian Essentialism', *Political Theory* 20(2): 202–46.

—— (2000). *Women and Human Development: The Capabilities Approach*. Cambridge: Cambridge University Press.

Parfit, D. (1984). *Reasons and Persons*. Oxford: Oxford University Press.

Paris, J.J., M.D. Schreiber, et al. (1993). 'Beyond autonomy—physicians' refusal to use life-prolonging extracorporeal membrane oxygenation', *N Engl J Med* 329(5): 354–7.

—— —— —— (2007). 'Parental refusal of medical treatment for a newborn', *Theor Med Bioeth* 28(5): 427–41.

Pignotti, M. and G. Donzelli (2008). 'Perinatal care at the threshold of viability: an international comparison of practical guidelines for the treatment of extremely preterm births', *Pediatrics* 121(1): e193–8.

Pope, T.M. (2007). 'Medical futility statutes: no safe harbor to unilaterally refuse life-sustaining treatment', *Tennessee Law Review* 75(1): 1–81.

Poulton, B., S. Ridley, et al. (2005). 'Variation in end-of-life decision making between critical care consultants', *Anaesthesia* 60(11): 1101–5.

Randolph, A.G., M.B. Zollo, et al. (1999). 'Variability in physician opinion on limiting pediatric life support', *Pediatrics* 103(4): e46.

Ravenscroft, A.J. and M.D. Bell (2000). '"End-of-life" decision making within intensive care—objective, consistent, defensible?', *J Med Ethics* 26(6): 435–40.

Royal College of Paediatrics and Child Health (2004). *Withholding and Withdrawing Life-Saving Treatment in Children: A Framework for Practice*. London: Royal College of Paediatrics and Child Health.

Schneiderman, L.J., N.S. Jecker, et al. (1990). 'Medical futility: its meaning and ethical implications', *Ann Intern Med* 112(12): 949–54.

Sen, A. (1993). 'Capability and Well-being', in M.C. Nussbaum and A. Sen (eds), *The Quality of Life*. New York: Oxford Clarendon Press.

Stewart, C. (2011). 'Futility Determination as a Process: Problems with Medical Sovereignty, Legal Issues and the Strengths and Weakness of the Procedural Approach', *Journal of Bioethical Inquiry* 8(2): 155–63.

Turillazzi, E. and V. Fineschi (2009). 'How old are you? Newborn gestational age discriminates neonatal resuscitation practices in the Italian debate', *BMC Med Ethics* 10: 19.

Tyson, J. (1995). 'Evidence-based ethics and the care of premature infants', *The Future of children/Center for the Future of Children, the David and Lucile Packard Foundation* 5(1): 197–213.

Tyson, J.E., N.A. Parikh, et al. (2008). 'Intensive care for extreme prematurity—moving beyond gestational age', *N Engl J Med* 358(16): 1672–81.

Veatch, R.M. (1977). 'The technical criteria fallacy', *Hastings Cent Rep* 7(4): 15–16.

—— (1995). 'Abandoning informed consent', *Hastings Cent Rep* 25(2): 5–12.

Verhagen, A., J. Dorscheidt, et al. (2009). 'End-of-life decisions in Dutch neonatal intensive care units', *Arch Pediatr Adolesc Med* 163(10): 895–901.

—— M.A.H. van der Hoeven, et al. (2007). 'Physician medical decision-making at the end of life in newborns: insight into implementation at 2 Dutch centers', *Pediatrics* 120(1): e20–8.

—— and P. J. Sauer (2005a). 'End-of-life decisions in newborns: an approach from The Netherlands', *Pediatrics* 116(3): 736–9.

—— and P. J. Sauer (2005b). 'The Groningen protocol—euthanasia in severely ill newborns', *N Engl J Med* 352(10): 959–62.

Verloove-Vanhorick, S.P. (2006). 'Management of the neonate at the limits of viability: the Dutch viewpoint', *BJOG: an international journal of obstetrics and gynaecology* 113 Suppl 3: 13–16.

Weijer, C., S.H. Shapiro, et al. (2000). 'For and against: clinical equipoise and not the uncertainty principle is the moral underpinning of the randomised controlled trial', *BMJ* 321(7263): 756–8.

Wilkinson, A.R., J. Ahluwalia, et al. (2009). 'Management of babies born extremely preterm at less than 26 weeks of gestation: a framework for clinical practice at the time of birth', *Arch Dis Child Fetal Neonatal Ed* 94(1): F2–5.

Wilkinson, D. (2006). 'Is it in the best interests of an intellectually disabled infant to die?', *J Med Ethics* 32(8): 454–9.

—— (2010). '"We don't have a crystal ball": neonatologists views on prognosis and decision-making in newborn infants with birth asphyxia', *Monash Bioethics Review* 29(1): 5.1–5.19.

—— G. Kahane, et al. (2009). 'Functional neuroimaging and withdrawal of life-sustaining treatment from vegetative patients', *J Med Ethics* 35(8): 508–11.

—— and J. Savulescu (2011). 'Knowing when to stop: futility in the ICU', *Current Opinion in Anesthesiology* 24(2): 160–5.

Wolf, S. (1982). 'Moral Saints', *Journal of Philosophy* 79(8): 419–39.

Wunsch, H., D.A. Harrison, et al. (2005). 'End-of-life decisions: a cohort study of the withdrawal of all active treatment in intensive care units in the United Kingdom', *Intensive Care Med* 31(6): 823–31.

Youngner, S.J. (1988). 'Who defines futility?', *JAMA* 260(14): 2094–5.

Index

(for specific cases, both hypothetical and real, *see* case examples)

abortion 86, 89, 96, 130, 134–5, 149–50
acts versus omissions 214
adoption, impact on treatment decisions
    of 148–50, 278, 301
allowing to die, *see* withdrawing/
    withholding treatment
American Academy of Pediatrics
    guidelines 58–9, 219, 221–2, 297
Anencephaly 29, 69
asymmetrical harms 248–50
asymmetry
    conception and 250–2
    harm-benefit 95, 250–2
autonomy 30, 48–9, 187, 271

balance sheet (approach to best interests), *see*
    best interests
Benatar, David 98, 251–2
best interests 46–78, 125–50, 212–13, 223–4,
    228, 231, 237, 239, 242–50, 261–303;
    see also interests
    balance sheet approach to 61–2, **71–8**, 85,
        185, 244–50, 262
    definition of 48–50, 109–11
    intolerability approach to 55–6, 58–9,
        60–70, 73, 76, 185, 223, 244–50, 262,
        274, 276, 278
    uncertainty impact on 243–52
birth asphyxia 35–9, 167–78, 202–6, 263,
    291–4, 299
Boswell, John 106
Bradley, Ben 138–41, 146
brain death 52

Camosy, Charles 299, 301
capabilities approach, *see* wellbeing
Carmentis machine 46–78, 83–4, 102–3,
    108–9, 113, 143, 151–2, 194, 236, 255–6,
    276, 302
Carmentis/Carmenta 45
case examples
    Baby Jane Doe 223

Baby M 223–4
Baby Pearson 220
Bloomington Baby Doe 223
Case 1: Baby Amelia 50, 52, 69, 74,
    239, 287
Case 2: Angelos 50–1, 69, 74–5, 77, 237–8
Case 3: Phillip 51–2, 66–7, 69
Case 4: Baby Chloe 51–2, 54, 69,
    276–7, 295
Charlotte Wyatt 60–2, 76
Christine 82, 83, 85, 89, 91, 98–9, 102–3
Henry 263, 264, 293, 296
Michael 263, 264, 295
Re J 56–8, 63, 67, 70
Re MB 71–2, 77, 241
Re RB 112–14
Teratogen case 85–6, 88–9, 93, 101, 252
Transplant Choice 132, 135–9, 142–4, 146
cerebral palsy 26, 36–8, 50, 52, 57, 61, 68,
    74–5, 79, 85, 89, 98, 163, 171, **173**, 184,
    186–9, 203, 260, 263, 292–3
Cicero 22, 159
conception (causing an individual to exist) 84,
    87, 90–1, 96, 98–100, 103, 250–2
contraception 90, 96, 106

death, harm of 27, 131–6, 138–9, 141–2, 151,
    246, 248, 269
desire theories, *see* wellbeing
disability **53–5**, 59, 63, 65, 70, 88–9, 119,
    121, **171–4**, 190, 239–40, 246
    cognitive, intellectual 54, 56–7, 66–71,
        76–7, 144, 148, 172–4, 187–9, 191, 195,
        203, 210, 223, 238–40, 249, 254, 257,
        276, 292–6
    motor/physical 54, 71–2, **74–6**, 113, 144,
        148, 173, 187, 190–1, 239, 293
    paradox 28, 75, 89, 186, 190
    sensory 52, **71–2**, 76
    social model 53–4, 75, 79, 119–23
discrimination 53–4, 122–3
doctrine of double effect 210–17, 220–1

INDEX

Down syndrome 70, 85, 89, 119, 123, 222–3, 228, 249, 275, 284
dynamic choices 137

encephalopathy, hypoxic-ischaemic (HIE); *see* birth asphyxia
equipoise 281–3
ethics committee 284–6, 290
euthanasia
　active 33–4, 231, 297–8
　passive 33; *see also* withdrawing or withholding treatment
extraordinary/ordinary treatment 220
extremely premature infants
　quality of life 188–94, 254
　resuscitation 31, 55–6, 57, 59–60, 83, 133, 179–80, 183, 184, 202–4, 272–3, 279, 287, 290–1

fetus 134, 143–4, 146, 149–50, 248
futility 25, 180, 270, 279–80, 284–5, 301

Golden, Mark 22
grey zone 267, 273
Groningen protocol, *see* active euthanasia

handicap, *see* disability
Hare, RM 83, 94–5, 99, 101
hedonism, *see* wellbeing
human flourishing 295
hydranencephaly 114–15
hypoxic-ischaemic encephalopathy (HIE), *see* birth asphyxia

impairment, *see* disability
infanticide 89, 106, 159–60
intensive care 23–4; *see also* withdrawing/withholding treatment
interests
　in future life 128–50
　of newborn infants 128–50, 246–50, 299
　of parents/families 56, **113–24**, 126–7, 145, 147–51, 236–43, 254, 258, 262, 272–8, 288, 294, 299, 301
　of the child, *see* best interests
　time-relative 134–50
intolerability (test for best interests), *see* best interests

Kaposy, Chris 131, 145–7

law 47, *see also* case examples
letting die *see* withdrawing/withholding treatment
life not worth living, *see* life worth living
life-sustaining treatment, *see* withdrawing/withholding treatment
life worth living (LWL) **28**, 62, **85**, 86, 88, 99–100, 125, 127, 131, 138, 148, 185, 217, 228, 230–1, 237–8, 240, 243, 244–6, 248–50, 252, 264–5, 274–8, 293, 296, 298, 301
locked-in syndrome 71, 190

McMahan, Jeff 90–1, 134–45
magnetic resonance imaging (MRI) 37–9, 167–71, 175–8, 205, 292, 302
maximin 249–50
moral status 88–90, 109–12, 152, 239
morphine, treatment of dying patients with 210–11, 216–17

next child, implications for decisions, *see* replacement
non-identity problem 85–8
Nuffield council of bioethics report 55–6, 62–3, 67, 219
Nussbaum, Martha 191, 295

objective list theories, *see* wellbeing
One Tattered Angel 114–16, 237, 295
ordinary versus extraordinary treatment 220
Ovid 45

parents
　discretion in decisions, *see* threshold framework
　interests, *see* interests of parents/families
Parfit, Derek 86–7, 98–9
Paulus 107
persistent vegetative state, (PVS) 11, 27, 52, 70, 178, 203, 204, 219, 222, 256, 275, 297
personal identity 128–30,
　see also non-identity problem
personhood 130–2
Philo of Alexandria 107
plasticity 164, 166
preferences, *see* wellbeing
premature newborn infants, *see* extremely premature infants
prenatal testing 89

procreative beneficence 93, 100
prognosis 34–9, 47, 59, 167–78, 180, 195, 206, 208, 303 *see also* uncertainty, prognostic
prophecies, *see* self-fulfilling prophecies

quality of life **26–30**, 39, 52, 55, 57, 59, 63, 66, 68, 184–95, 207–10, 213–4, 216–7, 227, 229, 231, 244, 247, 254–5, 256, 264, 268, 272, 280–1, 292, 295, 298, 300, 302
  research measuring 185–94
quantity of life 25–6

Rawls, John 249–50
reasons
  impersonal 87–8, 90–1, 93–4, 96–9, 102–3, 252
  individual affecting 87–9, 97, 99–100, 102–3, 252
relativism 267
religion/religious views 27, 240–1, 255–7, 267, 285–6
replacement 82–103
  arguments against 88–90
  definition 84
  the insubstantial reason argument against 90–4, 96–102
resilience 163
resources, role in treatment limitation 30–1, 97, 121, 123, 144, 147, 237, 257, 299–301
rights 109, 253, 255
Royal College of Paediatrics and Child Health (RCPCH) guideline 25, 51–2, 62, 64–5, 67, 219
rubella 87

self-fulfilling prophecies 170, 178–84, 280
Seneca the Elder 22, 160
Singer, Peter 83, 88–90, 94, 96, 128–31, 134, 136, 141
slippery slope 227–8
Soranus of Ephesus 159–60
sorites paradox 265–7
spina bifida 94, 160, 223, 290–1
spinal muscular atrophy 71, 113
substituted judgement 30, 49, 63, 65–7, 73
substitution 84–5, 88–9, 93, 98, 100
supererogation 276–7

Tertullian 105, 107

threshold framework, *see* withdrawing/withholding treatment
tolerability paradox 67–9, 76, 187–8
Tooley, Michael 130
treat until certainty strategy 202
trisomy (13/18) 179
trisomy (21), *see* Down syndrome

uncertainty
  causes of 162–201
  effect on interests 236–50
  moral 242, **253–9**, 262, 272–3, 277, 281, 283–4, 296, 303
  prognostic 58, 163–7, 207, 231, 253–6, 262, 273, 303
  strategies for managing 202–32
  types of 253

Veatch, Robert 291
vegetative state, persistent, *see* persistent vegetative state
vitalism 27, 240, 257

waiting, strategy under uncertainty 202–4
wellbeing **84–5**, 88, 90–3, 97–9, **109–12**, 121, 124, 126, 128, 131–2, 139, 141–2, 144, 149, 185–7, 190–3, 244, 247, 249, 255, 268, 272, 281, 292–6, 299–300
  capabilities approach to 191, 295
  desire theories of 110, 128, 131, 139, 140–1, 191, 237–8, 296
  hedonism theories of 110, 131, 141
  objective list theories 110, 131, 141, 191, 237–8, 295–6
  preference theories of, *see* desire theories
When the Bough Breaks 117
window of opportunity 204–17, 221, 229–30
withdrawing or withholding treatment
  artificial nutrition/feeding 206, 217–32, 248, 297
  distinction between 32
  mechanical ventilation 26, 33, 50, 57, 61, 69, 71, 169, 205, 209–10, 217–18, 220, 221–2, 224, 226–31, 294, 297
  reasons in favour of 25–31
  threshold framework for decisions about 261–304
  timing, *see* window of opportunity

zero-point of wellbeing 244–50, 252, 255, 271, 272, 274–5, 277–8, 287, 292–3, 297, 301

Printed and bound by CPI Group (UK) Ltd, Croydon, CR0 4YY